FATTY ACID METABOLISM AND ITS REGULATION

New Comprehensive Biochemistry

Volume 7

General Editors

A. NEUBERGER
London

L.L.M. van DEENEN
Utrecht

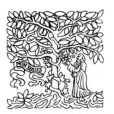

ELSEVIER
AMSTERDAM·NEW YORK·OXFORD

Fatty Acid Metabolism and Its Regulation

Editor

Shosaku NUMA

*Department of Medical Chemistry, Kyoto University Faculty of Medicine, Kyoto 606
(Japan)*

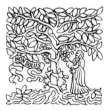

1984

ELSEVIER
AMSTERDAM·NEW YORK·OXFORD

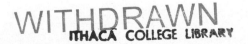

ISBN for the series: 0444 80303 3
ISBN for the volume: 0444 80528 1

Published by:
Elsevier Science Publishers B.V.
P.O. Box 1527
1000 BM Amsterdam, The Netherlands

Sole distributors for the U.S.A. and Canada
Elsevier Science Publishing Company Inc.
52 Vanderbilt Avenue
New York, NY 10017, U.S.A.

Library of Congress Cataloging in Publication Data
Main entry under title:

Fatty acid metabolism and its regulation.

   (New comprehensive biochemistry ; v. 7)
   Includes bibliographical references and index.
   1. Acids, Fatty--Metabolism--Regulation. I. Numa,
Shōsaku, 1929-   . II. Series. [DNLM: 1. Fatty acids
--Metabolism. 2. Fatty acids--Enzymology. Wl NE372F
v.7 / QU 90 F2519]
QD415.N48 vol. 7 [QP752.F35]   574.19'2s   83-25471
ISBN 0-444-80528-1 (U.S.)   [574.1'33]

Printed in The Netherlands

Preface

Since the topic of fatty acid metabolism was last treated in a previous volume of this series, the main emphasis of research in this field has shifted towards the molecular characterization of the enzymes involved and their regulation. Biochemical, molecular-biological and genetic studies carried out during the last decade or so have provided considerable information as to the molecular and catalytic properties and the control of the fatty acid-synthesizing and -degrading enzymes.

This volume is devoted to the recent progress in the field of fatty acid metabolism and its regulation. The first three chapters cover the structural, functional, regulatory and genetic aspects of acetyl-coenzyme A carboxylase and fatty acid synthetase from animal, yeast and bacterial sources, which are responsible for fatty acid synthesis de novo. Chapter 4 concerns the enzymology and control of desaturation and elongation of preformed fatty acids in mammals. In Chapter 5, the animal enzymes involved in fatty acid oxidation and the regulation of this enzyme system are extensively treated. The two final chapters deal with fatty acid synthesis and degradation and the control of these processes in higher plants. It is hoped that all the chapters, contributed by leading scientists in the specific areas, will serve those who teach as well as those engaged in research.

Although the recent studies described have improved the understanding of fatty acid metabolism and its regulation, many questions remain to be answered. In the near future, some of the genes encoding the enzymes responsible for fatty acid metabolism will be isolated and characterized by recombinant DNA techniques. This approach will be useful for elucidating the structure, catalytic and regulatory functions and evolution of the enzymes as well as the control of expression of the genes.

Shosaku Numa
Kyoto, December 1983

Contents

Chapter 4
The regulation of desaturation and elongation of fatty acids in mammals
by R. Jeffcoat and A.T. James (Bedford) 85

Chapter 5
Fatty acid oxidation and its regulation
Jon Bremer and Harald Osmundsen (Oslo) 113

Chapter 6
Fatty acid biosynthesis in higher plants

Chapter 7
Lipid degradation in higher plants

S. Numa (Ed.) Fatty Acid Metabolism and Its Regulation
© *1984 Elsevier Science Publishers B.V.*

CHAPTER 1

Acetyl-coenzyme A carboxylase and its regulation

SHOSAKU NUMA and TADASHI TANABE [1]

*Department of Medical Chemistry, Kyoto University Faculty of Medicine, Kyoto 606
and [1] Department of Biochemistry, National Cardiovascular Center Research Institute,
Suita 565, Japan*

1. Introduction

The living organism needs fatty acids for the hydrophobic parts of biological membranes or as an energy store in the form of triglycerides. The requirement for fatty acids can be met either by biosynthesis or by dietary supply. Because fatty acids are essential for the proper functioning of the living organism, their synthesis and degradation must be precisely regulated so as to respond to various metabolic conditions. For instance, fatty acid synthesis is reduced in fasted and in diabetic animals as well as in animals fed a high-fat diet; in all these metabolic conditions, carbohydrate utilization is restricted. On the other hand, when fasted animals are refed a fat-free high-carbohydrate diet, more fatty acids are synthesized than in normally fed animals to replenish triglycerides which have been depleted during starvation. The first step in the pathway of long-chain fatty acid biosynthesis is mediated by acetyl-CoA carboxylase [acetyl-CoA:carbon-dioxide ligase (ADP-forming), EC 6.4.1.2], a biotin-containing enzyme which catalyzes the carboxylation of acetyl-CoA to form malonyl-CoA, the activated donor of 2-carbon units for the elongation of fatty acids catalyzed by fatty acid synthetase. Because malonyl-CoA has no apparent metabolic alternative, it would be of teleonomic significance to regulate fatty acid synthesis at this carboxylation step. In fact, accumulated evidence indicates that acetyl-CoA carboxylase plays a critical role in the regulation of this biosynthetic process. The cellular content of the enzyme varies with the rate of fatty acid synthesis in different nutritional, hormonal, developmental and genetic conditions, and the catalytic activity of the enzyme is modulated by a number of metabolites and by phosphorylation/dephosphorylation of the enzyme.

Since acetyl-CoA carboxylase was last treated in a previous volume of this series [1], extensive studies have been made on this enzyme, particularly on its regulation. Not only biochemical but also molecular–biological and genetic approaches have been applied to this field and have made important contributions to the understanding of the structure and function of the enzyme as well as the molecular mechanisms underlying the regulation of the enzyme. As acetyl-CoA carboxylase from plants is discussed in Chapter 6, this article deals with the enzyme from animals, yeasts and bacteria. The yeast enzyme is partly covered in Chapter 3. Various aspects of acetyl-CoA carboxylase have been reviewed previously [2–14].

2. Purification

Acetyl-CoA carboxylase is located in the cytoplasm and has been purified from liver [15–24], mammary gland [25–29], adipose tissue [30,31], uropygial gland [32], plants [33–36], yeast [37–40] and bacteria [41–44]. The purification procedures used include precipitation with ammonium sulfate or polyethylene glycol, ion-exchange column chromatography with DEAE-cellulose or phosphocellulose, calcium phosphate or alumina C_γ gel adsorption, hydroxyapatite column chromatography and gel filtration or sucrose density-gradient centrifugation. Recently, avidin–agarose affinity chromatography has been effectively utilized (see below). As the enzyme is sensitive to proteolytic attack by endogenous proteases in crude preparations, purified preparations sometimes contain proteolytically modified forms of the enzyme. Analysis by sodium dodecylsulfate–polyacrylamide gel electrophoresis has shown that rat-liver acetyl-CoA carboxylase, unlike the bacterial enzymes, has one kind of subunit with a molecular weight of 230 000 and contains 1 molecule of biotin [45]. In some purified enzyme preparations, the native subunit was proteolytically cleaved into polypeptides with molecular weights of 124 000 and 118 000; the prosthetic group biotin was contained in the larger polypeptide, but not in the smaller one. However, the [^{14}C]biotin-labeled enzyme in crude rat liver extracts, when immunoprecipitated with specific antibody, invariably exhibits only the native subunit. Treatment of the native enzyme with trypsin or chymotrypsin results in cleavage of the native subunit into 2 nonidentical polypeptides such as observed with modified preparations. Purified acetyl-CoA carboxylase from rabbit mammary gland contains a major polypeptide with a molecular weight of 240 000 and 2 minor polypeptides with molecular weights of 230 000 and 220 000 [46]. Formation of 2 minor polypeptides with similar molecular weights by limited trypsin treatment of the major polypeptide has been demonstrated. Proteolytic modification of the chicken liver enzyme has also been observed [47].

One of the catalytic components of acetyl-CoA carboxylase from *Escherichia coli*, biotin carboxyl carrier protein (see Section 3a), was initially purified as a polypeptide with a molecular weight of 9100 or 10 400 [48], which has subsequently been shown to be a proteolytic product of the native polypeptide with a molecular weight of 22 500 [42]. The carboxyltransferase component of acetyl-CoA carboxylase (see Section 3a) from *E. coli* [43] as well as from *Pseudomonas citronellolis* [44] has been shown to be composed of 2 different polypeptides with similar molecular weights. Possible conversion of the larger polypeptide into the smaller one has been suggested by the fact that the stoichiometry of the complex isolated from *P. citronellolis* is somewhat variable in different preparations [44].

In general, it is very difficult to obtain intact acetyl-CoA carboxylase without exercising due caution against proteolytic modification. Recently, an effective affinity adsorbent using monomeric avidin, a unique biotin-specific binding protein, has been developed for the isolation of biotin-dependent enzymes [49–51]. The application of avidin-agarose affinity chromatography in combination with protease inhibitors has successfully minimized proteolytic modification of acetyl-CoA carboxylase during its purification [18,23,24,32,47,52,53]. It is also noteworthy that acetyl-CoA carboxylase from animal sources is phosphorylated and that the presence of protein phosphatase inhibitors during purification affects the phosphate content and specific activity of the enzyme (see Section 5b).

3. Structure

(a) Subunit structure

The carboxylation reaction by acetyl-CoA carboxylase proceeds in 2 steps according to the following reactions as is the case for other biotin-dependent carboxylases:

$$E\text{-biotin} + ATP + HCO_3^- \overset{Mg^{2+}}{\rightleftharpoons} E\text{-biotin} \sim CO_2 + ADP + P_i \qquad (1)$$

$$E\text{-biotin} \sim CO_2 + \text{acetyl-CoA} \rightleftharpoons E\text{-biotin} + \text{malonyl-CoA} \qquad (2)$$

$$\text{Overall: } ATP + HCO_3^- + \text{acetyl-CoA} \rightleftharpoons ADP + P_i + \text{malonyl-CoA} \qquad (3)$$

where E-biotin denotes acetyl-CoA carboxylase.

The first step represents the carboxylation of the enzyme-bound biotin, and the second step the transfer of the "activated" carboxyl group to acetyl-CoA (see Section 4). Thus, 3 catalytic units, that is, biotin carboxyl carrier protein (CCP) which contains the enzyme-bound biotin, biotin carboxylase which catalyzes the first partial reaction (Eqn. 1), and carboxyltransferase which catalyzes the second partial reaction (Eqn. 2), are required for the carboxylation of acetyl-CoA.

In fact, acetyl-CoA carboxylase from *E. coli* has been shown to consist of 3 corresponding dissociable components [10,54,55]. The *E. coli* CCP component is a dimer of an identical polypeptide with a molecular weight of 22 500 which contains 1 mole of biotin per mole of polypeptide [42]. A partial amino acid sequence of this polypeptide has been determined [56]. The amino acid sequence around the biotinyl lysine is homologous with that of transcarboxylase from *Propionibacterium shermanii* as well as with those of pyruvate carboxylases from sheep, chicken and turkey (see ref. 9). According to the sequence of *E. coli* CCP, the pentapeptide derivative Boc–Glu–Ala–Met–Bct–Met (Boc, tertiary butoxycarbonyl; Bct, biotinyl lysine) has been chemically synthesized and tested for the ability to act as a substrate for biotin carboxylase [57]. The K_m value for the pentapeptide is about one-tenth the value for free biotin, but is 10^5- and 10^3-fold higher than the values for the native and modified CCP, respectively [42,48,57]. This indicates that a fairly broad region of the protein structure including the biotinyl lysine is required for the recognition of CCP by biotin carboxylase. The *E. coli* biotin carboxylase component is a dimer of an apparently identical polypeptide with a molecular weight of 51 000 [42]. The *E. coli* carboxyltransferase component consists of 4 polypeptides, that is, 2 moles of a polypeptide with a molecular weight of 30 000 and 2 moles of a polypeptide with a molecular weight of 35 000 [43]; the possibility that the smaller polypeptide may arise from the larger one by proteolytic modification has been suggested (see Section 2).

In crude extracts of *E. coli,* acetyl-CoA carboxylase exists as 2 dissociated components, that is, a complex of CCP and biotin carboxylase, and carboxyltransferase [54,55]. In the case of acetyl-CoA carboxylase from *P. citronellolis,* which has a subunit structure similar to that of the *E. coli* enzyme, an enzyme complex composed of 3 catalytic components has been isolated in the presence of high salt and exhibits an average molecular weight of approximately 250 000 as estimated by gel filtration in high salt medium [44]. Thus, the bacterial acetyl-CoA carboxylases may function as an enzyme complex in the cell.

Accumulated evidence, including protein-chemical [45], immunochemical [45,58] and genetic analysis [59], indicates that acetyl-CoA carboxylase from yeasts (see Chapter III), birds, mammals and probably higher plants (see Chapter VI), unlike the bacterial enzymes, is composed of one kind of subunit. The subunit molecular weight of acetyl-CoA carboxylase from *Saccharomyces cerevisiae* [38] and *Candida lipolytica* [39] is 189 000–230 000, while that of the enzyme from rat [23,45,52,53] and chicken liver [18,47], rat [25] and rabbit mammary gland [26] and goose uropygial gland [32] ranges from 220 000 to 260 000. Because no suitable marker polypeptides are available for estimating molecular weights of this range by sodium dodecylsulfate–polyacrylamide gel electrophoresis, it is not clear whether the different molecular weight values reported reflect experimental errors or species differences. The single subunit of eukaryotic acetyl-CoA carboxylase carries the functions of CCP, biotin carboxylase and carboxyltransferase as well as the regulatory function [45]. Thus, the eukaryotic enzyme exhibits a highly integrated structure, representing a multifunctional polypeptide [45,60,61].

Thus, prokaryotic and eukaryotic acetyl-CoA carboxylase have different structural organizations in that the former consists of multiple unifunctional component polypeptides, whereas the latter is composed of a single, integrated multifunctional polypeptide. It is noteworthy in this context that some biotin-dependent carboxylases are composed of 2 nonidentical polypeptides with molecular weights of 58 000–78 000 and 67 000–96 000, the larger of which contains the biotinyl prosthetic group. They include acyl-CoA carboxylase from the nematode *Tubatrix aceti* [62], propionyl-CoA carboxylase from *Streptomyces erythreus* [63], *Mycobacterium smegmatis* [64], bovine kidney mitochondria [65] and human liver [51], and 3-methylcrotonyl-CoA carboxylase from Achromobacter IVS [66], *P. citronellolis* [67] and bovine kidney mitochondria [65]. The two polypeptides of Achromobacter 3-methylcrotonyl-CoA carboxylase have been dissociated from each other, and their catalytic functions have been studied [66]. The larger biotin-containing polypeptide catalyzes the carboxylation of free biotin. The smaller polypeptide alone shows no enzymic activity, but its addition to the larger polypeptide restores the overall catalytic activity. Thus, it is apparent that the CCP component has been integrated into the biotin carboxylase component in this group of carboxylases, which exhibit a structural organization halfway between those of prokaryotic and eukaryotic acetyl-CoA carboxylase. Future studies on the primary structures and genes of biotin enzymes will shed light on the mechanism by which the multifunctional polypeptides evolved by gene fusion [60,61].

(b) Molecular forms

Acetyl-CoA carboxylase from animal species exhibits an absolute requirement for citrate or isocitrate and is inactive in the absence of these activators [68–71]. The activation of the enzyme by citrate is accompanied by an increase in the sedimentation coefficient of the enzyme [72]. The citrate-induced increase in the sedimentation coefficient of the enzyme is abolished either by the specific inhibitor long-chain acyl-CoA [73] or by exposure to cold [74], which annuls the activation by citrate. The close correlation observed between the sedimentation coefficient and the catalytic activity of the enzyme indicates that the "large" molecular form (40–60 S) represents the active conformation, whereas the "small" molecular form (13–25 S) represents the inactive conformation (see ref. 6). Electron-microscopic [30,75,76] and light-scattering [77] studies have shown that the 40–60 S form of the enzyme represents a large filamentous polymer with a molecular weight of 4 000 000–11 000 000. Centrifugation of the enzyme in an analytical ultracentrifuge under conditions of high pH and high salt concentration, which favor depolymerization of the enzyme, exhibits an $s_{20,w}$ of 13–16 S [78,79]; the 13–16 S form represents a mixture of the monomeric subunit (molecular weight, 230 000) and its dimer [45]. Biotin may be essential for the polymerization, because the apoenzyme fails to aggregate even in the presence of citrate [80]. An attempt to determine whether the polymerization is a prerequisite for the activation of the enzyme or merely a consequence of the activation has been made by using the enzyme immobilized on agarose [81], but at present no definite conclusion has been drawn because protein molecules attached to agarose can move through distances larger than 20 nm [49].

Indirect evidence for the occurrence of the filamentous polymeric form of acetyl-CoA carboxylase in vivo has been obtained with cultured chicken liver cells [82], using the "digitonin-rapid-stop" technique. Digitonin, which perforates the plasma membrane, rendering it immediately permeable to cytosolic enzymes such as lactate dehydrogenase, causes a release of acetyl-CoA carboxylase at a rate inversely related to the cellular concentration of citrate and the apparent state of polymerization. The extent of polymerization was estimated by exploiting the fact that the "small" molecular form of the enzyme is rapidly inactivated by avidin, whereas the "large" molecular form is resistant to it [83]. It has also been reported that the cellular content of the "large" molecular form of the enzyme is proportional to the ratio of the cellular concentration of the activator citrate to that of the inhibitor long-chain acyl-CoA [84].

4. Reaction mechanism

The acetyl-CoA carboxylase reaction proceeds in 2 steps through the carboxy-lated enzyme intermediate as described above (see Section 3a). There are 3 types of evidence supporting this reaction mechanism. The first has been provided by isotope exchange studies [69,85]. ATP-^{32}P_i exchange is demonstrable in the absence of acetyl-CoA, indicating the reaction represented by Eqn. 1. Evidence for the reaction represented by Eqn. 2 is the occurrence of malonyl-CoA–[^{14}C]acetyl-CoA exchange in the absence of ATP, ADP, P_i, HCO_3^- and Mg^{2+}. Secondly, the carboxylated enzyme intermediate (E-biotin $\sim CO_2$) has been isolated and shown to be active in transferring its carboxyl group to the carboxyl acceptor acetyl-CoA [86]. The active carboxyl group is bound to the $N1'$-atom of biotin, which is linked to the ϵ-amino group of a lysyl residue in the enzyme protein [86] (see below). Finally, detailed kinetic analysis has indicated that the 2-step mechanism in fact represents the principal pathway of the reaction as described below.

The results of initial velocity studies as well as product and dead-end inhibition studies have led to the conclusion that the acetyl-CoA carboxylase reaction proceeds through an ordered bi-bi-uni-uni ping-pong mechanism [20,87] as shown in Fig. 1; the order of addition of substrates to the enzyme is ATP, HCO_3^- and acetyl-CoA in the forward reaction, and malonyl-CoA, P_i and ADP in the reverse reaction. Moreover, studies of malonyl-CoA–[^{14}C]acetyl-CoA exchange, in conjunction with the inhibition pattern produced by malonyl-CoA, reveals that malonyl-CoA forms a dead-end complex with the inactive species of the carboxylated form of the enzyme [87].

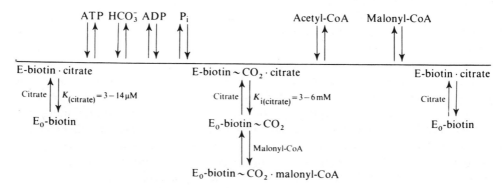

Fig. 1. Kinetic analysis of acetyl-CoA carboxylase reaction and citrate activation. $K_{(citrate)}$ and $K_{i(citrate)}$ denote the dissociation constants of the uncarboxylated and carboxylated forms of the enzyme for citrate, respectively. Data taken from refs. 20 and 87.

Accumulated evidence, including the subunit structures of biotin-dependent enzymes (see Section 3a), indicates that acetyl-CoA carboxylase possesses dual sites for the covalently bound biotin, which are located adjacent to the two substrate sites responsible for the partial reactions (Eqns. 1 and 2). Thus, the reaction mechanism of this enzyme appears to involve a shuttling of the biotin ring between the two sites. Consideration of this structure of biotin-dependent enzymes, together with the observed kinetics of the oxaloacetate transcarboxylase reaction, has led to the proposal of a novel mechanism for this enzymic reaction [88,89]. This is designated as a hybrid ping-pong mechanism to indicate that it involves the intermediate formation of a substituted form of the enzyme and allows independent binding of substrates to two distinct sites of the enzyme. The pyruvate carboxylase reaction proceeds through a similar 2-site ping-pong mechanism [90,91]. Several findings also indicate the hybrid character of the reaction catalyzed by acetyl-CoA carboxylase from rat liver [79,87]. These include a stimulatory effect of acetyl-CoA on the rate of ATP-^{32}P$_i$ exchange. The results of recent kinetic studies on chicken liver acetyl-CoA carboxylase are most consistent with an ordered ter-ter mechanism involving a quaternary complex of the carboxylated enzyme, ADP, P$_i$ and acetyl-CoA; the order of addition is ATP, HCO$_3^-$ and acetyl-CoA [18].

The mechanism underlying the carboxylation of the enzyme-bound biotin has been studied with biotin-dependent enzymes and chemically synthesized model compounds. Earlier studies have been reviewed in detail [2,4,6,10,92]. Biotin, which is covalently attached to the ϵ-amino group of a lysine residue by an amide bond, plays an essential role in the carboxylation reaction. The ureido ring of biotin is the center of the catalytic reaction. It has been proved with acetyl-CoA carboxylase from liver [86] and *E. coli* [93] and with other biotin enzymes [94–97] that the carboxylation site of biotin is the 1'-nitrogen of the ureido group and that the carboxyl group attached to the 1'-nitrogen can be transferred to acetyl-CoA or other specific acceptors. The crystal structure of $N1'$-methoxycarbonyl-D-biotin methyl ester, a derivative of $N1'$-carboxybiotin, has been determined [98] as shown in Fig. 2. The ureido carbonyl bond in the carboxybiotin derivative exhibits more double-bond (keto) character than does the corresponding bond in free biotin, while the $C2'-N1'$ bond in the carboxylated compound shows more single-bond character than in free biotin. The free-energy change for the decarboxylation of the carboxylated trans-carboxylase at pH 7 and 25°C has been estimated to be -4.74 kcal [96] and is sufficiently high to allow the carboxybiotin enzyme to act as a carboxylating agent with suitable acceptors.

E. coli biotin carboxylase, the component of acetyl-CoA carboxylase that carries out the ATP-dependent carboxylation of biotin (see Section 3a), catalyzes phosphoryl transfer from carbamyl phosphate to ADP to form ATP [99]. The latter reaction is dependent on biotin. This implies two possible reaction mechanisms. One is a "concerted mechanism" where carboxyphosphate is an intermediate and carbamyl phosphate is considered to be an analogue of carboxyphosphate. The other is an "O-phosphorylation mechanism" where O-phosphobiotin is an intermediate and carbamyl phosphate is thought to be an analogue of O-phosphobiotin. The

8

"concerted mechanism" for the carboxylation of biotin has been deduced from the results of isotope exchange and kinetic studies with propionyl-CoA carboxylase [100] and pyruvate carboxylase [101], as previously reviewed in detail [2,4,10].

The "O-phosphorylation mechanism" has been proposed on the basis of the fact

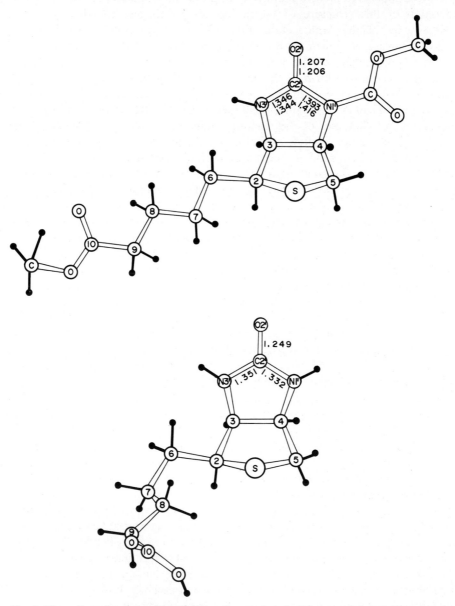

Fig. 2. Three-dimensional structure of N1'-methoxycarbonyl-D-biotin methyl ester (above) and D-biotin (below). The numbers in the figure are bond lengths expressed in Å. Data taken from ref. 98.

that ATP–ADP exchange is catalyzed by purified biotin-dependent enzymes in the absence of HCO_3^- [102]. This is further supported by the finding that the intramolecular reaction of a phosphonate ester and a covalently connected urea occurs readily, suggesting that the oxygen of the ureido moiety of biotin is nucleophilic toward phosphate derivatives [103,104]. Accurate three-dimensional crystal structure analysis of D-biotin shows a lengthening of the ureido carbonyl bond to 1.25 Å and a shortening of the carbonyl carbon–nitrogen bond to 1.33 and 1.35 Å, suggesting a partial delocalization of electronic charge within the ureido group, namely an increased nucleophilicity of carbonyl oxygen [105]. Recently, the reactions of oxy- and thio-phosphoric acid diesters with carbodiimides have been studied, and an analogue of O-phosphobiotin has successfully been isolated as an intermediate [106]. It is worthy of note that this intermediate is susceptible to nucleophilic attack. Furthermore, it has been found that E. coli biotin carboxylase in the presence of N1'-substituted biotin, which is masked at the enzymic carboxylation site, shows phosphoryl transfer activity from carbamyl phosphate to ADP [99]. These results may indicate that the ATP-dependent carboxylation of biotin proceeds through O-phosphobiotin as an intermediate. However, the actual carboxylation mechanism still remains to be elucidated. In this context, resolution of the 3-dimensional structure of biotin-dependent enzymes, especially at the active center, deserves special interest.

Prior to the transfer of the active carboxyl group to an acceptor such as acetyl-CoA, the carboxybiotin must be shifted to the active site of carboxyltransferase or the corresponding domain of eukaryotic enzymes. As the valeryl side chain of biotin linked to the lysyl residue extends from the polypeptide blackbone by 14 Å [107], the process of biotin translocation between the two active sites was originally envisioned as a movement of the prosthetic group over a distance of about 28 Å on the "swinging arm". It has been demonstrated, however, that the active sites of P. shermanii transcarboxylase, although located on different subunits, are separated by no more than 7 Å [108,109]. In accord with this finding are the results of diffraction studies of biotin and its vitamers suggesting that the translocation involves rotation about 1, or at most 2, bonds in the valeryl chain of biotin [110]. The rotations are energetically economical gauche ⇌ trans rotations about the 2 valeryl bonds nearest to the biotin bicyclic ring, moving the carbon atom of the CO_2 moiety bound at N-1' by approximately 7 Å.

The mechanism of the carboxyl transfer reaction has been studied with chemically synthesized compounds [111]. 1-Carboxy-2-ethoxy-2-imidazoline is decarboxylated in alkaline solution 5 times as fast as 1-carboxy-2-imidazolidone. This indicates the involvement of the enol form of biotin in decarboxylation of the carboxyl transfer reaction. The importance of protonation prior to carboxyl transfer has been suggested by the finding that intramolecular transcarboxylation occurs in N-methyl-N-carbomethoxy-2-phenacylthioimidazolinium fluoroborate [112]. The half-life of free carboxybiotin at pH 6.8 and 20°C is 140 min, whereas the half-life of the enzyme-bound carboxybiotin in the absence of substrate is 10–20 min [4,113]. Furthermore, the enzyme-bound carboxybiotin is even more unstable in the presence of a carboxyl acceptor. These facts suggest that the protein moiety of the enzyme may contribute to the stabilization of the enol form of biotin and also to the protonation of the ureido ring so as to facilitate carboxyl transfer from carboxybiotin. The carboxylation reaction catalyzed by acetyl-CoA carboxylase is a stereochemically retained reaction [114] as is the case for the reactions of other biotin-dependent enzymes, and this may indicate a cyclic mechanism. However, the cyclic mechanism in which O-acetylation of the carbonyl oxygen is involved [112] is excluded by the fact that the terminal methyl group of acetonyldethio-CoA can be carboxylated [115]; the apparent K_m value of rat liver acetyl-CoA carboxylase for acetonyldethio-CoA is approximately 5 times as high as that for acetyl-CoA, while the V_{max} value for this analogue is approximately one-seventh that for acetyl-CoA.

It has been shown with rat adipose tissue acetyl-CoA carboxylase that the apoenzyme lacking biotin fails to catalyze the carboxylation of acetyl-CoA [116]. Accumulation of apo-acetyl-CoA carboxylase in the adipose tissue of biotin-deficient rats has been demonstrated by immunochemical titration with specific antibody before and after treatment with biotin [117] and by separation of the apoenzyme with an avidin-agarose column [118]. The apoenzyme to holoenzyme ratio is much lower in the adipose tissue than in the liver. Studies with crude and partially purified enzyme systems have indicated that the biotinylation of apo-acetyl-CoA carboxylase proceeds through the same mechanism as that of other biotin-dependent enzymes [4,80,119]. The reaction of holo-acetyl-CoA carboxylase synthetase requires the apoenzyme, biotin, ATP and Mg^{2+}. It has been shown with propionyl-CoA carboxylase that D-biotinyl 5'-adenylate can replace biotin, ATP and Mg^{2+} [120]. Recently, S. cerevisiae mutants defective in holo-acetyl-CoA carboxylase synthetase have been isolated, and this holoenzyme synthetase is responsible for the biotinylation of at least 2 biotin-dependent enzymes, that is, acetyl-CoA carboxylase and pyruvate carboxylase [59] (see Chapter III). It has also been reported that human fibroblasts from patients with biotin-responsive, multiple carboxylase deficiency exhibit low levels of acetyl-CoA carboxylase, pyruvate carboxylase, propionyl-CoA carboxylase and 3-methylcrotonyl-CoA carboxylase and contain an abnormal holocarboxylase synthetase with a decreased V_{max} value and an elevated K_m value for biotin [121]. These results suggest that one holocarboxylase synthetase is responsible for the biotinylation of multiple biotin-dependent enzymes. This view is supported by the fact that the primary structure of the region surrounding the biotinylation site is similar in different enzymes (see ref. 10).

5. Regulation of acetyl-CoA carboxylase

It is generally accepted that acetyl-CoA carboxylase represents the rate-limiting enzyme for the regulation of fatty acid synthesis [3,122,123]. In support of this view is the fact that the tissue concentration of malonyl-CoA varies in parallel with the rate of fatty acid synthesis [84,124]. The regulation of acetyl-CoA carboxylase is effected by changes both in the catalytic efficiency and in the cellular content of the enzyme. Principally, two mechanisms are known to control the catalytic efficiency of the enzyme; activation and inhibition by metabolites and phosphorylation/dephosphorylation of the enzyme. It is possible to regulate the enzyme content by changes either in the rate of synthesis or in the rate of degradation of the enzyme. In general, the enzyme content is controlled by accelerated or diminished synthesis of the enzyme.

(a) Activation and inhibition

Acetyl-CoA carboxylase from animal tissues requires a hydroxy tricarboxylic acid activator such as citrate or isocitrate for its catalytic activity [68–71]. Because citrate is a precursor of acetyl-CoA, it appears to function as a positive feed-forward activator [6,125]. On the other hand, long-chain fatty acyl-CoA , the end product of fatty acid synthesis, specifically counteracts the activation by hydroxy tricarboxylic acid as a negative feedback inhibitor [73,126,127].

Studies on the specificity of the activation with a variety of carboxylic acids indicate that hydroxy tricarboxylic acids, such as citrate, isocitrate, hydroxycitrate, and fluorocitrate, and the dicarboxylic acid malonate are most effective [69,72,85,128,129]. For the activation by citrate, its hydroxyl group is essential, because tricarballylate and *O*-acetylated citrate are ineffective [69,85,128]. Isocitrate lactone, which has no free hydroxyl group as a result of intramolecular ester bond formation, shows no activation [128]. The absolute configuration of isocitrate does not affect the stimulatory action [69].

Prior incubation with citrate at higher temperature (25–37°C) is required for the enzyme to exhibit full activity when subsequently assayed in the presence of citrate [69,72,74,85]. The activation by preincubation is dependent on temperature and enzyme concentration [72,74]. The rat-liver enzyme that has previously been activated by citrate at 25°C is inactivated upon exposure to low temperature [74]; this process is largely reversible. Proteolytic modification of the liver and mammary gland enzymes results in partial loss of its citrate dependency [46,47,130].

Both of the partial reactions (Eqns. 1 and 2) involved in the overall carboxylation require a hydroxy tricarboxylate activator as shown by isotope exchange experiments [69,85] as well as by experiments with model substrates [131]. The kinetic data indicate that, of the obligatory enzyme forms, only the carboxylated form of the enzyme (E-biotin $\sim CO_2$) is dependent on the presence of citrate, the dissociation constant of the E-biotin $\sim CO_2 \cdot$ citrate complex being 3–6 mM (Fig. 2). On the other hand, it is well established that the effect of citrate is also exerted on the uncarboxylated form of the enzyme (E-biotin) to induce polymerization of the enzyme molecule (see Section 3b). In fact, equilibrium dialysis and other experiments indicate that the uncarboxylated form of liver acetyl-CoA carboxylase exhibits a dissociation constant of 2–14 μM for citrate [87,132]. This value is 3 orders of magnitude lower than the dissociation constant of the E-biotin $\sim CO_2 \cdot$ citrate complex estimated by kinetic studies [87], so that the effect of citrate on the uncarboxylated enzyme (E-biotin) is not apparent upon kinetic analysis of the carboxylation reaction. These findings indicate that the carboxylation of the biotinyl

12

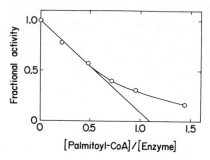

Fig. 3. Titration of rat liver acetyl-CoA carboxylase with palmitoyl-CoA. Data taken from ref. 135.

prosthetic group induces a conformational change, resulting in a marked decrease in the affinity of the enzyme for citrate. Thus, the main role of citrate in the catalysis is to keep the carboxylated form of the enzyme in active conformation by shifting the equilibrium between the active and inactive species of this enzyme form [87].

In addition to hydroxy tricarboxylic acids, CoA has been shown to activate acetyl-CoA carboxylase from rat liver [133]. The enzyme contains one CoA-binding site per subunit, and the CoA binding is not affected by the presence of citrate.

Long-chain acyl-CoA thioesters inhibit acetyl-CoA carboxylase from liver [73,126,127,134,135], mammary gland [136] and adipose tissue [137]. This inhibition is competitive with respect to the activator citrate and is noncompetitive with respect to the substrates acetyl-CoA, bicarbonate and ATP [73]. On the basis of the kinetics of tight-binding inhibitors [138], it has been demonstrated that 1 mole of palmitoyl-CoA completely inhibits 1 mole of rat liver acetyl-CoA carboxylase, the inhibition constant being 5.5 nM [135] (Fig. 3); this value is about 3 orders of magnitude smaller than the critical micellar concentration of palmitoyl-CoA [139,140]. The

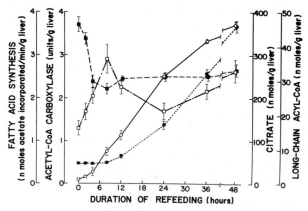

Fig. 4. Effects of fat-free refeeding on fatty acid synthesis in rat liver slices (O———O) and on the levels of hepatic acetyl-CoA carboxylase (●------●), citrate (□·—·—·□) and long-chain acyl-CoA (■— — —■). Results are given as means ± S.D. per gram of wet tissue. For each point, 6–8 rats were used. Data taken from ref. 145.

binding of [^{14}C]palmitoyl-CoA to the enzyme has been studied by sucrose density gradient centrifugation [135]. The enzyme, when preincubated with palmitoyl-CoA in low molar ratios (inhibitor/enzyme ≤ 5), is associated with an equimolar amount of the inhibitor, assuming the "small" molecular form. The equimolar enzyme–inhibitor complex is formed even in the presence of phosphatidylcholine, which is known to bind palmitoyl-CoA. The activator citrate, which competes kinetically with palmitoyl-CoA, not only prevents this equimolar association but also dissociates the equimolar enzyme–inhibitor complex in the presence of an acceptor for long-chain acyl-CoA, such as alkylated cyclodextrin or phosphatidylcholine. The enzyme thus freed of the inhibitor assumes the "large" molecular form and regains its full activity. In contrast, the enzyme, when preincubated with palmitoyl-CoA in high molar ratios (inhibitor/enzyme ≥ 20), binds a large molar excess of the inhibitor and is further dissociated into the monomeric subunit as is the enzyme treated with sodium dodecylsulfate. Phosphatidylcholine protects the enzyme from binding an excess of palmitoyl-CoA. When the enzyme associated with a large excess of palmitoyl-CoA is deprived of the inhibitor by treatment with citrate and alkylated

TABLE 1

K_i values of rat liver acetyl-CoA carboxylase for long-chain acyl-CoA and its analogues [a]

Inhibitor	K_i (nM)
Palmitoyl-CoA	6.5
Palmitoyl-CoA(L)	22
Palmitoyl-keto-CoA	21
Palmitoyl-1,N^6-etheno-CoA	15
Palmitoyl-inosino-CoA	14
Palmitoyl-dephospho-CoA	260
Palmitoyl-4′-phosphopantetheine	650
S-Cetyl-CoA	10
Palmitate	– [b]
Lauroyl-CoA	– [c]
Myristoyl-CoA	680
Stearoyl-CoA	1.3
Arachidoyl-CoA	< 1
Docosanoyl-CoA	40
Tetracosanoyl-CoA	150
Palmitoleoyl-CoA	130
Oleoyl-CoA	44
Linoleoyl-CoA	27
Linolenoyl-CoA	66
Arachidonoyl-CoA	48

[a] Taken from refs. 135 and 141.
[b] No inhibition is observed at concentrations up to 15 μM.
[c] No inhibition is observed at concentrations up to 10 μM.

cyclodextrin, the enzyme becomes nonspecifically aggregated as in the case of the sodium dodecylsulfate-treated enzyme and does not regain activity. Thus, it is concluded that palmitoyl-CoA binds tightly and reversibly to hepatic acetyl-CoA carboxylase in an equimolar ratio to inhibit the enzyme.

The specificity of inhibition of rat liver acetyl-CoA carboxylase by long-chain acyl-CoA has been studied with various structural analogues of palmitoyl-CoA, and the inhibition constants (K_i), determined with the use of the kinetics of tight-binding inhibitors [138,141], are listed in Table 1. The 3'-phosphate of the CoA moiety is essential for the inhibition of the enzyme by palmitoyl-CoA. Modification of the pantoic acid, adenine or thioester moiety of palmitoyl-CoA does not appreciably influence its inhibitory effect. The CoA thioesters of saturated fatty acids with 16–20 carbon atoms inhibit the enzyme more effectively than those of saturated fatty acids of shorter and longer chain lengths. The CoA thioesters of unsaturated fatty acids are less inhibitory than those of saturated fatty acids of corresponding chain lengths. The rather strict structural requirement for the inhibitory effect of long-chain acyl-CoA indicates that the inhibitor binds to a specific site on the enzyme molecule. This, together with the reversible formation of the equimolar enzyme–inhibitor complex, supports the concept that long-chain acyl-CoA is a physiological regulator of acetyl-CoA carboxylase.

In addition to long-chain acyl-CoA, a number of naturally occurring or chemically synthesized compounds have been reported to inhibit liver acetyl-CoA carboxylase. They include metabolites of tryptophan such as kynurenate and xanthrenate [87], polyphosphoinositides such as phosphatidylinositol 4,5-bisphosphate [142] as well as hypolipidemic agents such as 2-methyl-2-[p-(1,2,3,4-tetrahydro-1-naphthyl)phenoxy]propionate and 2-(p-chlorophenoxy)-2-methylpropionate [143]. The apparent inhibition constants for these compounds are 2–5 orders of magnitude higher than those for long-chain acyl-CoA.

The intracellular concentrations of positive and negative allosteric regulators, namely citrate and long-chain acyl-CoA, have been studied in relation to the physiological regulation of fatty acid synthesis. The cellular concentrations of citrate and long-chain acyl-CoA in various metabolic conditions, determined for whole tissues, are generally consistent with the changes in the rate of fatty acid synthesis (see ref. 6). Recently, the "digitonin-rapid-stop" technique has been applied to the determination of citrate in liver cells, and 50–75% of the cellular citrate is found in the cytoplasm [144], where acetyl-CoA carboxylase is localized. The estimated cytoplasmic concentrations of citrate in various metabolic conditions are in the range of 0.33–1.9 mM, which is close to the concentration required for half-maximal activation of acetyl-CoA carboxylase. Moreover, glucagon or dibutyryl cyclic AMP, which inhibits fatty acid synthesis, decreases the cytoplasmic concentration of citrate by an order of magnitude in cultured chicken liver cells [82]. This decrease appears to shift the equilibrium between the "large" and the "small" molecular form toward the latter to lower the catalytic efficiency of acetyl-CoA carboxylase (see Section 3b). On the other hand, the cytoplasmic concentration of long-chain acyl-CoA has not been reported. Owing to interactions with intracellular proteins and membrane lipids, it seems difficult to assess the effective concentration of long-chain acyl-CoA regulating the catalytic efficiency of acetyl-CoA carboxylase in vivo.

Fig. 4 shows an experiment designed to evaluate the relative contributions of the cellular content and the catalytic efficiency of acetyl-CoA carboxylase to increased fatty acid synthesis that occurs upon refeeding fasted rats with a fat-free diet [145]. For this purpose, the time course of changes in the hepatic contents of acetyl-CoA carboxylase, citrate and long-chain acyl-CoA as well as in the rate of fatty acid synthesis in liver slices was followed. The rate of fatty acid synthesis from acetate begins to increase within 2 h of realimentation and keeps rising during the whole period of 48-h refeeding. The long-chain acyl-CoA content falls sharply within 4 h and changes little thereafter. The citrate content increases during the first 8 h, decreases thereafter to some extent, and increases again after 24 h. On the other hand, the acetyl-CoA carboxylase content remains unchanged during the initial 8 h. Only after this time, it begins to increase and keeps rising during the whole experimental period. These results indicate that the initial rise in the rate of fatty acid synthesis observed within 8 h of refeeding cannot be ascribed to an increased quantity of acetyl-CoA carboxylase but may rather be due to changes in the concentrations of allosteric effectors such as citrate and long-chain acyl-CoA. After the lapse of 8 h, the content of acetyl-CoA carboxylase begins to increase, thus contributing also to the elevated rate of fatty acid synthesis. Thus, the modulation of the catalytic efficiency of acetyl-CoA carboxylase makes a greater contribution to the short-term regulation of fatty acid synthesis, whereas the change of the enzyme content plays an important role in the long-term regulation (see Section 5c).

Acetyl-CoA carboxylase from S. cerevisiae is inhibited by long-chain fatty acyl-CoA, but is not activated by citrate in contrast to the animal enzymes [146]. Reversibility of the inhibition has been demonstrated by removing long-chain acyl-CoA with phosphatidylcholine. Acetyl-CoA carboxylase from C. lipolytica is markedly activated by polyethylene glycol [39]. The activation is due principally to a decrease in the K_m values for substrates. In a myo-inositol-deficient strain of S. carlsbergensis, fatty acid synthesis from acetate is markedly augmented [147], and this increase can be ascribed to activation of acetyl-CoA carboxylase by fructose 1,6-bisphosphate, which increases the V_{max} value for ATP [148]. Citrate counteracts the activation by fructose bisphosphate, but has no inhibitory effect in the absence of the activator.

In E. coli, the synthesis of phospholipids as well as RNA is under the control of the rel locus [9,149]. Amino acid starvation of stringent (rel^+) strains, but not of relaxed (rel^-) strains, results in a 2–4-fold decrease in phospholipid synthesis. Guanine-5'-diphosphate-3'-diphosphate (ppGpp) accumulates (up to 4 mM) during amino acid starvation. Acetyl-CoA carboxylase [150] and β-hydroxydecanoyl thioester dehydrase [151], which are involved in fatty acid synthesis, as well as glycerophosphate acyltransferase and phosphatidylglycerol phosphate synthetase [152], which are involved in phospholipid synthesis, are inhibited by physiological concentrations of ppGpp. Of the two catalytic components of the acetyl-CoA carboxylase system of E. coli (see Section 3a), only carboxyltransferase is inhibited;

50–60% inhibition occurs at saturating concentrations of ppGpp or pppGpp (1.0–1.2 mM) [150]. The acetyl-CoA carboxylase system from *P. citronellolis* is inhibited by 70% at 1 mM ppGpp [44].

(b) Phosphorylation and dephosphorylation

Intraperitoneal injection of [^{32}P]phosphate into rats results in the incorporation of ^{32}P into adipose tissue acetyl-CoA carboxylase [153]. Administration of adrenaline stimulates the ^{32}P incorporation and decreases the activity of the enzyme. Similar observations have been made with rat adipose tissue [154], fat cells [155] and liver cells [154,156] incubated with adrenaline, glucagon or cyclic nucleotides. This suggests that the reduced activity of acetyl-CoA carboxylase may be due, at least partly, to the phosphorylation of the enzyme (see refs. 10 and 12).

A number of studies on the modulation of acetyl-CoA carboxylase activity by phosphorylation have been reported with purified or partially purified acetyl-CoA carboxylase preparations from liver [53,157–165] and mammary gland [166–168]. 3–6 moles of phosphate are contained in purified enzyme preparations [22–24,28,29,31,47,52,53,169]. Acetyl-CoA carboxylase from rabbit mammary gland purified in the presence of sodium fluoride has a specific activity of 1.2 units/mg protein and 6.2 moles of covalently bound phosphate per mole of subunit [169]. On the other hand, the enzyme purified in the absence of sodium fluoride exhibits a specific activity of 3.0 units/mg protein and a phosphate content of 4.8 moles/mole of subunit [169]. When the purified enzyme from liver [53,165] and mammary gland [166,167] is incubated with [γ-^{32}P]ATP and a protein kinase, 1–2 moles of phosphate per subunit are incorporated into the carboxylase; the catalytic subunit of cyclic AMP-dependent protein kinase from bovine heart or cyclic AMP-independent protein kinase from rat liver (see below) was used. This increase in the phosphate content is accompanied by a decrease in the enzyme activity by more than 80%.

It is noteworthy that an apparently homogeneous acetyl-CoA carboxylase preparation from rabbit mammary gland can be phosphorylated both in the cyclic AMP-dependent and -independent manner without addition of an exogenous protein kinase [166]. This may indicate that the enzyme preparation used contains traces of protein kinases. Recently, a cyclic AMP-independent protein kinase that catalyzes phosphorylation of acetyl-CoA carboxylase has been purified from rat liver; the K_m of the protein kinase for acetyl-CoA carboxylase is 90 nM [165]. This protein kinase is also capable of phosphorylating protamine and histone, but not hydroxymethylglutaryl-CoA reductase and phosphorylase *b*.

When rabbit mammary gland acetyl-CoA carboxylase is phosphorylated in vitro with [γ-^{32}P]ATP and endogenous protein kinases in the presence and absence of cyclic AMP, two different spots are observed in the 2-dimensional maps of the tryptic digests [13]. These spots are due to two different sites, one of which is specifically phosphorylated with cyclic AMP-dependent protein kinase. Multiple spots are also seen in the 2-dimensional maps of the tryptic digests of the immunochemically precipitated acetyl-CoA carboxylase from homogenates prepared from rat fat cells incubated in medium containing [^{32}P]phosphate in the presence or absence of adrenaline [170].

When highly phosphorylated acetyl-CoA carboxylase from rabbit mammary gland (containing 5.9 moles of phosphate per mole of subunit) is dephosphorylated with protein phosphatase-1 from rabbit muscle, 1.5 moles of the protein-bound phosphate are lost [169]. The carboxylase thus treated exhibits a 4-fold higher activity than does the untreated enzyme when assayed at physiological citrate concentrations (0.3–1.0 mM); the increase in activity is 2.3-fold at 10 mM citrate. This activation is completely dependent on Mn^{2+} and is prevented by a protein phosphatase inhibitor. A protein phosphatase has been highly purified from rat adipose tissue; the phosphatase is copurified with acetyl-CoA carboxylase up to the ethanol precipitation step [171]. This protein phosphatase shows a K_m value of 1.5 μM for acetyl-CoA carboxylase and has a broad substrate specificity.

Limited trypsin treatment of highly phosphorylated acetyl-CoA carboxylase from rabbit mammary gland results in a decrease of its subunit molecular weight from 250 000 to 225 000 and in a 2-fold increase in its activity [46]. The trypsin-treated enzyme undergoes no further activation when subsequently treated with protein phosphatase-1. When the enzyme dephosphorylated by protein phosphatase is subjected to limited trypsin treatment, the cleavage of the subunit polypeptide occurs at the same rate, but no activation is observed. Treatment with either trypsin or protein phosphatase causes the loss of about 1 mole of phosphate per mole of subunit. Similar results have been obtained with chicken liver acetyl-CoA carboxylase [47]. This finding suggests that acetyl-CoA carboxylase contains a domain or region near one end of the polypeptide chain, which is inhibitory when the enzyme is phosphorylated.

In contrast to protein phosphatase treatment, alkaline phosphatase treatment of highly phosphorylated liver acetyl-CoA carboxylase does not affect the enzyme activity despite the fact that 2–3 moles of phosphate per mole of subunit are removed [23,47]. Thus, acetyl-CoA carboxylase from animal species has multiple phosphorylation sites, one or at most two of which seem to be responsible for modulating the catalytic efficiency of the enzyme.

It has been reported that the extent of phosphorylation as well as the activity of acetyl-CoA carboxylase in cultured chick liver cells is not altered by addition of dibutyryl cyclic AMP to culture medium [172]. The discrepancy between this experiment and other analogous studies with rat liver cells and fat cells may be due to the difference in species or cell type or in experimental conditions.

(c) Synthesis and degradation

In addition to the regulation by changes in the catalytic efficiency per enzyme molecule brought about by allosteric effectors and by phosphorylation/dephosphorylation, the regulation by changes in the enzyme quantity, that is, the number of enzyme molecules, plays an essential role in the control of the acetyl-CoA carboxylation reaction (see Section 5a). The tissue level of acetyl-CoA carboxylase activity varies in accord with the rate of fatty acid synthesis in a variety of dietary, hormonal, developmental and genetic conditions (see refs. 6 and 7). Fasted rats and alloxan-diabetic rats exhibit about one-fourth and one-half, respectively, the normal level of hepatic acetyl-CoA carboxylase activity, whereas rats fasted and subsequently refed a fat-free diet and genetically obese mice show enzyme levels about 4-fold higher than the normal level [19,123,173–177]; in normal and obese mice, comparison is made in terms of unit liver weight. The enzyme level in chick liver increases drastically after hatching [178–180]. Immunochemical titrations with specific antibody indicate that, in all these conditions, the level of acetyl-CoA carboxylase activity reflects the quantity of the enzyme protein [19,176,177,180]. On the other hand, control and adrenaline-treated rat adipose tissues have been shown by immunochemical titrations to contain an equal amount of the enzyme with different catalytic efficiencies; the reduced catalytic efficiency of the enzyme from the hormone-treated tissue is attributable to phosphorylation of the enzyme [181] (see Section 5b).

The quantity of an enzyme is affected by changes in the rates of its synthesis and/or degradation. Under steady-state conditions, the content of an enzyme is related to these rates as follows:

$$E = k_s / k_d \qquad (4)$$

where E is the content of enzyme per mass, k_s is a zero-order rate constant of synthesis per mass, and k_d is a first-order rate constant of degradation expressed as reciprocal of time (see ref. 182). Combined immunochemical and isotopic techniques have been used to determine whether the observed variations in the hepatic acetyl-CoA carboxylase content in different metabolic conditions are due to changes in the rate of synthesis or in the rate of degradation of the enzyme (see ref. 7). The rate of synthesis is measured by injecting animals with a dose of [^{3}H]leucine and shortly thereafter determining the extent of isotope incorporation into the enzyme precipitated with specific antibody. The rate of degradation is measured by following the loss of isotope from the prelabeled enzyme. These studies have shown that the increase or decrease in the enzyme content in refed or diabetic rats is ascribed solely to a corresponding change in the rate of synthesis of the enzyme, whereas the decrease in the enzyme content in fasted rats is due to both diminished synthesis and accelerated degradation of the enzyme [19,176]; the half-life ($t_{1/2}$) for degradation of the enzyme is 50–59 h in control, fat-free refed and alloxan-diabetic rats and 18–31 h in fasted rats. The increased enzyme content in obese mice is due mainly to elevated synthesis of the enzyme and, in a minor degree, to diminished degradation of the enzyme [177] ($t_{1/2} = 67$ and 115 h in normal and obese mice, respectively). The increase in the enzyme content in growing chicks is attributable to accelerated synthesis of the enzyme [180]; the enzyme in 9-day-old chicks is degraded with a $t_{1/2}$ of 46 h, whereas no apparent degradation is observed in 1-day-old chicks.

It is evident from the results described above that the cellular content of acetyl-CoA carboxylase is regulated principally by changes in the rate of synthesis of

TABLE 2

Correlation between the hepatic content of acetyl-CoA carboxylase-synthesizing polysomes and the rate of hepatic acetyl-CoA carboxylase synthesis in vivo

Animal	Content of specific polysomes [a]	Rate of enzyme synthesis in vivo [b]
Rat		
Normal [c]	1	1
Fasted	1/2–1/3	1/2
Refed	3–4	4
Alloxan-diabetic	1/2	1/2
Mouse		
Normal [c]	1	1
Obese	2	3

[a] Taken from refs. 183–185.
[b] Taken from refs. 19 and 177.
[c] Values for normal animals are taken as unity.

the enzyme. In an attempt to assess the question, at which step the rate of acetyl-CoA carboxylase synthesis is regulated, the hepatic content of specific polysomes synthesizing this enzyme have been estimated by determining the binding of ^{125}I-labeled antibody to isolated liver polysomes [183,184] and by translating liver polysomes in a cell-free protein-synthesizing system [185] ("run-off" experiments). The results of these experiments, summarized in Table 2, show that the hepatic content of polysomes synthesizing acetyl-CoA carboxylase varies in accord with the rate of synthesis in vivo of the enzyme as estimated by combined immunochemical and isotopic techniques [19,176,177]. Thus, the different rates of acetyl-CoA carboxylase synthesis in various metabolic conditions can be ascribed to changes in the amount of translatable mRNA coding for the enzyme.

A next important question is what metabolite is responsible for the regulation of acetyl-CoA carboxylase synthesis. A plausible candidate would be fatty acid or some compound metabolically related to it. In fact, the rate of synthesis of the enzyme (measured by combined immunochemical and isotopic techniques) in cultured hepatocytes [186] as well as in yeasts [187,188] is diminished when fatty acid is added to the culture medium. For studying the mechanism responsible for the repression of acetyl-CoA carboxylase, the hydrocarbon-utilizing yeast *Candida lipolytica* represents a useful eukaryotic system because this yeast is capable of utilizing fatty acid (or *n*-alkane) as well as glucose as a sole carbon source and thus exhibits large variations in the rate of synthesis of the enzyme [188]. Recently, complete acetyl-CoA carboxylase (subunit molecular weight, 230 000) has successfully been synthesized by translating mRNA from *C. lipolytica* in a cell-free protein-synthesizing system derived from rabbit reticulocytes [189]. With the use of this assay system, it has been demonstrated that the level of acetyl-CoA carboxylase mRNA in *C.*

lipolytica cells decreases with increasing concentrations of fatty acid in culture medium in parallel with the cellular content of the enzyme [189], as shown in Fig. 5. It is therefore concluded that the repression of acetyl-CoA carboxylase is effected at the pretranslational level.

In an attempt to determine whether the repressive effect is mediated by fatty acid itself or a metabolite derived from it, mutant strains of *C. lipolytica* that exhibit apparently no activity of long-chain acyl-CoA synthetase [acid:CoA ligase (AMP-forming), EC 6.2.1.3] were isolated [190]. The mutants were selected by their inability to grow in the presence of exogenous fatty acid under conditions where the cellular synthesis de novo of fatty acids was blocked by cerulenin, a specific inhibitor of fatty acid synthetase. Because the activation of exogenous fatty acid is an obligatory step for its further metabolism, it was unexpected that these mutants were capable of growing on fatty acid (or *n*-alkane) as a sole carbon source. This phenotype has been understood, however, by the finding that the mutant strains, unlike the wild-type strain, cannot incorporate exogenous fatty acid as a whole into cellular lipids, but are able to degrade it to yield acetyl-CoA, from which cellular fatty acids are synthesized de novo [190]. Moreover, this finding has led to the discovery of a second long-chain acyl-CoA synthetase, which occurs in the mutant strains as well as in the wild-type strain [191]. This enzyme is designated as acyl-CoA synthetase II, while the enzyme missing in the mutant strains is designated as acyl-CoA synthetase I. The two enzymes have been purified to homogeneity and are protein-chemically and immunochemically distinguishable from each other. Thus, it has been concluded that acyl-CoA synthetase I is responsible for the production of long-chain acyl-CoA to be utilized for the synthesis of cellular lipids, whereas acyl-CoA synthetase II provides long-chain acyl-CoA that is exclusively degraded via β-oxidation. Consistent with this conclusion is the fact that acyl-CoA synthetase II, in contrast to acyl-CoA synthetase I, is induced by fatty acid and exhibits a broad substrate specificity with respect to fatty acid [191]. In further support of the

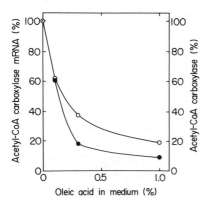

Fig. 5. Levels of acetyl-CoA carboxylase (○) and its mRNA (●) in *C. lipolytica* cells grown in the presence of oleic acid. Cells were grown in media containing oleic acid at the indicated concentrations and 2% glucose. Data taken from ref. 189.

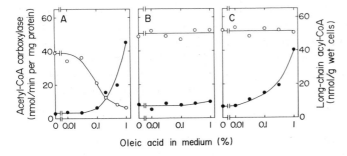

Fig. 6. Effect of the two long-chain acyl-CoA pools on acetyl-CoA carboxylase. Cells of *C. lipolytica* strain A-633-7 defective in acyl-CoA synthetase II (A), strain LA-633 defective in both acyl-CoA synthetase I and II (B) and strain LB-742 defective in acyl-CoA synthetase I (C) were grown in media containing oleic acid at the indicated concentrations and 2% glucose. The cells harvested were divided into 2 portions for determination of the levels of long-chain acyl-CoA (●) and acetyl-CoA carboxylase (○). Data taken from ref. 193.

different physiological roles of the two long-chain acyl-CoA synthetases, their subcellular localizations are different [192]. Acyl-CoA synthetase I is distributed among various subcellular fractions, including microsomes and mitochondria where glycerophosphate acyltransferase, the initial enzyme responsible for glycerolipid synthesis, is located, whereas acyl-CoA synthetase II is localized in microbodies where the acyl-CoA-oxidizing system of this yeast is located.

From the findings described above, it may be inferred that the cell of *C. lipolytica* has 2 independent long-chain acyl-CoA pools, one destined for lipid synthesis and the other for β-oxidation. In order to prove this hypothesis, additional mutant strains of *C. lipolytica* that are defective in acyl-CoA synthetase II and that completely fail to grow on fatty acid as a sole carbon source were isolated [193]. This phenotype, in conjunction with that of the acyl-CoA synthetase I mutants mentioned above, indicates clearly that the long-chain acyl-CoA produced by acyl-CoA synthetase I is utilized solely for lipid synthesis, whereas that produced by acyl-CoA synthetase II is destined exclusively for β-oxidation.

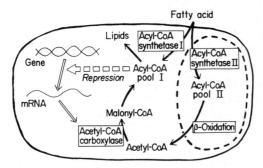

Fig. 7. Mechanism of repression of acetyl-CoA carboxylase.

As described above, the wild-type strain of *C. lipolytica* exhibits the repression of acetyl-CoA carboxylase when it is grown in the presence of fatty acid. In contrast, the acetyl-CoA carboxylase content in the mutants defective in acyl-CoA synthetase I is hardly decreased by exogenous fatty acid [193]. The mutants defective in acyl-CoA synthetase II as well as the revertants derived from an acyl-CoA synthetase I mutant respond normally to exogenous fatty acid. Thus, it is evident that the activity of acyl-CoA synthetase I, but not that of acyl-CoA synthetase II, is required for the repression of acetyl-CoA carboxylase.

In the experiment represented in Fig. 6, an attempt has been made to measure separately the two independent long-chain acyl-CoA pools provided by acyl-CoA synthetase I and acyl-CoA synthetase II, using appropriate mutant strains [193]. When fatty acid is added to culture medium at increasing concentrations, the mutant defective in acyl-CoA synthetase II (Fig. 6A) should accumulate the long-chain acyl-CoA to be utilized for lipid synthesis, whereas the mutant lacking acyl-CoA synthetase I (and also the acyl-CoA-oxidizing system) (Fig. 6C) should accumulate the long-chain acyl-CoA destined for β-oxidation. On the other hand, the mutant defective in both acyl-CoA synthetases (Fig. 6B) should produce no long-chain acyl-CoA from exogenous fatty acid. The repression of acetyl-CoA carboxylase is observed in the mutant defective in acyl-CoA synthetase II, but not in the other two mutants. These results clearly indicate that the long-chain acyl-CoA to be utilized for lipid synthesis is causally related to the repression of acetyl-CoA carboxylase, whereas the long-chain acyl-CoA to be degraded via β-oxidation is not involved in this repression. It is intriguing to hypothesize that a similar regulatory mechanism is valid for other lipogenic enzymes such as fatty acid synthetase (see Chapter 2), citrate cleavage enzyme, hexose monophosphate shunt dehydrogenases and malic enzyme. The cellular contents of these enzymes, together with acetyl-CoA carboxylase, undergo coordinate changes in accord with the rate of fatty acid synthesis in various metabolic conditions (see refs. 6 and 7).

The regulatory mechanism discussed above is obviously of teleological significance in view of the homeostasis of lipid synthesis, as schematically shown in Fig. 7. The long-chain acyl-CoA destined for lipid synthesis is supplied both by fatty acid synthesis de novo, the rate of which is regulated by acetyl-CoA carboxylase, and by the activation of exogenous fatty acid catalyzed by acyl-CoA synthetase I. It seems probable that the long-chain acyl-CoA to be utilized for lipid synthesis, or a compound metabolically related to it, acts as a corepressor or its eukaryotic equivalent to suppress the expression of the acetyl-CoA carboxylase gene. In view of the fact that long-chain acyl-CoA is a specific and potent inhibitor of acetyl-CoA carboxylase (see Section 5a), this fatty acid derivative plays a dual role in the regulation of the rate-limiting enzyme for fatty acid biosynthesis.

6. Concluding remarks

During the last decade or so, considerable progress has been made in studies on the structure, function and regulation of acetyl-CoA carboxylase, which plays a critical role in controlling the rate of fatty acid biosynthesis. Different levels of structural organization of the enzyme have been elucidated, and this may imply that gene fusion occurred in the course of evolution of the gene encoding the enzyme. Different modes of regulation of the enzyme have been discussed with special emphasis on the dual regulatory role of long-chain acyl-CoA in the repression and inhibition of the enzyme. In the future, the acetyl-CoA carboxylase gene will be cloned by recombinant DNA techniques, and this certainly will promote studies on the structure, function and evolution of the enzyme as well as on the regulation of expression of the gene.

References

1 Wakil, S.J. and Barnes Jr., E.M. (1971) in: M. Florkin and E.H. Stotz (Eds.), Comprehensive Biochemistry, Vol. 18S, Elsevier, Amsterdam, pp. 57–104.

2 Lynen, F. (1967) Biochem. J. 102, 381–400.

3 Numa, S., Nakanishi, S., Hashimoto, T., Iritani, N. and Okazaki, T. (1970) Vitam. Horm. 28, 213–243.

4 Moss, J. and Lane, M.D. (1971) Adv. Enzymol. 35, 321–442.

5 Volpe, J.J. and Vagelos, P.R. (1973) Annu. Rev. Biochem. 42, 21–60.

6 Numa, S. (1974) Ergebn. Physiol. 69, 53–96.

7 Numa, S. and Yamashita, S. (1974) in: B.L. Horecker and E.R. Stadtman (Eds.), Current Topics in Cellular Regulation, Vol. 8, Academic Press, New York, pp. 197–246.

8 Numa, S. (1975) Naturwissenschaften 62, 80–86.

9 Bloch, K. and Vance, D. (1977) Annu. Rev. Biochem. 46, 263–298.

10 Wood, H.G. and Barden, R.E. (1977) Annu. Rev. Biochem. 46, 385–413.

11 Kim, K.-H. (1983) in: B.L. Horecker and E.R. Stadtman (Eds.), Current Topics in Cellular Regulation, Vol. 22, Academic Press, New York, pp. 143–176.

12 Lane, M.D., Watkins, P.A. and Meredith, M.J. (1979) CRC Crit. Rev. Biochem. 7, 121–142.

13 Hardie, D.G. (1980) in: P. Cohen (Ed.), Molecular Aspects of Cellular Regulation, Vol. 1, Recently Discovered Systems of Enzyme Regulation by Reversible Phosphorylation, Elsevier/North-Holland Biomedical Press, Amsterdam, pp. 32–62.

14 Numa, S. (1981) Trends Biochem. Sci. 6, 113–115.

15 Goto, T., Ringelmann, E., Riedel, B. and Numa, S. (1967) Life Sci. 6, 785–790.

16 Numa, S. (1969) Methods Enzymol. 14, 9–16.

17 Gregolin, C., Ryder, E. and Lane, M.D. (1968) J. Biol. Chem. 243, 4227–4235.

18 Beaty, N.B. and Lane, M.D. (1982) J. Biol. Chem. 257, 924–929.

19 Nakanishi, S. and Numa, S. (1970) Eur. J. Biochem. 16, 161–173.

20 Hashimoto, T. and Numa, S. (1971) Eur. J. Biochem. 18, 319–331.

21 Tanabe, T., Nakanishi, S., Hashimoto, T., Ogiwara, H., Nikawa, J. and Numa, S. (1981) Methods Enzymol. 71, 5–16.

22 Inoue, H. and Lowenstein, J.M. (1972) J. Biol. Chem. 247, 4825–4832.

23 Song, C.S. and Kim, K.-H. (1981) J. Biol. Chem. 256, 7786–7788.

24 Witters, L.A. and Vogt, B. (1981) J. Lipid Res. 22, 364–369.

25 Manning, R., Dils, R. and Mayer, R.J. (1976) Biochem. J. 153, 463–468.

26 Hardie, D.G. and Cohen, P. (1978) Eur. J. Biochem. 92, 25–34.

27 Miller, A.L. and Levy, H.R. (1969) J. Biol. Chem. 244, 2334–2342.

28 Ahmad, F., Ahmad, P.M., Pieretti, L. and Watters, G.T. (1978) J. Biol. Chem. 253, 1733–1737.

29 Hardie, D.G. and Guy, P.S. (1980) Eur. J. Biochem. 110, 167–177.

30 Moss, J., Yamagishi, M., Kleinschmidt, A.K. and Lane, M.D. (1972) Biochemistry 11, 3779–3786.

31 Brownsey, R.W. and Denton, R.M. (1982) Biochem. J. 202, 77–86.

32 Rainwater, D.L. and Kolattukudy, P.E. (1982) Arch. Biochem. Biophys. 213, 372–383.

33 Wolpert, J.S. and Ernst-Fonberg, M.L. (1975) Biochemistry 14, 1095–1102.

34 Nielsen, N.C., Adee, A. and Stumpf, P.K. (1979) Arch. Biochem. Biophys. 192, 446–456.

35 Egin-Buler, B., Loyal, R. and Edel, J. (1980) Arch. Biochem. Biophys. 203, 90–100.

36 Mohan, S.B. and Kekwick, R.G.O. (1980) Biochem. J. 187, 667–676.

37 Sumper, M. and Riepertinger, C. (1972) Eur. J. Biochem. 29, 237–248.

38 Sumper, M. (1981) Methods Enzymol. 71, 34–37.

39 Mishina, M., Kamiryo, T., Tanaka, A., Fukui, S. and Numa, S. (1976) Eur. J. Biochem. 71, 295–300.

40 Mishina, M., Kamiryo, T. and Numa, S. (1981) Methods Enzymol. 71, 37–44.

41 Alberts, A.W., Gordon, S.G. and Vagelos, P.R. (1971) Proc. Natl. Acad. Sci. (U.S.A.) 68, 1259–1263.

42 Fall, R.R. and Vagelos, P.R. (1972) J. Biol. Chem. 247, 8005–8015.

43 Guchhait, R.B., Polakis, S.E., Dimroth, P., Stoll, E., Moss, J. and Lane, M.D. (1974) J. Biol. Chem. 249, 6633–6645.

44 Fall, R.R. (1976) Biochim. Biophys. Acta 450, 475–480.

45 Tanabe, T., Wada, K., Okazaki, T. and Numa, S. (1975) Eur. J. Biochem. 57, 15–24.

46 Guy, P.S. and Hardie, D.G. (1981) FEBS Lett. 132, 67–70.

47 Wada, K. and Tanabe, T., (1983) Eur. J. Biochem. 135, 17–23.

48 Fall, R.R. and Vagelos, P.R. (1973) J. Biol. Chem. 248, 2078–2088.

49 Green, N.M. and Toms, E.J. (1973) Biochem. J. 133, 687–700.

50 Henrikson, K.P., Allen, S.H.G. and Maloy, W.L. (1979) Anal. Biochem. 94, 366–370.

51 Gravel, R.A., Lam, K.F., Mahuran, D. and Kronis, A. (1980) Arch. Biochem. Biophys. 201, 669–673.

52 Kubo, T. and Numa, S., Unpublished results.

53 Tippers, J.P. and Witters, L.A. (1982) Biochim. Biophys. Acta 715, 162–169.

54 Alberts, A.W. and Vagelos, P.R. (1968) Proc. Natl. Acad. Sci. (U.S.A.) 59, 561–568.

55 Alberts, A.W., Nevri, A.M. and Vagelos, P.R. (1969) Proc. Natl. Acad. Sci. (U.S.A.) 63, 1320–1326.

56 Sutton, M.R., Fall, R.R., Nevri, A.M., Alberts, A.W. and Vagelos, P.R. (1977) J. Biol. Chem. 252, 3934–3940.

57 Kondo, H., Uno, S., Moriuchi, F., Sunamoto, J., Ogushi, S. and Tsuru, D. (1983) Bull. Chem. Soc. Jpn. 56, 1176–1180.

58 Mackall, J.C. and Lane, M.D. (1977) Biochem. J. 162, 635–642.

59 Mishina, M., Roggenkamp, R. and Schweizer, E. (1980) Eur. J. Biochem. 111, 79–87.

60 Obermayer, M. and Lynen, F. (1976) Trends Biochem. Sci. 1, 169–171.

61 Kirschner, K. and Bisswager, H. (1976) Annu. Rev. Biochem. 45, 143–166.

62 Meyer, H. and Meyer, F. (1978) Biochemistry 17, 1828–1833.

63 Hunaiti, A.R. and Kolattukudy, P.E. (1982) Arch. Biochem. Biophys. 216, 362–371.

64 Henrikson, K.P. and Allen, S.H.G. (1979) J. Biol. Chem. 254, 5888–5891.

65 Lau, E.P., Cochran, B.C., Muson, L. and Fall, R.R. (1979) Proc. Natl. Acad. Sci. (U.S.A.) 76, 214–218.

66 Schiele, U., Niedermeiyer, R., Sturzer, M. and Lynen, F. (1975) Eur. J. Biochem. 60, 259–266.

67 Fall, R.R. and Hecter, M.L. (1977) Biochemistry 16, 4000–4005.

68 Matsuhashi, M., Matsuhashi, S., Numa, S. and Lynen, F. (1962) Fed. Proc. 21, 288.

69 Matsuhashi, M., Matsuhashi, S. and Lynen, F. (1964) Biochem. Z. 340, 263–289.

70 Martin, D.B. and Vagelos, P.R. (1962) J. Biol. Chem. 237, 1787–1792.

71 Waite, M. and Wakil, S.J. (1962) J. Biol. Chem. 237, 2750–2757.

72 Vagelos, P.R., Alberts, A.W. and Martin, D.B. (1963) J. Biol. Chem. 238, 533–540.

73 Numa, S., Ringelmann, E. and Lynen, F. (1965) Biochem. Z. 343, 243–257.

74 Numa, S. and Ringelmann, E. (1965) Biochem. Z. 343, 258–268.

75 Gregolin, C., Ryder, E., Kleinschmidt, A.K., Warner, R.C. and Lane, M.D. (1966) Proc. Natl. Acad. Sci. (U.S.A.) 56, 148–155.

76 Kleinschmidt, A.K., Moss, J. and Lane, M.D. (1969) Science 166, 1276–1278.

77 Henniger, G. and Numa, S. (1972) Hoppe-Seyler's Z. Physiol. Chem. 353, 545–548.

78 Numa, S., Ringelmann, E. and Riedel, B. (1966) Biochem. Biophys. Res. Commun. 24, 750–757.

79 Numa, S., Hashimoto, T., Nakanishi, S. and Okazaki, T. (1972) in: J. Ganguly and R.M.S. Smellie (Eds.), Current Trends in the Biochemistry of Lipids, Academic Press, New York, pp. 27–39.
80 Landman, A.D. and Dakshinamurti, K. (1975) Biochem. J. 145, 545–548.
81 Landman, A.D. and Lampert, J. (1978) Biochem. J. 169, 255–256.
82 Watkins, P.A., Tarlow, D.M. and Lane, M.D. (1977) Proc. Natl. Acad. Sci. (U.S.A.) 74, 1497–1501.
83 Gregolin, C., Ryder, E., Warner, R.C., Kleinschmidt, A.K. and Lane, M.D. (1966) Proc. Natl. Acad. Sci. (U.S.A.) 56, 1751–1758.
84 Clarke, B.A. and Clarke, S.D. (1982) Arch. Biochem. Biophys. 218, 92–100.
85 Lynen, F., Matsuhashi, M., Numa, S. and Schweizer, E. (1963) in: J.K. Grant (Ed.), The Cellular Control of Fatty Acid Synthesis, Academic Press, New York, pp. 43–56.
86 Numa, S., Ringelmann, E. and Lynen, F. (1964) Biochem. Z. 340, 228–242.
87 Hashimoto, T., Isano, H., Iritani, N. and Numa, S. (1971) Eur. J. Biochem. 24, 128–139.
88 Northrop, D.B. (1969) J. Biol. Chem. 244, 5808–5819.
89 Northrop, D.B. and Wood, H.G. (1969) J. Biol. Chem. 244, 5820–5827.
90 McClure, W.R., Lardy, H.A., Wagner, M. and Cleland, W.W. (1971) J. Biol. Chem. 246, 3579–3583.
91 Barden, R.E., Fung, C.H., Utter, M.F. and Scrutton, M.C. (1972) J. Biol. Chem. 247, 1323–1333.
92 Wood, H.G. (1976) Trends Biochem. Sci. 1, 4–6.
93 Guchhait, R.B., Polakis, S.E., Hollis, D., Fenselau, C. and Lane, M.D. (1974) J. Biol. Chem. 249, 6646–6656.
94 Knappe, J., Wenger, B. and Wiegand, U. (1963) Biochem. Z. 337, 232–246.
95 Lane, M.D. and Lynen, F. (1963) Proc. Natl. Acad. Sci. (U.S.A.) 49, 379–385.
96 Wood, H.G., Lochmuller, H., Riepertinger, C. and Lynen, F. (1963) Biochem. Z. 337, 247–266.
97 Scrutton, M.C., Keech, D.B. and Utter, M.F. (1965) J. Biol. Chem. 240, 574–581.
98 Stallings, W.C., Monti, C.T., Lane, M.D. and Detitta, G.T. (1980) Proc. Natl. Acad. Sci. (U.S.A.) 77, 1260–1264.
99 Polakis, S.E., Guchhait, R.B. and Lane, M.D. (1972) J. Biol. Chem. 247, 1335–1337.
100 Kaziro, Y., Haas, L.F., Boyer, P.D. and Ochoa, S. (1962) J. Biol. Chem. 237, 1460–1468.
101 Ashman, L.K. and Keech, D.B. (1975) J. Biol. Chem. 250, 14–21.
102 Retey, J. and Lynen, F. (1965) Biochem. Z. 342, 256–271.
103 Kluger, R. and Adwadkar, P.D. (1976) J. Am. Chem. Soc. 98, 3741–3742.
104 Kluger, R., Davis, P.P. and Adwadkar, P.D. (1979) J. Am. Chem. Soc. 101, 5995–6000.
105 DeTitta, G.T., Edmonds, J.W., Stallings, W. and Donohue, J. (1976) J. Am. Chem. Soc. 98, 1920–1926.
106 Blonski, C., Gasc, M.-B., Klaebe, A., Perie, J.-J., Roques, R., Declercq, J.P. and Germain, G. (1982) J. Chem. Soc. (Perkin Trans. 2), 7–13.
107 Mildvan, A.S., Scrutton, M.C. and Utter, M.F. (1966) J. Biol. Chem. 241, 3488–3498.
108 Fung, C.H., Feldmann, R.J. and Mildvan, A.S. (1976) Biochemistry 15, 75–84.
109 Fung, C.H., Gupta, R.K. and Mildvan, A.S. (1976) Biochemistry 15, 85–92.
110 DeTitta, G.T., Parthasarathy, R., Blessing, R.H. and Stallings, W. (1980) Proc. Natl. Acad. Sci. (U.S.A.) 77, 333–337.
111 Kondo, H., Miura, K. and Sunamoto, J. (1982) Tetrahedron Lett. 23, 659–662.
112 Kohn, H. (1976) J. Am. Chem. Soc. 98, 3690–3694.
113 Lynen, F., Knappe, J., Lorch, E., Jütting, G., Ringelmann, E. and Lachance, J.-P. (1961) Biochem. Z. 335, 123–167.
114 Sedgwick, B., Cornforth, J.W., French, S.J., Gray, R.T., Kelstrup, E. and Willadsen, P. (1977) Eur. J. Biochem. 75, 481–485.
115 Nikawa, J., Numa, S., Shiba, T., Stewart, C.J. and Wieland, T. (1978) FEBS Lett. 91, 144–148.
116 Dakshinamurti, K. and Desjardins, P.R. (1969) Biochim. Biophys. Acta 176, 221–229.
117 Jacobs, R., Kilburn, E. and Majerus, P.W. (1970) J. Biol. Chem. 245, 6462–6467.
118 Landman, A.D. and Dakshinamurti, K. (1973) Anal. Biochem. 59, 191–195.
119 Desjardins, P.R. and Dakshinamurti, K. (1971) Can. J. Biochem. 46, 989–991.
120 Lane, M.D., Rominger, K.L., Young, D.L. and Lynen, F. (1964) J. Biol. Chem. 239, 2865–2971.

121 Sweetman, L. and Burri, B.J. (1982) in: International Symposium on Biotin-Dependent Enzymes, Glenelg, Australia, 1982, Abstr.
122 Ganguly, J. (1960) Biochim. Biophys. Acta 40, 110–118.
123 Numa, S., Matsuhashi, M. and Lynen, F. (1961) Biochem. Z. 334, 203–217.
124 Foerster, E.-C. (1979) Ph.D. Thesis, University of Munich.
125 Lowenstein, J.M. (1968) in: T.W. Goodwin (Ed.), The Metabolic Roles of Citrate, Academic Press, New York, pp. 61–86.
126 Bortz, W.M. and Lynen, F. (1963) Biochem. Z. 337, 505–509.
127 Numa, S., Bortz, W.M. and Lynen, F. (1965) Adv. Enzymol. Regul. 3, 407–423.
128 Tanabe, T., Ogiwara, H., Nikawa, J. and Numa, S., Unpublished results.
129 Hackenschmidt, J., Garth, C. and Decker, K. (1972) FEBS Lett. 27, 131–133.
130 Iritani, N., Nakanishi, S. and Numa, S. (1969) Life Sci. 8, 1157–1165.
131 Stoll, E., Ryder, E., Edwards, J.B. and Lane, M.D. (1968) Proc. Natl. Acad. Sci. (U.S.A.) 60, 976–981.
132 Gregolin, C., Ryder, E., Warner, R.C., Kleinschmidt, A.K., Chang, H.-C. and Lane, M.D. (1968) J. Biol. Chem. 243, 4236–4245.
133 Yeh, L.-A., Song, C.-S. and Kim, K.-H. (1981) J. Biol. Chem. 256, 2289–2296.
134 Goodridge, A.G. (1972) J. Biol. Chem. 247, 6946–6952.
135 Ogiwara, H., Tanabe, T., Nikawa, J. and Numa, S. (1978) Eur. J. Biochem. 89, 33–41.
136 Miller, A.L., Geroch, M.E. and Levy, H.R. (1970) Biochem. J. 118, 645–657.
137 Halestrap, A.P. and Denton, R.M. (1973) Biochem. J. 132, 509–517.
138 Dixon, M. (1972) Biochem. J. 129, 197–202.
139 Zahler, W.L., Barden, R.E. and Cleland, W.W. (1968) Biochim. Biophys. Acta 164, 1–11.
140 Barden, R.E. and Cleland, W.W. (1969) J. Biol. Chem. 244, 3677–3684.
141 Nikawa, J., Tanabe, T., Ogiwara, H., Shiba, T. and Numa, S. (1979) FEBS Lett. 102, 223–226.
142 Blytt, H.J. and Kim, K.-H. (1982) Arch. Biochem. Biophys. 213, 523–529.
143 Maragoudakis, M.E. and Hankin, H. (1971) J. Biol. Chem. 246, 348–358.
144 Siess, E.A., Brocks, D.G. and Wieland, O.H. (1978) Hoppe-Seyler's Z. Physiol. Chem. 359, 785–798.
145 Nishikori, K., Iritani, N. and Numa, S. (1973) FEBS Lett. 32, 19–21.
146 Sumper, M. (1974) Eur. J. Biochem. 49, 469–475.
147 Hayashi, E., Hasegawa, R. and Tomita, T. (1976) J. Biol. Chem. 251, 5759–5769.
148 Tomita, T., Hasegawa, R. and Hayashi, E. (1979) J. Nutr. Sci. Vitaminol. 25, 59–66.
149 Cashel, M. (1975) Annu. Rev. Microbiol. 29, 301–318.
150 Polakis, S.E., Guchhait, R.B. and Lane, M.D. (1973) J. Biol. Chem. 248, 7957–7966.
151 Stein Jr., J.P. and Bloch, K.E. (1976) Biochem. Biophys. Res. Commun. 73, 881–884.
152 Merlie, J.P. and Pizer, L.I. (1973) J. Bacteriol. 116, 355–366.
153 Lee, K.-H. and Kim, K.-H. (1979) J. Biol. Chem. 254, 1450–1453.
154 Witters, L.A., Kowaloff, E.M. and Avruch, J. (1979) J. Biol. Chem. 254, 245–248.
155 Brownsey, R.W., Hughes, W.A. and Denton, R.M. (1979) Biochem. J. 184, 23–32.
156 Ly, S. and Kim, K.-H. (1982) Arch. Biochem. Biophys. 217, 251–256.
157 Carlson, C.A. and Kim, K.-H. (1974) Arch. Biochem. Biophys. 164, 478–489.
158 Carlson, C.A. and Kim, K.-H. (1974) Arch. Biochem. Biophys. 164, 490–501.
159 Carlson, A.C. and Kim, K.-H. (1973) J. Biol. Chem. 248, 378–380.
160 Lee, K.-H. and Kim, K.-H. (1977) J. Biol. Chem. 252, 1748–1751.
161 Lent, B.A., Lee, K.-H. and Kim, K.-H. (1978) J. Biol. Chem. 253, 8149–8156.
162 Yeh, L.-A., Lee, K.-H. and Kim, K.-H. (1980) J. Biol. Chem. 255, 2308–2314.
163 Shiao, M.-S., Drong, R.F. and Porter, J.W. (1981) Biochem. Biophys. Res. Commun. 98, 80–87.
164 Shiao, M.-S., Drong, R.F., Dugan, R.E., Baker, T.A. and Porter, J.W. (1981) in: O.M. Rosen and E.G. Krebs (Eds.), Protein Phosphorylation, Book A, Cold Spring Harbor Laboratory, Cold Spring Harbor, NY.
165 Lent, B. and Kim, K.-H. (1982) J. Biol. Chem. 257, 1897–1901.
166 Hardie, D.G. and Cohen, P. (1978) FEBS Lett. 91, 1–7.
167 Hardie, D.G. and Guy, P.S. (1980) Eur. J. Biochem. 110, 167–177.

168 Brownsey, R.W. and Hardie, D.G. (1980) FEBS Lett. 120, 67–70.

169 Hardie, D.G. and Cohen, P. (1979) FEBS Lett. 103, 333–338.

170 Brownsey, R.W. and Denton, R.M. (1982) Biochem. J. 202, 77–86.

171 Krakower, G.R. and Kim, K.-H. (1981) J. Biol. Chem. 256, 2408–2413.

172 Pekala, P.H., Meredith, M.J., Tarlow, D.M. and Lane, M.D. (1978) J. Biol. Chem. 253, 5267–5269.

173 Wieland, O., Neufeldt, I., Numa, S. and Lynen, F. (1963) Biochem. Z. 336, 455–459.

174 Allman, D.W., Hubbard, D.D. and Gibson, D.M. (1965) J. Lipid Res. 6, 63–74.

175 Chang, H.-C., Seidman, I., Teebor, G. and Lane, M.D. (1967) Biochem. Biophys. Res. Commun. 28, 682–686.

176 Majerus, P.W. and Kilburn, E. (1969) J. Biol. Chem. 244, 6254–6262.

177 Nakanishi, S. and Numa, S. (1971) Proc. Natl. Acad. Sci. (U.S.A.) 68, 2288–2292.

178 Ryder, E. (1970) Biochem. J. 119, 929–930.

179 Arinze, J.-C. and Minstry, S.P. (1970) Proc. Soc. Exp. Biol. Med. 135, 553–556.

180 Teraoka, H. and Numa, S. (1975) Eur. J. Biochem. 53, 465–470.

181 Lee, K.-H. and Kim, K.-H. (1978) J. Biol. Chem. 253, 8157–8161.

182 Schimke, R.T. and Doyle, D. (1970) Annu. Rev. Biochem. 39, 929–976.

183 Nakanishi, S., Tanabe, T., Horikawa, S. and Numa, S. (1976) Proc. Natl. Acad. Sci. (U.S.A.) 73, 2304–2307.

184 Tanabe, T., Horikawa, S., Nakanishi, S. and Numa, S. (1976) FEBS Lett. 66, 70–72.

185 Horikawa, S., Nakanishi, S. and Numa, S. (1977) FEBS Lett. 74, 55–58.

186 Kitajima, K., Tashiro, S. and Numa, S. (1975) Eur. J. Biochem. 54, 373–383.

187 Kamiryo, T. and Numa, S. (1973) FEBS Lett. 38, 29–32.

188 Mishina, M., Kamiryo, T., Tanaka, A., Fukui, S. and Numa, S. (1976) Eur. J. Biochem. 71, 301–308.

189 Horikawa, S., Kamiryo, T., Nakanishi, S. and Numa, S. (1980) Eur. J. Biochem. 104, 191–198.

190 Kamiryo, T., Mishina, M., Tashiro, S. and Numa, S. (1977) Proc. Natl. Acad. Sci. (U.S.A.) 74, 4947–4950.

191 Mishina, M., Kamiryo, T., Tashiro, S. and Numa, S. (1978) Eur. J. Biochem. 82, 347–354.

192 Mishina, M., Kamiryo, T., Tashiro, S., Hagihara, T., Tanaka, A., Fukui, S., Osumi, M. and Numa, S. (1978) Eur. J. Biochem. 89, 321–328.

193 Kamiryo, T., Nishikawa, Y., Mishina, M., Terao, M. and Numa, S. (1979) Proc. Natl. Acad. Sci. (U.S.A.) 76, 4390–4394.

S. Numa (Ed.) Fatty Acid Metabolism and Its Regulation
© 1984 Elsevier Science Publishers B.V.

CHAPTER 2

Animal and bacterial fatty acid synthetase: structure, function and regulation

ALFRED W. ALBERTS and MICHAEL D. GREENSPAN

Merck Institute for Therapeutic Research, Merck Sharp and Dohme Research Laboratories, Rahway, NJ 07065, U.S.A.

1. Introduction

Fatty acid synthetase is the designation given to the enzyme system which catalyzes the synthesis of long-chain fatty acids from a short-chain acyl-CoA primer. Acetyl-CoA forms the methyl end of the fatty acid and malonyl-CoA (or in some circumstances methylmalonyl-CoA) contributes the remaining carbon atoms of the molecule. Prior to the mid-1950s it was generally assumed that fatty acid synthesis from acetyl-CoA occurred by direct reversal of the mitochondrial β-oxidation pathway of degradation of long fatty acids to acetyl-CoA [1]. This view became suspect when it was found that de novo synthesis of fatty acids from [^{14}C]acetate was catalyzed by the $100\,000 \times g$ supernatant fraction obtained by centrifugation of the cytoplasm prepared from homogenates of pigeon liver. The cofactors, ATP, Mn, bicarbonate and NADPH were required for the conversion of acetyl-CoA to long-chain fatty acids and were different from those to be expected for the reversal of β-oxidation [2]. Two key observations gave great impetus to studies on the mechanism of fatty acid biosynthesis: the discovery by Wakil [3] that acetyl-CoA was carboxylated to malonyl-CoA in a system containing a protein fraction obtained from the pigeon-liver extract as well as ATP, Mn and bicarbonate, and the additional finding that malonyl-CoA was an intermediate in fatty acid biosynthesis [4,5]. Subsequent progress was quite rapid. It was soon established that the reactions of fatty acid biosynthesis occurred with the substrates and intermediates covalently bound to the enzyme [1,6]. This provided the basis for much of the research on FAS from a wide variety of sources.

In this chapter, we will present a survey of the current state of knowledge of the bacterial and animal fatty acid synthetase systems. Plant and yeast fatty acid synthetases are described in other chapters of this volume. Particular emphasis will be placed on structure, reaction mechanisms and regulation of enzyme quantity, especially at the molecular level. No attempt is made to cover all the research that has been reported since the previous edition in this series was published [7]. A number of excellent reviews have appeared which detail many of the earlier studies. Of special note are those by Numa and Yamashita [8], Volpe and Vagelos [9], Bloch and Vance [10], Katiyar and Porter [11] and Stoops et al. [12].

2. Reaction sequence

Fatty acid synthetases are soluble cytoplasmic enzyme complexes found in bacteria and animal tissues which bring about the sequential condensation of acyl-CoA and malonyl-CoA (or methylmalonyl-CoA) in the presence of NADPH to form long-chain fatty acids. The stoichiometry for the synthesis of palmitate, the major fatty acid produced by most biosynthetic systems, is shown in Eqn. 1.

$$\text{Acetyl-CoA} + 7 \text{ malonyl-CoA} + 14 \text{ NADPH} + 14 \text{ H}^+ \rightarrow$$

$$\text{palmitate} + 8 \text{ CoA} + 7 \text{ CO}_2 + 6 \text{ H}_2\text{O} + 14 \text{ NADP}^+ \quad (1)$$

Brindley et al. [13] have classified fatty acid synthetases on the basis of their structural organization. Type I synthetases are classified as multienzyme complexes because they behave as single units: the individual partial reactions catalyzed by the complex cannot be separated from each other. This type includes the animal synthetases and synthetases from higher bacteria and yeast.

Type II synthetases also catalyze the multistep metabolic pathway but the constituent enzymes show no signs of physical interaction in vitro. This system occurs in lower bacteria and plants and has been most extensively studied in *E. coli*, where each of the monofunctional units has been purified and characterized.

Although the type I and type II synthetases differ markedly in their physical organization, both catalyze similar partial reactions resulting in the continuous addition of carbon units, usually derived from malonyl-CoA and finally ending with the completed long-chain fatty acid. The general outline of the sequence of reactions that result in the synthesis of long-chain fatty acids is illustrated by reactions 2–9 [9]. The central role of 4′-phosphopantetheine is indicated in the reactions. It is a constituent portion of the coenzyme A molecule and is covalently linked to a peptide. In type II synthetases this peptide is an individual protein with a molecular weight of approximately 9000 and has been designated as the acyl-carrier protein (ACP). In type I synthetase it is found as an integral part of the type I multienzyme synthetase complex. The structural features of ACP, the component enzymes of the type II system and the type I complex will be described in detail below.

The general description of the individual reactions catalyzed by both types of fatty acid synthetase will be discussed. In this discussion it is to be understood that ACP refers to an individual component of type II fatty acid synthetase and to a discrete segment of type I synthetases. The same distinctions can be made for each of the component enzymes of fatty acid synthetase; i.e. the individual reactions are catalyzed by distinct isolatable enzymes of the type II synthetase and by segments of the type I synthetase complex.

The reaction sequence that has been elucidated for type I and type II synthetases is as follows (reactions 2–9).

$$CH_3\overset{O}{\underset{\|}{C}}-SCoA + ACP-SH \;\underset{transacylase}{\overset{Acetyl}{\rightleftharpoons}}\; CH_3\overset{O}{\underset{\|}{C}}-S-ACP + CoA-SH \quad (2)$$

$$CH_3\overset{O}{\underset{\|}{C}}-S-ACP + HS-E_{cond.} \;\underset{enzyme}{\overset{Condensing}{\rightleftharpoons}}\; CH_3\overset{O}{\underset{\|}{C}}-S-E_{cond.} + ACP-SH \quad (3)$$

$$COOHCH_2\overset{O}{\underset{\|}{C}}-S-CoA + ACP-SH \;\underset{transacylase}{\overset{Malonyl}{\rightleftharpoons}}\; COOHCH_2\overset{O}{\underset{\|}{C}}-S-ACP + CoA-SH \quad (4)$$

$$CH_3\overset{O}{\underset{\|}{C}}-S-E_{cond.} + COOHCH_2\overset{O}{\underset{\|}{C}}-S-ACP \;\underset{enzyme}{\overset{Condensing}{\rightleftharpoons}}\; CH_3\overset{O}{\underset{\|}{C}}CH_2\overset{O}{\underset{\|}{C}}-S-ACP + CO_2 + HS-E_{cond.}\; E \quad (5)$$

$$CH_3\overset{O}{\underset{\|}{C}}CH_2\overset{O}{\underset{\|}{C}}-S-ACP + NADPH + H^+ \;\underset{reductase}{\overset{\beta-keto-}{\rightleftharpoons}}\; CH_3\overset{OH}{\underset{D(-)}{\underset{|}{C}H}}CH_2\overset{O}{\underset{\|}{C}}-S-ACP + NADP^+ \quad (6)$$

$$CH_3\overset{OH}{\underset{|}{C}H}CH_2\overset{O}{\underset{\|}{C}}-S-ACP \;\underset{dehydrase}{\overset{\beta-hydroxy-}{\rightleftharpoons}}\; CH_3\overset{H}{\underset{\underset{H}{|}}{C}}=C\overset{O}{\underset{\|}{C}}-S-ACP + H_2O \quad (7)$$

$$CH_3\overset{H}{\underset{\underset{H}{|}}{C}}=C\overset{O}{\underset{\|}{C}}-S-ACP + NADP + H^+ \;\underset{reductase}{\overset{Enoyl}{\rightleftharpoons}}\; CH_3CH_2CH_2\overset{O}{\underset{\|}{C}}-S-ACP + NADP^+ \quad (8)$$

X 6 repeats of cycle

$$CH_3(CH_2)_{14}\overset{O}{\underset{\|}{C}}-S-ACP$$

$$CH_3(CH_2)_{14}\overset{O}{\underset{\|}{C}}-S-ACP + H_2O \;\underset{thioesterase}{\overset{Palmityl}{\rightleftharpoons}}\; ACP-SH + \quad (9)$$

$$CH_3(CH_2)_{14}\overset{O}{\underset{\|}{C}}-OH$$

In the first reaction, a short-chain fatty acyl group is transferred from the sulfhydryl of the 4'-phosphopantetheine moiety of coenzyme A to the sulfhydryl group of the 4'-phosphopantetheine covalently associated with ACP in a reaction catalyzed by acetyl-CoA transacylase (reaction 2). The formation of fatty acyl-ACP is the primer reaction of fatty acid synthesis. The fatty acyl group utilized in this reaction provides the methyl end of the final fatty acid synthesized. The acyl group is transferred from ACP to a cysteine SH of β-keto-acyl-ACP synthase (condensing enzyme) liberating free ACP (reaction 3). The liberated SH group of ACP is then available to accept a malonyl group from malonyl-CoA in a reaction catalyzed by malonyl transacylase forming malonyl-ACP (reaction 4). This reaction is analogous to the acyl transacylase reaction.

The critical elongation reaction of fatty acid synthesis is catalyzed by the condensing enzyme, β-keto-acyl-ACP synthase. In this reaction the acyl group linked to a cysteine sulfhydryl linkage on the enzyme (reaction 3) is condensed with malonyl-ACP (reaction 5) resulting in the decarboxylation of malonyl-ACP with the formation of a β-keto-acyl-ACP derivative. β-Keto-acyl-ACP reductase catalyzes the NADPH-dependent reduction of β-keto-acyl-ACP to form specifically D-(−)-β-hydroxy-acyl-ACP (reaction 6). The latter is dehydrated by β-hydroxy-acyl-ACP dehydrase (reaction 7) to form an enoyl-ACP; this is then normally reduced in a second NADPH-dependent reaction by enoyl-ACP reductase (reaction 8) forming an acyl-ACP derivative 2 carbons longer than the original one.

In the usual sequence of de novo fatty acid synthesis the acyl group from the newly formed acyl-ACP derivative is transferred to the condensing enzyme (reaction 3), it reacts with another mole of malonyl-ACP and the reaction sequence continues as above. This process is repeated until the long-chain fatty acid, normally palmitate, is formed and then liberated from ACP. This last reaction (reaction 9) is catalyzed by specific fatty acid thioesterases. As it is most frequently described then, fatty acid synthetases catalyze a reaction in which the acetyl group derived from acetyl-CoA is sequentially condensed with 7 moles of malonyl-CoA to form the long-chain fatty acid, palmitate. Energy for the condensations is derived from the decarboxylations of malonyl ACP and the reducing equivalents are usually derived from NADPH.

3. Substrate specificity and cofactor requirements

Although acetyl-CoA is normally considered to be the acyl primer for fatty acid synthesis, it has long been known that various branched and straight-chained saturated acyl-CoA derivatives could also serve in this role. Thus, Horning et al. [14] demonstrated with a partially purified fatty acid synthetase derived from rat adipose tissue that isobutyryl-CoA, isocaproyl-CoA, isovaleryl-CoA or α-methyl-butyryl-CoA could replace acetyl-CoA in the formation of a corresponding long-chain iso or anti-iso fatty acid. Similarly, propionyl-CoA or butyryl-CoA also could serve as primers for fatty acid synthesis and were often more effective than acetyl-CoA. As would be expected, when propionyl-CoA was the primer, odd-chain fatty acids were formed.

A detailed investigation of the primer specificity of fatty acid synthetase preparations prepared from rat, rabbit, cow and goat mammary glands have been carried out by Knudsen and Grunnet [15]. They found that commercial preparations of malonyl-CoA were often contaminated with significant amounts of acetyl-CoA, thus making it difficult to determine substrate specificity unless scrupulously pure malonyl-CoA was used. This observation could explain earlier findings that acetyl-CoA was not very effective in stimulating malonyl-CoA-dependent NADPH oxidation [16,17]. However, the malonyl-CoA-dependent oxidation of NADPH showed an absolute requirement for acetyl-CoA or other short-chain acyl-CoAs when pure malonyl-CoA was used. The previous observation that butyryl-CoA was superior to acetyl-CoA as a primer for the rat and rabbit mammary gland enzymes could not be confirmed [18,19]; acyl-CoAs longer than 4 carbons were also inefficient primers for the rat and rabbit. Synthetases from ruminant mammary gland on the other hand preferentially utilized butyryl-CoA as a primer. Furthermore, as opposed to the rat and rabbit enzymes, cow and goat synthetases were able to use longer-chain acyl-CoA effectively as primers.

The primer specificity of bacterial fatty acid synthetases has been studied in the laboratory of Kaneda [20–23]. In a number of species of bacteria, branch-chain fatty acids of the iso and anti–iso series with 13–17 carbons occur as major cellular species accounting for 60–95% of the total fatty acids of the organisms [22]. These were produced using the branched acyl-CoA primers, isobutyryl-CoA, isovaleryl-CoA and 2-methylbutyryl-CoA, which are synthesized from the α-keto acids derived from valine, leucine and isoleucine [20,21]. The ability of acetyl-, propionyl- and butyryl-CoA to serve as substrates for straight-chain fatty acids was examined by Kaneda and Smith in a number of microorganisms [23]. In addition they examined the incorporation of α-keto-β-methyl butyrate into branched-chain fatty acids. As shown in Table 1, fatty acid synthetases derived from *Bacillus subtilis, Corynebacterium cyclohexanicum, Micrococcus luteus,* and *Pseudomonas maltophilia* efficiently utilize α-keto-β-methyl butyrate for fatty acid synthesis. These organisms, which contain predominantly branch-chain fatty acids, also incorporate butyryl-CoA preferentially to either acetyl or propionyl-CoA. On the other hand, synthetases from *Escherichia coli* and *Pseudomonas fluorescens,* bacteria which were essentially devoid of branch-chain fatty acids, could not utilize α-keto-β-methyl butyrate for fatty acid synthesis; acetyl-CoA was the preferred primer for synthesis with the synthetases from these organisms. These results indicated that fatty acid synthetase from organisms containing predominantly straight-chain fatty acids show decreased activity with increased chain length of the primer. Furthermore, they lack a system for supplying branch-chain primers.

Whereas a number of short-chain fatty acyl-CoAs could serve as a primer for fatty acid synthesis, purified fatty acid synthetases from most, if not all species, showed a high degree of specificity for malonyl-CoA. As has been indicated above, fatty acid synthetases catalyze the synthesis of mainly straight-chain fatty acids when acetyl-, propionyl-, or butyryl-CoA was used as the primer, and iso or anti–iso fatty acids when the appropriate short branch-chain acyl-CoA was condensed with malonyl-CoA. Other fatty acids containing 1–4 methyl groups are produced by the

TABLE 1

Primer specificity of fatty acid de novo synthetase from bacteria [a]

Microorganism	Fatty acid synthesized (pmoles mg protein^{-1} min^{-1})			
	Acyl CoA ester			α-Keto-β-methyl-butyrate
	Acetyl	Propionyl	Butyryl	
B. subtilis	0.038	0.81	4.4	16.2
C. cyclohexanicum	0.058	0.85	4.7	25.4
M. luteus	0.039	0.77	1.35	65.2
P. maltophilia (Bryan)	0.088	1.51	8.97	7.10
E. coli B	500	277	57	0.0
P. fluorescens	23.1	3.0	0.88	0.08

[a] From ref. 23.

sebaceous glands of guinea pigs [24] and water fowl [25–28]. The mechanism of synthesis of these methyl-branched acids has been extensively studied by Kolattukudy with fatty acid synthetase from the uropygial gland of the goose [25–28] and by Yamazaki and coworkers with the fatty acid synthetase derived from the Harderian gland of the guinea pig [24].

The synthesis of multibranched fatty acids involves the substitution of methylmalonyl-CoA for malonyl-CoA. It has been shown that methylmalonyl-CoA is a competitive inhibitor of malonyl-CoA with fatty acid synthetases from rat [29] and human liver [29,30] and the goose uropygial gland [28] with K_i values of 10–30 mM. The goose uropygial gland is unique in that it produces large amounts of multimethyl-branched fatty acids [25,26]. There was a paradox of how this fatty acid synthetase could have synthesized so much of the branch-chain fatty acids when the necessary substrate, methylmalonyl-CoA was less efficiently incorporated into fatty acids than malonyl-CoA. It was resolved by the discovery that there was a very active malonyl-CoA decarboxylase present in the gland [31], which prevented the accumulation of malonyl-CoA. Furthermore, propionyl-CoA was carboxylated by acetyl-CoA carboxylase to form the necessary substrate, methylmalonyl-CoA, for branched fatty acid synthesis. The predominant fatty acid formed, 2,4,6,8-tetramethyldecanoic acid, was also synthesized by the isolated purified fatty acid synthetase from the gland when methylmalonyl-CoA was the only available substrate [26].

That the formation of these multibranched-chain fatty acids was controlled by the presence of malonyl-CoA decarboxylase, and that the uropygial gland enzyme was not unique, was shown by the fact that goose liver and both the rat mammary gland and liver synthetase also catalyzed the incorporation of [^{14}C]methylmalonyl-CoA into 2,4,6,8-tetramethyl decanoic acid with acetyl-CoA as the primer [28]. This is in contrast to the studies cited above [29,30] which reported that methylmalonyl-CoA was not a substrate for rat or human FAS. It should also be noted that the goose uropygial gland synthetase can synthesize fatty acids containing straight and branched regions in the presence of methylmalonyl-CoA and small amounts of malonyl-CoA [26].

A somewhat different situation was found in the guinea pig [24]. The Harderian gland of the guinea pig secretes a large amount of lipids primarily in the form of 1-o-alkyl-2,3-diacylglycerol with 82% of the fatty acid at the 2-position consisting of saturated methyl-branched acids. The methyl branches in these fatty acids are mostly located at the even-numbered carbon atoms. Fatty acid synthetase isolated from the Harderian gland produced more than 19 different fatty acids when acetyl-CoA, malonyl-CoA and methylmalonyl-CoA were used as substrates; most of these fatty acids were methyl-branched and reflected the makeup of the lipid secreted by the gland [32]. Omission of methylmalonyl-CoA resulted in the synthesis of only straight-chain saturated fatty acids while no synthesis occurred upon omission of malonyl-CoA. Thus, the availability of substrates, especially methylmalonyl-CoA, regulated the composition of the fatty acids produced by the gland. As opposed to the systems studied by Kolattukudy and coworkers [28], there appeared to be organ-specific differences in fatty acid synthetases isolated from the guinea pig. Whereas both the uropygial gland and liver of the goose could synthesize branch-chain fatty acids when only methylmalonyl-CoA was used as the substrate, the fatty acid synthetase isolated from the liver of the guinea pig could not utilize methylmalonyl-CoA either alone or in the presence of malonyl-CoA as a substrate for fatty acid synthesis [24]. As with other fatty acid synthetases, the synthetase from the Harderian gland of the guinea pig was inhibited by methylmalonyl-CoA but it itself was incorporated in the presence of malonyl-CoA resulting in the synthesis of fatty acids methylated primarily at the 4th and 8th carbon. The structural features of the enzyme systems allowing for the condensation of methylmalonyl-CoA with the growing fatty acid chain and the specificity of the incorporation could give insight into the mechanism of biosynthesis of the methylated, fatty-acid-related macrolide antibiotics [33].

FAS from animal sources show a marked specificity for NADPH [11]. NADH was either poorly utilized or not utilized at all. Dual reduced pyridine nucleotide requirements have been documented for synthetases derived from bacteria [34–39]. With purified enzymes from *E. coli*, Weeks and Wakil [34] demonstrated that there was a specific requirement for NADPH for the reduction catalyzed by β-ketoacyl-ACP reductase while the enoyl-ACP reductase could utilize both NADPH and NADH. This apparent dual specificity was shown to be the result of at least two separate enoyl reductases, one specific for NADPH and the other for NADH. Higher bacteria such as Mycobacterium [35], Corynebacterium [36] and Brevibacterium [37] also showed a dual reduced pyridine nucleotide requirement. These organisms have a type I FAS where the enzyme activities are associated with multifunctional polypeptide chains. Nevertheless, as with the type II system of *E. coli*, the β-ketoacyl reductase domain was shown to be specific for NADPH and the enoyl reductase was specific for NADH [35,36]. It was found that the stereochemistry of the enoyl reductase was dependent on the source of the enoyl reductase. Thus the stereochemistry of hydrogen incorporation from reduced pyridine nucleotides involved re-attack of hydride from NADPH with the rat liver enzyme and si-attack of hydride from NADH with the *B. ammoniagenes* FAS [37].

In addition to the reduced pyridine nucleotide requirements, FAS from yeast required FMN as a cofactor [38]. FMN was not a cofactor for animal synthetases or for *E. coli* FAS but was a cofactor in some other bacteria such as *C. kluyveri* [39], *M. smegmatis* [40] and *C. diphtheriae* [36]. The FMN requirement in these systems was believed to be at the level of the enoyl reductase step [38].

4. Chain termination

It is generally acknowledged that free palmitic acid formed by the hydrolysis of a palmityl-enzyme complex is the typical final product of isolated animal fatty acid synthetase (see ref. 41 for review). The hydrolytic cleavage of the fatty acid chain is carried out by a thioesterase, shown to be an integral part of the multienzyme complex. However, fatty acids with chain lengths of 4–24 carbons are found in vivo in various animal tissues. Several factors have been discovered which are responsible for regulating the chain length of the fatty acids in vivo. Studies involving chain length regulation have been primarily performed with enzymes purified from animal mammary glands or the sebaceous gland of waterfowl.

The triglyceride composition of fatty acids found in mammalian milk varies considerably between species [42]. Rat and rabbit milk triglycerides were composed predominantly of medium-chain fatty acids ($C_{8:0}$–$C_{10:0}$) [43], guinea pig contained long-chain fatty acids ($C_{14:0}$–$C_{18:1}$) [43], cow has short-chain ($C_{4:0}$–$C_{6:0}$) [44] and goat contained all three — short-, medium- and long-chain fatty acids [45]. Since all three types were synthesized de novo, these variations in chain length must be found in the fatty-acid- or triglyceride-synthesizing system. The existence of medium-chain fatty acids in the rat and rabbit mammary gland was particularly interesting since the isolated fatty acid synthetase complex from the lactating glands synthesized only short- and long-chain fatty acids [43].

Research on chain termination has involved: (a) identification of the end product fatty acids from a particular tissue, (b) isolation and characterization of fatty acid synthetase from the tissue, (c) comparison of the in vivo products with those of the isolated enzyme, and (d) identification and characterization of factors present in the tissue extract which explain differences between the end products of the two systems.

In 1971 Smith and Abraham [18] reported that the isolated rat mammary gland FAS produced C_{16} and C_{18}, whereas in vivo, the mammary gland produced mostly medium-chain fatty acids ($C_{6,8,10}$) [18]. Furthermore, the rat liver and mammary gland enzyme were immunologically identical [46].

It was possible to separate an active thioesterase from the purified mammary gland FAS by mild treatment with trypsin [47]. This was referred to as "thioesterase I" and was an integral part of the multienzyme complex. The properties of this enzyme were investigated by Lin and Smith [48]. Although this thioesterase cleaved long-chain acyl-CoA esters off the enzyme complex, the question of how medium-chain fatty acids were formed in the mammary gland and not the liver still remained unanswered, particularly since the liver and the mammary gland enzymes appeared to be identical. In 1978, Libertini and Smith [49,50] found a "factor" in the cytoplasm of rat mammary gland which when added to FAS, shifted the specificity from long- to medium-chain fatty acids. Purified of this cytoplasmic factor — referred to as "thioesterase II" — and subsequent addition of this enzyme to a mammary gland FAS in which the bound thioesterase I was inhibited by trypsin resulted in the release of medium-chain acyl groups. It was further shown that thioesterase II acted by cleaving the acyl-4-phosphopantetheine bond, not an acylcysteine linkage [51].

Substantiation that thioesterase II played an essential role in chain termination came from the synchronous appearance of thioesterase II and medium-chain fatty acids in the lactating mammary gland [52].

Rabbit mammary gland, which likewise produces medium-chain fatty acids, was also shown to contain a soluble thioesterase which catalyzed the release of medium-chain fatty acids from the FAS [53]. The partially purified hydrolase terminated the chain at 8–12 carbons; it had a molecular weight of 29000 and could hydrolyze acyl-CoA esters [54,55]. In addition, this enzyme was induced in the rabbit mammary gland coincident with the appearance of medium-chain fatty acids in the tissue of the pregnant rabbit [55]. No medium-chain hydrolase was found in the cytosol of the rabbit liver [55].

In contrast, goat mammary gland, which produced short-, medium- and long-chain fatty acids did not contain a soluble medium-chain thioesterase like rat and rabbit [56]. Partially purified goat FAS produced only short- and long-chain fatty acids, although short-, medium- and long-chain fatty acyl-CoA esters were hydrolyzed by the enzyme [57]. However, when the incubation was supplemented with microsomes and a high speed supernatant from the goat gland, medium-chain fatty acids were produced [58]. Further analysis of the lactating goat mammary gland FAS showed that the enzyme possessed both thioesterase and transacylase activity. The addition of microsomes, ATP, and glycerol 3-phosphate in the incubation stimulated the incorporation of medium-chain fatty acids ($C_{8:0}$, $C_{10:0}$, $C_{12:0}$) into triglycerides. More recent experiments have shown that addition of albumin, β-lactoalbumin or cyclodextran to the incubation increased the amount of C_{10} fatty acids incorporated into triacylglycerols whereas that of C_{14} and C_6 decreased [59]. These compounds were thought to facilitate the removal of the acyl-CoA esters from the enzyme.

The fatty acids present in the sebaceous gland of waterfowl also indicated that an unusual method of chain determination exists. While the goose liver and uropygial gland fatty acid synthetase appeared to be identical, the end product fatty acids were very different. The goose uropygial gland produced mainly 2,4,6,8-tetramethyl decanoic acid and 2,4,6-trimethyl lauric acid; whereas, the liver made the normal straight-chain saturated fatty acids. The sebaceous glands of Muscovy and mallard ducks synthesized monomethyl hexanoic and dimethyl octanoic acid [25]. As previously mentioned, these branched-chain fatty acids found in the sebaceous glands resulted from the incorporation of methylmalonyl-CoA as substrate because of the presence of a highly active malonyl-CoA decarboxylase [26,31]. The glands of the Muscovy and mallard ducks synthesized fatty acid chains which were not only branched, but were shorter ($C_{6:0}$) than those found in goose; on investigation, an acyl-fatty acid synthetase hydrolase was isolated from the duck gland [60,61]. This enzyme had a molecular weight of 29000 and was similar to the thioesterase II discovered in the rat and rabbit mammary gland. This acyl-fatty acid synthetase hydrolase caused production of short, branched-chain fatty acids when incubated together with purified fatty acid synthetase and methylmalonyl-CoA. The evidence also indicated that this hydrolase functions as such in vivo since (a) the addition of the purified hydrolase to a FAS preparation in which the thioesterase was inhibited by PMSF regenerated FAS activity and (b) the hydrolase was not found in the uropygial gland of the goose which produced only long branched-chain fatty acids.

Although the product of animal FAS is free palmitic or stearic acid, some recent studies by Linn and Srere [62] have suggested that CoA was needed for hydrolysis of the fatty acyl chain from the enzyme, since the addition of a CoA scavenger system inhibited the enzyme. Their conclusion was that the acyl group was cleaved from the enzyme as an acyl-CoA, which was further hydrolyzed to the free fatty acid and CoASH. However, Stern et al. [63] showed this apparent dependence of the FAS activity on addition of CoA was probably due to the need to unload bound acetyl or malonyl groups from common binding sites on the synthetase in order to facilitate the continuation of the reaction.

The factors which regulate the length of the acyl chain in *Escherichia coli* have also been investigated. Greenspan et al. [64] showed that purified β-ketoacyl-ACP synthetase was unable to elongate palmitoyl and *cis*-vaccenyl acyl carrier proteins although shorter chain lengths could be further elongated. Cronan et al. [65] indicated however that fatty acids of longer chain lengths (*cis*-13-eicosenoic and arachidic acids) accumulated in glycerol starved cells, suggesting that chain elongation continued if acyl transfer was blocked by a lack of *sn*-glycerol-3-phosphate. Thus, acyl transfer to form phospholipids was an important factor in determining chain length in *E. coli*. This study also suggested that fatty acid synthesis may also play a role in chain termination, since the chains that accumulated during glycerol starvation were only about 30% longer than normal. Barnes and Wakil [66,67] have purified two thioesterases from *E. coli* which hydrolyzed both acyl-ACP and CoA derivatives. CoA was present in the reaction mixture so it was difficult to determine whether the product was terminated as the free fatty acid or the acyl-CoA, which was subsequently hydrolyzed.

The chain termination step of the fatty acid synthetase from *Mycobacterium smegmatis* involves transacylation with CoA [68–80] rather than hydrolysis of the free fatty acid as found with the animal enzyme. The products of the *M. smegmatis* synthetase were the C_{16}–C_{24} acyl-CoA esters. Mycobacterium polysaccharides stimulated the rate of transacylation, which became greater as the chain length of the substrate increased [68]. The presence of the polysaccharide appeared to facilitate the diffusion of the acyl-CoA esters from the synthetase rather than promoting acyl transfer from the enzyme to CoA [69,70].

Finally, the fatty acid synthetase from *Brevibacterium ammoniagenes* also produced CoA derivatives but of 16–18 carbon atoms in length. The unique feature of the synthetase from this organism was that it produced oleic as well as stearic and palmitic acid [71,72]. The ratio of unsaturated to saturated fatty acids formed depended on the temperature of the enzyme reaction rather than the growth temperature of the microorganism [71]; the relative proportion of stearic to palmitic acid was dependent on the malonyl-CoA concentration and the ratio of malonyl-CoA to acetyl-CoA [72].

It is not clear as yet why the products of the animal synthetase for the most part are the free fatty acids and the bacterial (and yeast) the CoA esters. Both products are ultimately esterified as either phospholipids or triglycerides. In one case the acceptor of the acyl chain is water — in the other case it is CoA. The final products are also dependent on the substrate as in Brevibacterium where the ratio of malonyl-CoA to acetyl-CoA controlled the proportion of palmitate to stearate, or in the sebaceous gland of waterfowl where methylmalonyl-CoA replaced malonyl-CoA as the substrate for elongation.

5. Purification, physical properties and reaction mechanism

Animal fatty acid synthase (FAS) has been purified and characterized from a wide variety of animal sources [16,23,27,29,73–96]. A partial listing is presented in Table 2. In most cases, standard procedures were utilized and will not be discussed. Several of these systems deserve comment, however, either because of the extremely high levels of enzyme present or because of the novel means of purification that was used.

The goose uropygial gland is a highly specialized organ producing large amounts of fatty acids [16,27]. FAS comprises 1/6–1/3 of the total soluble protein in this gland. Homogeneous enzyme was obtained by gel filtration on a Sepharose 4B column of a high-speed supernatant prepared from homogenates of the gland. Up to 200 mg of enzyme was obtained from one gland from a mature Chinese white goose.

A convenient source for the isolation of human FAS is the human mammary gland epithelial cell line, SKBr3 [90]. This aberrant epithelial cell line contains prodigious amounts of this enzyme; FAS accounts for 22–28% of the cytosolic proteins of the SKBr3 cell. Human FAS has been purified to homogeneity from extracts of this cell line and has been characterized.

Rat-liver FAS has been obtained in high yield and with high specific activity by

TABLE 2

Sources of animal fatty acid synthetase

Species	Source	Reference
Rat	Liver	73–76
	Adipose tissue	75
	Lactating mammary gland	77–81
	Red blood cells	82, 83
Rabbit	Lactating mammary gland	78, 79, 81, 84
Guinea pig	Liver	23
	Harderian gland	23
Pig	Liver	85, 86
Human	Liver	29, 87, 88
	Chang liver cells	89
	Mammary epithelial cell line (SKBr$_3$)	90
Goat	Lactating mammary gland	78
Bovine	Lactating mammary gland	78, 91, 92
Chicken	Liver	74, 93–95
	Oviduct	95
Pigeon	Liver	96
Goose	Uropygial gland	16, 27

substituting polyethylene glycol precipitation for conventional purification methods [76]. Enzyme prepared by this means readily crystallized. It appears that this method may be a useful one for the rapid purification of FAS from other sources.

The immunological cross-reactivity between fatty acid synthetases derived from different species has been studied. Using rabbit antiserum prepared against purified lactating rat mammary gland FAS, cross-reactivity was determined by immunodiffusion and immunoprecipitation tests [97]. No differences in the immunological cross-reactivity were found between liver, mammary gland and adipose enzyme from the same species. FAS from the rat and mouse gave reactions of incomplete identity whereas no cross-reactivity was found between rat and pigeon enzymes. Partial antigenic identity between rat and human liver enzyme was indicated with antibody against rat FAS [29] and between rat, mouse and human enzyme using antibody against either rat or mouse FAS [90] while antibody against human FAS, which gave a strong reaction with human FAS, cross-reacted poorly with synthases from the rat and mouse. Very little reaction occurred between goose uropygial enzyme and antisera from the three mammalian sources [90]. Similarly, antibody prepared against chicken and pigeon FAS gave precipitin reactions with FAS from avian but not rat liver, and antibody against the rat enzyme did not react with avian synthetases. These results indicated that there are very few common antigenic determinants on the avian and mammalian enzymes, whereas the common inter-species antigenic determinants are present on mammalian enzyme.

The structure of animal FAS obtained from bovine, human, rodent and avian species are similar (see Table 2 for refs.). It is a homodimer with a molecular weight of between 450000 and 550000. Complete conversion of the dimer to monomeric units was accomplished in low-ionic-strength buffers at alkaline pH or low temperature [11,16,79,94,99–101]. The dissociated enzyme was inactive in catalyzing the overall FAS reaction. Reassociation with recovery of enzymatic activity was achieved by dialysis against high-ionic-strength buffer. Under these conditions, the native enzyme was found to have a sedimentation constant of 13.3 S and the subunit was 9.9 S. These observations universally apply, with only small differences in detail, to every animal FAS that has been studied regardless of the source.

The question of whether FAS is a homodimer, a heterodimer or a multisubunit enzyme system where the subunits are held together by strong non-covalent bonds was a matter of considerable dispute for a number of years. It is now generally agreed that the synthetase is in fact a homodimer; thus, it consists of two identical very large polypeptide subunits each of which contains a complete complement of catalytic domains [9,11,12,16,74,75]. The evidence for this comes from several lines of research.

As indicated above, the synthase readily dissociated into monomeric species as determined by ultracentrifugal analysis. When FAS was subjected to electrophoresis on SDS-polyacrylamide, a peptide with a molecular weight of about 240000 were found [12,16,74,75,89]. The presence, in some cases, of lower molecular bands on the gels led to the conclusion that FAS of animal origin was composed of multiple subunits [87,102]. However, when synthases were isolated with appropriate precautions, such as the inclusion of protease inhibitors, only the 240 000-dalton peptide was observed on SDS-polyacrylamide gels [16,74,89].

Further evidence for the homodimeric structure of FAS came from studies on the localization of the prosthetic group 4'-phosphopantetheine in animal FAS (Fig. 1). Workers in several laboratories had reported the isolation from animal FAS of low molecular weight peptides containing 4'-phosphopantetheine [103–105]. However, when [³H]- or [¹⁴C]pantothenic acid was used to label the FAS prosthetic group in human Chang liver cells grown in culture [89] or in vivo in chicken liver [74] and goose uropygial gland [16], the homogeneous fatty acid synthetase contained radioactivity derived from the labeled pantothenic acid. When these synthetase preparations were subjected to electrophoresis on SDS-polyacrylamide gels, it was found that the radioactivity was associated only with a peptide of molecular weight of 220 000–240 000, if steps were taken to inactivate proteases that may have been present. When the protease was not inactivated, the FAS was degraded and numerous radiolabeled peptides were detected [16]. Evidence that each FAS subunit contains 1 mole of 4'-phosphopantetheine was obtained by direct determination of the cysteamine and β-alanine content of FAS. These components comprise a portion of 4'-phosphopantetheine and were obtained by acid hydrolysis of the protein. Careful analysis of FAS derived from several different sources revealed the presence of approximately 2 moles of 4'-phosphopantetheine per mole of enzyme [16,74,94].

Additional support for the homodimeric nature of FAS has come from studies on the thioesterase domain (reaction 9) of the synthetase. When FAS was subjected to limited digestion with trypsin or elastase, an enzymatically active thioesterase component was released [106–110]. Fatty acid synthetase activity was lost, yet all partial reactions except the thioesterase were retained. Intact FAS treated with ¹⁴C- or ³²P-labeled diisopropylphosphofluoridate, which binds to a serine residue on the thioesterase domain [111], was found to bind a maximum of 1 mole of inhibitor per

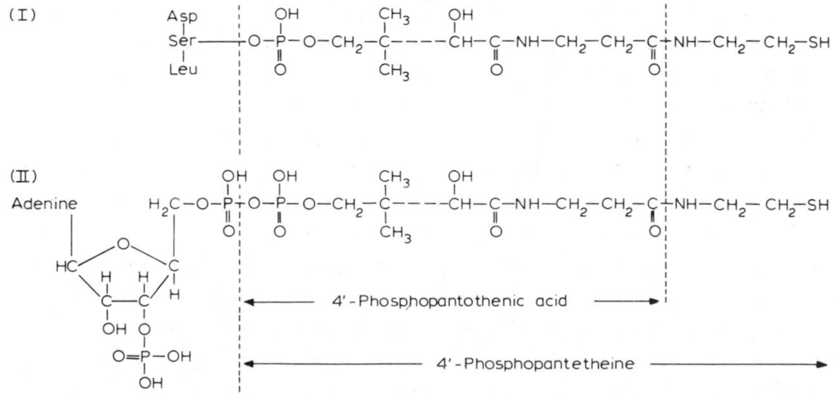

Fig. 1. Structures of ACP (I) and CoA (II) showing the common 4'-phosphopantetheine prosthetic group. In ACP it is in phosphodiester linkage to serine 36 [132].

mole of subunit [107,108,112]. SDS gel electrophoresis of the labeled FAS demonstrated that the radioactivity was associated with a polypeptide of molecular weight of approximately 240 000. After digestion with trypsin, the radioactivity was associated predominantly with a fragment with a molecular weight of 35 000. In the absence of inhibitor, this 35 000 dalton fragment contained the thioesterase activity [106,107,109]. These results lend credence to the concept that animal FAS is composed of 2 equal subunits containing 2 thioesterase domains per dimer as well as 2 phosphopantetheine domains.

Delineation of the domains of FAS has been aided by the use of specific ligands which bind covalently to sites on the FAS molecule. These include the substrates, acetyl-CoA and malonyl-CoA as well as site-specific inhibitors. Radioactivity derived from [14C]acetyl-CoA or [14C]malonyl-CoA is incorporated with either of these substrates and is associated with a peptide that has a molecular weight of 220 000, the subunit molecular weight of FAS [74]. By labeling FAS with either [14C]acetate or [14C]malonate followed by proteolysis and purification of the resulting labeled peptides, it was possible to define the binding sites for each of the substrates [113–115]. Thus it was found that there were 3 groups of [14C]acetyl peptides and 2 of [14C]malonyl peptides. One of the [14C]acetyl and one of the [14C]malonyl groups was bound to the sulfhydryl group of the 4-phosphopantetheine moiety of FAS; this is the ACP site. One site for each group was a non-thiol site which identified as a serine hydroxyl group. Presumably this was the transacylase site or sites. The observation that both groups were associated with a single peptide suggested that this may be a common site for the acetyl and malonyl transacylase. Alternatively there could be 2 separate domains on the enzyme, one specific for acetyl transfer and the other specific for malonyl transfer, each with identical peptides at their respective active sites. Definitive evidence for either hypothesis is lacking. The third acetyl binding site was shown to be a cysteine-SH at the condensing site of FAS.

Detailed studies involving inhibitors which covalently react with sulfhydryl groups have been carried out in the laboratories of Kumar, Wakil and Porter. Kumar et al. [116] demonstrated that the substrate analog, chloroacetyl-CoA inhibited overall rat liver FAS and that this inhibition was localized to the β-ketoacyl-ACP site. There was no inhibition of either transacylase or the thioesterase. With [2-14C]chloroacetyl-CoA it was shown that complete inactivation occurred when 2 moles of the chloroacetyl group was bound per mole of enzyme or 1 per subunit. Peptide maps of the labeled FAS indicated that most of the [14C]chloroacetate was covalently associated with a peptide which mapped on the region of the cysteine sulfhydryl site.

Katiyar et al. [117] have demonstrated that S-(4-bromo-2,3-dioxobutyl)-CoA inhibited FAS activity. This inhibitor was selectively and irreversibly bound to the enzyme with a stoichiometry of 4 moles of inhibitor bound per mole of enzyme. Under these conditions, β-ketoacyl-ACP synthetase and acetyl transacylase were inhibited whereas the remaining partial reactions were unaffected. The inhibitor prevented the binding of [14C]acetate derived from [14C]acetyl-CoA to the cysteine-SH of the condensing enzyme site and to the 4′-phosphopantetheine-SH of the ACP site.

In a series of elegant experiments, Stoops and Wakil [101,118,119] studied the reaction of FAS with monofunctional and bifunctional sulfhydryl reagents. The monofunctional alkylating agent, iodoacetamide, completely inhibited chicken-liver FAS with a rate constant of 0.033 min^{-1} and $t_{1/2}$ of 21 min [101]. Inhibition was prevented by preincubation of the synthetase with acetyl-CoA prior to the addition of iodoacetamide, whereas preincubation with malonyl-CoA accelerated the in- activation with an apparent first-order rate constant of 0.17 min^{-1}. It was indicated that the protective effect of acetyl-CoA was because the acetyl group was bound to the sulfhydryl site of β-ketoacyl-ACP synthase and this prevented the binding of the alkylating agent. The reason for the enhancement of inhibition by malonyl-CoA was not known. Direct confirmation that iodoacetamide was bound to a cysteine sulfhydryl was obtained by reacting FAS with [^{14}C]iodoacetamide followed by acid hydrolysis of the resulting labeled peptide. Over 80% of the ^{14}C label was recovered as S-[^{14}C]carboxy-methylcysteine indicating that inhibition was due to alkylation of an active cysteine sulfhydryl group.

As indicated, overall FAS activity is catalyzed only by the dimeric form of the enzyme and not by the monomers. It was found, however, that the monomeric species catalyzed each of the partial reactions except the β-ketoacyl-ACP synthase reaction [75,115]. The loss of activity upon dissociation suggested that a close association between the 2 subunits was required for synthase activity. It was further proposed that the interaction between the subunits involved 2 essential thiol groups, one from each of the 2 FAS monomers. Evidence for this proposal has been obtained through the use of the bifunctional reagents, dibromopropanone [101,118] and 5,5'-dithiobis-(2-nitrobenzoic acid) [119].

Chicken liver FAS was irreversibly inhibited when 2 moles of dibromopropanone were bound per mole of enzyme indicating 2 reactive centers in the dimer [101,118]. The only partial reaction of the synthetase that was inhibited was β-ketoacyl synthetase. Inhibition of the overall reaction was prevented by prior incubation of the enzyme with acetyl-CoA but not with malonyl-CoA. As a consequence of inhibition by dibromopropanone, the FAS dimer was cross-linked, as demonstrated by SDS-polyacrylamide gel electrophoresis of the inhibited enzyme. Under these conditions a peptide was found with an apparent molecular weight of 440 000 indicating that the bifunctional reagent reacted intermolecularly with the 2 subunits of FAS and resulted in the cross-linking of the monomers.

Preincubation with acetyl-CoA but not malonyl-CoA prevented the inhibition by dibromopropanone and preincubation with both substrates prevented the cross-link- ing. These somewhat anomalous results were explained when it was determined that the cross-linking reaction involved the cysteine-SH site of β-ketoacyl synthetase and the pantetheine-SH site of ACP. Since the acetyl group of acetyl-CoA is transferred to both sites, preincubation with it prevented inactivation and cross-linking. As would be expected, the malonyl group of malonyl-CoA was bound to the pan- tetheine-SH site, thus preventing cross-linking. However, since the cysteine-SH site remained unoccupied, it allowed for the binding and inactivation by di- bromopropanone. In similar fashion, 5,5'-dithiobis-(2-nitrobenzoic acid) [119] was covalently bound to a pantetheine-SH on one subunit and to a cysteine-SH on the other subunit of FAS thus cross-linking the two subunits. On the basis of the results with dibromopropanone, Stoops and Wakil [101,118] concluded that the pantetheine residue of one subunit was juxtaposed opposite a cysteine residue of the adjacent subunit. This vicinal arrangement of sulfhydryl groups was originally suggested by Brady et al. [120] in their studies on the effects of arsenite on rat adipose FAS.

The two reductase domains of FAS, β-ketoacyl reductase and enoyl reductase, have been studied with the enzyme systems derived from the goose uropygial gland [121–123] and rat mammary gland [124] using specific chemical probes. FAS was inactivated by the arginine modifying reagents, phenylglyoxal [121,124] and 2,3-butanedione [121]. Of the 7 different reactions catalyzed by FAS, only the ketoacyl and enoyl reductase activities were inhibited by these reagents. With [2-^{14}C]phenylglyoxal, the number of arginine residues modified was determined to be 4 out of a total of 106 arginines in the subunit of goose FAS [121]. Of these, 2 per 106 residues were found by Scatchard analysis to be involved in the overall activity of the enzyme. Both reductases and the overall FAS activity could be protected from inhibition by phenylglyoxal and 2,3-butanedione by NADP and analogs containing the 2'-phosphate group; NAD and NADH had no effect on the reaction. These results suggested that the guanidine group of an essential arginine residue at the active site of each reductase domain interacts with the 2'-phosphate of NADPH.

FAS was also reversibly inhibited by pyridoxal phosphate [122,124]. Of the partial reactions of FAS, the only one inhibited by this reagent was enoyl reductase. The inhibition was made irreversible by reduction with borohydride which suggested that a Schiff base was formed with an ϵ-amino group of lysine. Inhibition by pyridoxal phosphate could be partially protected by NADPH or 2'-monophospho-ADP-ribose but not by 2'-AMP, 5'-AMP, ADP ribose or NADH. This indicated that the ϵ-amino group of lysine modified by pyridoxal phosphate interacted with the 5'-pyrophosphoryl group of NADPH and that the 2'-phospho group was necessary for binding of the coenzyme to synthetase.

Identification of the group on the enzyme interacting with pyridoxal phosphate was obtained by either reducing the pyridoxal phosphate-treated protein with NaB_3H_4 or by reacting the enzyme directly with [4-^{3}H]pyridoxal phosphate. In each case, ^{3}H was incorporated into protein and after hydrolysis it was found in N^6-pyridoxal lysine. When [4-^{3}H]pyridoxal phosphate was used, it was found that incorporation of 2 moles/subunit resulted in complete loss of enoyl-CoA reductase activity. In the presence of NADPH, only 1 mole of [^{3}H]pyridoxal was bound per subunit and the inactivation was prevented.

6. Bacterial fatty acid synthase

FAS in bacteria may be of the Type I or Type II form. Type I synthases, those that contain multiple catalytic functions in a single polypeptide chain, are found in the higher bacteria. Type II synthases are those in which the constituent enzymes fail to show any physical interaction and exist as monofunctional units readily separable by conventional protein fractionation techniques. Because of the relative ease by which the component proteins could be isolated, studies on Type II synthases, particularly from *E. coli*, have provided many of the salient features of the general mechanisms involved in fatty acid synthesis in general. Most of the studies on these enzymes have been reviewed in detail in the past [9,125] and will only be briefly summarized.

In 1961 Lynen discovered that yeast FAS [1] catalyzed the condensation of acetyl-CoA and malonyl-CoA to form protein-bound acetoacetate. Based upon this observation, Lynen proposed a mechanism of fatty acid biosynthesis in which all the intermediates are protein-bound. This observation was confirmed with a partially purified extract of *Clostridium kluyveri* [6] which catalyzed the condensation reaction of fatty acid biosynthesis (reaction 5). Upon further fractionation of this extract, a small peptide which was stable to boiling in 0.1 N HCl was isolated. It was shown to be a required component of the condensation reaction and for overall fatty acid biosynthesis.

This unique protein was shown to function as a specific acyl-group carrier in fatty acid synthesis [126]. Because of its role, it was called the acyl-carrier protein (ACP). It has been isolated from a number of bacterial species including *E. coli* [125,126], *C. butyricum* [127], Arthrobacter [128] and Propionobacterium [129]. It has been most extensively purified and characterized from extracts of *E. coli* [9,125,126].

E. coli ACP is a very acidic, heat- and acid-stable peptide with a molecular weight of approximately 10 000. Of prime importance was the finding that ACP contained the prosthetic group, 4′-phosphopantetheine which is in phosphodiester linkage to the hydroxyl group of a serine residue of the peptide [130]. The relationship between the prosthetic group of ACP and coenzyme A is shown in Fig. 1. It was discovered that the substrate binding site of ACP was the sulfhydryl of the prosthetic group, 4′-phosphopantetheine [131]. ACP from *E. coli* has been sequenced and found to contain 77 amino acid residues [132]. In addition, there was one mole each of β-alanine, pantoic acid, thioethanolamine and phosphate [130,132], the component parts of the prosthetic group linked to serine at residue 36 [132].

In addition to ACP, each of the components of the *E. coli* FAS system has been purified and characterized. Acetyl-CoA–ACP transacylase catalyzes the reversible transfer of the acetyl groups from the sulfhydryl of CoA to that of ACP (reaction 2) [133,134]. The requirement for a particular sulfhydryl compound was not absolute since pantetheine could replace ACP as an acceptor for the acetyl group [133]. However, there was a relatively high degree of specificity with regard to the acyl group; activity fell off sharply with increasing chain length of acyl-CoA [134]. This was reflected in the primer chain length specificity of *E. coli* FAS [22]. Experiments with [^{14}C]acetyl-CoA demonstrated that a [^{14}C]acetyl enzyme was formed and that the [^{14}C]-labeled group could be transferred to either CoA or ACP [134]. Apparently one or more sulfhydryl groups on the enzyme was involved at or near the active site since the enzyme was inhibited by the sulfhydryl poisons, *N*-ethylmaleimide and iodoacetamide [134]. However, the substrate binding site has not been directly identified.

The transfer of the malonyl group from the sulfhydryl of CoA to that of ACP is catalyzed by malonyl-CoA–ACP transacylase (reaction 4) [133,134]. As with acetyl transacylase, pantetheine can replace ACP as a malonyl acceptor [133]. Malonyl transacylase was stimulated by dithiothreitol and inhibited by a number of sulfhydryl inhibitors indicating the presence of reactive SH groups at or near the active site of the enzyme [133–137]. In addition, the enzyme was inhibited by phenylmethyl-sulfonyl fluoride, suggesting the presence of an active serine [137]. This led to the suggestion that an activated oxygen ester was involved in the *E. coli* malonyl transacylase reaction [137]. Confirmation of this proposal was obtained by reacting the enzyme with [^{14}C]malonyl-CoA and isolation of the resulting [^{14}C]malonyl enzyme [136]. The labeled enzyme was subjected to proteolysis and a [^{14}C]malonyl-peptide was isolated. This was identified as malonyl-*O*-serine. Thus the malonyl-CoA–ACP transacylase reaction can be visualized as shown in reactions 10 and 11.

$$\text{Malonyl-S-CoA} + \text{E-OH} \rightleftharpoons \text{Malonyl-O-E} + \text{CoA-SH} \tag{10}$$

$$\text{Malonyl-O-E} + \text{ACP-SH} \rightleftharpoons \text{Malonyl-S-ACP} + \text{E-OH} \tag{11}$$

β-Ketoacyl-ACP synthetase catalyzes the elongation of the fatty acyl chains in fatty acid biosynthesis in a two-step reaction (reactions 3 and 5). The enzyme has been purified to homogeneity [133,138–140], crystallized [140] and the mechanism of action extensively studied [141]. The involvement of a sulfhydryl group in the condensation reaction was suggested by the requirement of high levels of thiols for optimal enzyme activity; the inhibition by sulfhydryl reagents; and the prevention of this inhibition by prior incubation of the enzyme with acetyl-ACP [133,138,139]. β-Keto-acyl-ACP synthetase contained 8 moles of cysteine per mole of protein as determined by amino acid analysis and by titration of the enzyme with [1-^{14}C]iodoacetamide under denaturing conditions [139]. Under non-denaturing conditions however, it was found that inhibition occurred when approximately 1 mole of iodoacetamide was bound per mole of enzyme; preincubation with acetyl-ACP prevented the incorporation of labeled iodoacetamide into the enzyme. The amino acid residue to which iodoacetamide was bound was shown to be cysteine [139]. These result strongly suggested that an acetyl enzyme intermediate was involved in the overall reaction. This was evidenced by experiments which showed that the enzyme reacts with acetyl-ACP to form acetyl enzyme. This acetyl enzyme which behaved as a thioester, was itself enzymatically active in that it could react with free-ACP to form acetyl-ACP in the reversal of reaction 3 or react with malonyl-ACP to form acetoacetyl-ACP, reaction 5.

The condensation reaction of fatty acid synthesis was first described in extracts of *C. kluyveri* using a malonyl-CoA–CO_2 exchange reaction [142]. This reaction, which has become a primary assay for the condensation reaction in bacterial and animal systems [141,115] has been most extensively studied with the purified β-ketoacyl ACP synthase from *E. coli* [141]. The requirements for the reaction include in addition to $^{14}CO_2$, malonyl-CoA, ACP, malonyl transacylase, acetyl-ACP or a longer chain acyl-CoA. Acetyl-CoA did not substitute for acetyl-ACP [141]. However, CoA derivatives of longer chain fatty acids, especially hexanoate, octanoate and decanoate substituted for acetyl-ACP in the exchange of $^{14}CO_2$ into malonyl-CoA. In the absence of ACP, these acyl-CoA's were also effective in preventing inhibition of the synthase by the alkylating agent, iodoacetamide.

Further experiments revealed that purified β-ketoacyl-ACP synthase catalyzed a fatty acyl-CoA–ACP transacylase reaction analogous to the acetyl-CoA–ACP transacylase reaction and that formation of fatty acyl-ACP was required for the malonyl-CoA–$^{14}CO_2$ exchange [141]. A possible explanation for the mechanism of the transacylase reaction involves the specificity of this enzyme for fatty acyl groups. It had been shown that saturated and unsaturated fatty acyl-ACP thioesters from C_2 to C_{16} were effective substrates in the β-ketoacyl-ACP synthase reaction. This broad specificity suggested that there was a hydrophobic region on the enzyme that has affinity for the acyl group, in addition to a site specific for ACP. It was postulated that at the C_2 level the affinity of the enzyme was high for acetyl-ACP which contains the active site thiol, but that it was very low for acetyl-CoA because the 2-carbon acyl group was too small for adequate hydrophobic interaction with the acyl site of the enzyme. There is greater opportunity for hydrophobic interactions with longer acyl groups and therefore the enzyme had a high affinity for longer chain fatty acyl-CoA's as well as acyl-ACP's. It is likely that the transacylation catalyzed by β-ketoacyl-ACP synthase is a model for the physiological transfer of the elongating acyl group from acyl-ACP back to the synthase (reaction 3) in preparation for condensation with malonyl-ACP (reaction 5).

β-Ketoacyl-ACP synthase also catalyzes the decarboxylation of malonyl-ACP. This reaction is independent of fatty acyl-ACP and does not involve a thiol group on the enzyme. Two mechanisms had been proposed for the condensation–decarboxylation reaction catalyzed by the synthase. One involved a concerted condensation decarboxylation and the second a two-step reaction characterized by the initial formation of an enzymatically stabilized carbanion by decarboxylation of malonyl-ACP followed by condensation of the carbanion with acyl-enzyme. The former case would represent an abortive reaction of the enzyme while the latter would represent the actual formation of the carbanion.

This question was resolved by the studies of Arnstadt et al. [143]. Using deuteromalonyl-ACP they demonstrated that there was no kinetic isotope effect in the formation of acetoacetyl-ACP. In addition, no isotope effect was observed when the reaction was carried out in the presence of D_2O nor was there any incorporation of label when the reaction was carried out in the presence of tritiated water thus excluding proton exchange with the solvent. These results indicated that the condensation reaction between acetyl-ACP and malonyl-ACP followed a concerted mechanism with coupling of carbon–carbon bond formation and cleavage of the carboxyl bond of the malonyl group.

Two forms of β-ketoacyl-ACP synthetase (designated I and II) have been identified in extracts of *E. coli* by the isolation and characterization of a number of fatty acid biosynthetic mutants. Synthetase I corresponds to the enzyme studied earlier by Greenspan et al. [139]. Synthetase II was isolated by D'Agnolo et al. [144] as a homogeneous protein with a higher molecular weight, a lower pH optimum and a greater resistance to heat than synthetase I. Both enzymes were inhibited by iodoacetamide and prior incubation with fatty acyl thioesters protected against this inhibitor. Examination of the kinetics of these two enzymes indicated that the only difference was that synthetase II had a lower K_m and a higher V_{max} than synthetase I with palmitoyl-ACP as substrate [144].

Further confirmation of the existence of two synthetases was shown when Garwin et al. [145] demonstrated that an *E. coli* mutant unable to convert palmitoleic to *cis*-vaccenic acid was deficient in synthetase II. This mutant (Cvc −) was also deficient in its thermal regulation of membrane fatty acids. Reversion of the mutation resulted in normalization of the *cis*-vaccenate content and the β-ketoacyl-ACP synthetase II level. Synthetase II therefore appears to play an essential role in the thermal regulation of the fatty acid content of *E. coli*. Garwin et al. [146] also established that synthetase II had a greater molecular weight than synthetase I (85 000 vs. 80 000) and that gel electrophoresis of partial proteolytic digests demonstrated that the synthetases share few if any common peptides. The enzymes were shown to be immunologically distinct as well.

7. Regulation

A vast amount of literature has been published on the regulation of fatty acid synthetase (for reviews, see refs. 8–10). Studies on the regulation of this particular enzyme is especially interesting, applicable to many current problems and has proven to be very fruitful.

The connection between fatty acid synthesis and the metabolic problems of obesity, diabetes, and starvation is well recognized. Early studies indicated that the enzymes, acetyl-CoA carboxylase and fatty acid synthetase, were involved in the changes seen when animals were starved and refed or made diabetic [147–150]. Typically these studies were carried out by assaying the activity of the enzymes as measured in various cell-free systems and correlating this with the incorporation of radioactive precursors into fatty acids [151,152]. Research into the regulation of the synthetase gained momentum as the mechanism of its enzymatic reactions was elucidated in *E. coli* [126,131,139,153,154]. It became increasingly easy to purify the enzyme from a variety of sources so that with pure enzyme, antibodies against the synthetase could be made to clarify whether the activity or amount of enzyme protein changed with altered metabolic states. Finally, with the advent of new techniques in molecular biology, more basic questions could be asked on the nature of molecular factors which control the level of fatty acid synthetase.

Immunochemical methods indicated that the decrease in the activity of hepatic fatty acid synthetase on starvation and the subsequent increase with refeeding were due to changes in the actual amount of enzyme protein [155,156]. This was shown to be true for both rats [155] and pigeons [156]. Other experiments using isotope incorporation into the synthetase have also indicated that synthesis of the enzyme, not the activity, changed on starvation [157].

Volpe et al. [158] observed a 20-fold difference in fatty acid synthetase per gram of liver between starved and refed animals. Analysis of the enzyme by immunotitration showed that in the case of the refed animals, synthesis of the enzyme was increased; and in the case of the starved animals, the rate of degradation of the enzyme was increased. So, both synthesis and degradation of the enzyme can change to adjust the activity of fatty acid synthesis to different nutritional states.

Other studies by Volpe and Vagelos [159] comparing fatty acid synthetase in rat brain and liver indicated that the brain enzyme did not respond to nutritional stimuli in the same manner as the liver. Brain fatty acid synthetase did not change when the animal was fasted or refed a fat-free diet whereas the liver enzyme changed as expected. Liver synthetase increased on weaning due to an increased synthesis of enzyme protein. At the same time however, brain enzyme was decreased. The $t_{1/2}$ of brain and liver FAS was 6.4 and 2.8 days, respectively [159].

Feeding a fat-free diet stimulated synthesis of hepatic fatty acid synthetase; in the opposite situation, feeding fat-containing diets reduced the capacity of the liver for incorporating [^{14}C]glucose or [^{14}C]acetate into fatty acids [152]. Further studies showed that feeding rats methyl esters of linoleic, linolenic and arachidonic acid reduced the activity of fatty acid synthetase, as well as acetyl-CoA carboxylase, citrate cleavage enzyme, malic enzyme and glucose-6-phosphate dehydrogenase [160,161]. Flick et al. [162] looked at this more closely and determined that the rate of synthesis of the liver synthetase in animals fed a diet containing 15% safflower oil was about one-half that of control animals. The rate of degradation of the enzyme was also increased in the safflower-fed animals over the controls. The half-lives of the enzyme were 1.8 and 3.8 days, respectively.

The majority of studies on the regulation of fatty acid synthetase have pointed to long-term regulation controlled by synthesis or degradation of enzyme protein; there have also been some reports which suggested that there may be short-term regulation as well. Yu and Burton [163] have shown that the amount of immunoreactive FAS increased in the liver 1 h after refeeding previously starved rats, whereas an increase in its activity was not seen until 3 h after feeding. Experiments have shown that [^{14}C]pantetheine incorporation into the isolated synthetase followed the same course as enzyme activity, suggesting the existence of an enzymatically inactive precursor of the synthetase, possibly an apo-haloenzyme conversion.

In addition to regulation of fatty acid synthetase by the nutritional state of the animal, many studies have described changes of the synthetase in response to hormonal effects. Thus, experimentally induced diabetes caused a marked depression in the activities of enzymes involved in lipid biosynthesis, which can be subsequently reversed by insulin [155,164–168]. Lakshamanan et al. [169] and Volpe and Marasa [170] have shown that this decrease was due to a reduction in enzyme synthesis. However, the controlling mechanisms were not clear-cut since feeding of fructose to diabetic rats mimicked the effects of insulin in that it reversed the decrease in hepatic fatty acid synthetase. Interestingly, fructose feeding did not stimulate fatty acid synthetase in diabetic adipose tissue [168]. Adrenalectomy also restored liver FAS to normal in a diabetic animal in the absence of insulin [170]. Other hormonal effects on fatty acid synthetase have been noted. Thus, gluco-corticoids caused a decrease in both adipose tissue synthetase and acetyl-CoA carboxylase, whereas no effect was seen on the liver enzymes [170]. The converse experiment, adrenalectomy, resulted in an increase in the adipose tissue enzyme and again, no change in the liver synthetase or carboxylase [170]. Lastly, the gluco-corticoid effect in adipose tissue fatty acid synthetase was found to occur in hypophysectomized animals, indicating that pituitary hormones were not necessary for the effect. These changes in fatty acid synthetase induced by glucocorticoids were shown to be due to a reduction in the amount of enzyme, caused by a decrease in enzyme synthesis [170].

Administration of glucagon [169,170] or theophylline [170] to starved–refed rats inhibited the induction of the liver synthetase with no effect on the adipose enzyme. These responses also were due to a decrease in the synthesis of fatty acid synthetase [170].

Embryonic chicken liver contains very little fatty acid synthetase, but the enzyme could be induced by administration of insulin, hydrocortisone, growth hormone, glucagon or dibutyryl cyclic AMP [171,172]. Induction was blocked however by cyclohexamide, suggesting that the alteration in fatty acid synthetase was due to changes in the content of the enzyme. On one hand glucagon and cAMP inhibited a rise in liver FAS due to refeeding in starved rats; on the other hand these hormones stimulated the induction of FAS in embryonic chick liver. Whether or not there is a conflict in these results remains to be seen as the mechanism of cAMP's effect on the synthetase is more carefully elucidated.

Still other effects of hormonal action on fatty acid synthetase were found: Aprahamian et al. [173] showed that β-estradiol increased FAS in 1-month-old female chicks; Volpe and Marasa [174] noted that theophylline decreased the enzyme content in cultured glia cells; Fischer and Goodridge [175] demonstrated that incubation of insulin and triiodothyronine with cultured chick-liver cells gave a large stimulation of FAS, much greater than the effect of either hormone alone. Glucagon plus insulin had no effect, although glucagon did inhibit the increase in FAS when added with insulin and T_3. All of the above studies have shown by immunochemical techniques that the changes seen in FAS activity were due to increases or decreases in synthetase content brought about by modification of the rate of synthesis of the enzyme.

Developmental factors also play an important role in regulating the amount of fatty acid synthetase in chick liver [176], mammalian liver [177,178], mammalian brain [158,178] and mammary gland [179]. The synthetase increased in mammary glands during mid to late pregnancy and early in lactation [179]. FAS was induced after hatching in chick liver and appeared transiently at the time of birth and again after weaning [176]. On the other hand, fatty acid synthetase in brain was highest in fetal and neonatal rats, and decreased as the animals matured [158,178]. These changes in the liver enzyme were due to a rise in the synthesis of the enzyme [176];

in the case of the brain enzyme, an increase in the rate of its degradation was seen. The rate of degradation of the synthetase in the brain was approximately 3-fold greater than that in the mature brain [158].

Finally, differences in the regulation of fatty acid synthetase were seen in genetic mutants [179,180]. The obese hyperglycemic mouse had a higher hepatic activity than its non-obese litter mates when fed laboratory chow. Both animals responded to starvation by a decline in the rate of synthesis of the synthetase; however, there was also an increase in the hepatic degradation of the enzyme in the non-obese animals. The response of the mice to injection of triiodothyronine was quantitatively different as well; the hormone causes a much more marked rise in hepatic fatty acid synthetase in non-obese than in obese mice [180].

The regulation of fatty acid synthetase has also been studied in 3T3-L1 cells. These are a cloned cell line of 3T3 mouse embryo fibroblasts. The 3T3-L1 cells are capable of differentiating into adipocytes either spontaneously [181] or after treatment with hormones or drugs [182–186]. The induction of various lipogenic enzymes has been correlated with differentiation of the cells into adipocytes. In particular, it has been shown by Mackall et al. [184] that total fatty acid synthetase activity increased 40-fold after treatment of the cells with insulin. Further studies by Student et al. [187] and Weiss et al. [188] using immunochemical techniques indicated that this increase in fatty acid synthetase activity was due to enhanced synthesis of the enzyme. The rate of degradation of the enzyme was unaffected by differentiation.

A distinguishing feature of animal fatty acid synthetases is their response to nutritional and hormonal perturbations. As indicated above, FAS activity was depressed in starved or diabetic animals. Feeding a fat-free diet to starved animals or administration of insulin to diabetic animals resulted in a marked increase in the rate of synthesis of FAS leading to elevated levels of the enzyme. The mechanisms by which these changes in levels of FAS occur have been the subject of much interest in recent years. It was therefore not surprising that with the advent of modern molecular biology, these approaches would be used to define the mechanisms involved in regulation of synthetase synthesis. The approach that was taken initially involved the identification of polysomes synthesizing FAS [89,189]. Rat liver polysomes that synthesize FAS were identified by sucrose-gradient analysis of polysomes that had been treated with ^{125}I-labeled anti-FAS antibody. By quantitating the amount of binding of ^{125}I-labeled antibody to nascent FAS peptides it was demonstrated that the relative content of FAS mRNA-containing polysomes in rat liver increases dramatically during dietary induction. Correlative evidence that ^{125}I-labeled anti-FAS antibody was bound to the nascent chains of FAS on the polysomes was obtained by using an in vitro translation system with the polysomes [190]. In these studies, the nascent chains were completed in vitro in the presence of a radiolabeled amino acid, the products were precipitated with anti-FAS antibody, and identified by sodium dodecyl sulfate polyacrylamide gel electrophoresis. There was excellent agreement between the time of appearance of antibody precipitable FAS synthesized in vitro from nascent chains on polysomes and the binding to polysomes of ^{125}I-labeled anti-FAS antibody. There was also very good correlation between these molecular approaches and the actual changes in FAS-specific activity measured in extracts of the liver. These methods however did not distinguish whether changes in rate of synthesis of FAS were due to differences in the rate of initiation, of protein synthesis, quantity of translatable FAS, mRNA or both. They did show that a marked increase in the rate of in vitro translation of synthetase peptides from polysomes could be correlated with the induced synthesis of fatty acid synthetase after fat-free refeeding of starved rats.

As indicated, the synthesis of FAS may be regulated by transcriptional control, i.e. alteration in the amount of its messenger RNA or by translational control, i.e. mechanisms that determine the efficiency of mRNA translation. Therefore, in order to gain insight into the mechanism of regulation of fatty acid synthetase synthesis, it is necessary to directly measure levels of mRNA coding for this enzyme.

The approach used involved the isolation of mRNA followed by its translation into polypeptides with an in vitro protein-synthesizing system containing a radio-labeled amino acid [191–193]. Quantitation of the synthesis was achieved by immunoprecipitation of the labeled FAS peptide and subsequent electrophoresis on SDS–polyacrylamide gel. The counts migrating with FAS were compared with the mRNA-dependent incorporation into total protein. The quantity of translatable fatty acid synthetase mRNA in liver of rats subjected to modification of nutritional state or subjected to different hormonal states was determined by this procedure [191–193]. Although in these studies optimal translation efficiency was not obtained, relative changes in synthetase synthesis from mRNA consistent with changes in liver FAS levels were found. Thus, in rats starved for 48 h, very little translatable messenger RNA could be found; similarly, completion of FAS nascent chains on polysomes was very low [191]. By 12 h after refeeding a fat-free, high-carbohydrate diet, translatable messenger RNA activity increased approximately 10-fold from the fasting state. Completion of polysomal nascent FAS-nascent chains increased 13-fold and enzyme activity in the liver increased 7-fold. Similarly, very low FAS mRNA activity was found in starved diabetic rats that had been refed a low-fat diet for 12 h; insulin administration at times of refeeding resulted in an 11-fold increase in FAS mRNA activity [194]. Treatment of normal rats with either glucagon or dibutyryl cyclic AMP resulted in an approximate 3-fold decrease in the level of functional rat liver FAS mRNA. These results suggested that insulin and glucagon are involved in the regulation of some step in the production of mRNA for fatty acid synthetase.

The translation product of mRNA coding for full-length FAS was analyzed by copurification of the synthetic product with authentic enzyme [193]. Rat liver poly(A$^+$)-RNA was enriched 1270-fold with 27% translational purity as measured by the percentage of total translation product precipitated by anti-FAS antibody. The translation product was mixed with fatty acid synthetase from rat liver and subjected to sucrose-gradient centrifugation. It was found that radioactivity derived from the in vitro translation comigrated with a protein of molecular weight of 480 000, the same as native synthetase. Further proof that the radioactivity was associated with native enzyme was observed by immunoprecipitation of an aliquot of the fractions from the sucrose gradient followed by SDS gel electrophoresis. It was found that under these conditions the radioactivity migrated with the 240 000 molecular weight subunits of native fatty acid synthetase. These results indicated that fatty acid synthetase synthesized in vitro were assembled in vitro into dimers which were the native form of the enzyme.

FAS mRNA has been partially purified from rat liver [191,193,194], mammary gland [195] and goose uropygial gland [196–198]. It has been most extensively purified and characterized from the goose uropygial gland by Goodrich and his associates [197,198]. Poly(A$^+$)-RNA was prepared from 16 000 × g supernatants of homogenates of goose uropygial gland, precipitated at pH 5 with acetic acid, followed by chromatography of the resuspended precipitate on oligo-dT cellulose [197]. As might be expected, because of the very large size of the FAS peptide, it was found that FAS mRNA could be separated from the bulk of the poly(A$^+$)-RNA by sucrose gradient centrifugation sedimenting as a small distinct peak which migrated at about 36 S. For the uropygial gland this peak represented about 1% total poly(A$^+$)-RNA. 60–70% of the total protein synthesized in vitro in the presence of RNA from the 36-S region was immunoprecipitated by anti-FAS antibody.

Because difficulties had been encountered in early attempts to translate unfractionated FAS mRNA [197], conditions were developed to optimize the cell-free synthesis of FAS. It was found that addition of calf liver tRNA to the translation system stimulated FAS synthesis 9-fold while total polypeptide production was only slightly stimulated. Similar requirements have been found for in vitro synthesis of FAS with mRNA derived from the rat mammary gland [195]. Also found to be critical for maximal translation of goose FAS mRNA were the concentrations of potassium and magnesium and the time of the reaction [197]. Thus, synthesis of full-length immunoprecipable fatty acid synthetase did not appear until 60–90 min after initiation of the reaction and then increased for an additional 90 min. In contrast, total polypeptides that were synthesized increased in a linear fashion for about 60 min. Presumably differences in requirements for in vitro FAS synthesis compared with synthesis of total peptide were a reflection of the large size of the synthetase polypeptide chain.

To accurately measure the level and the turnover of FAS mRNA required the availability of complementary DNA (cDNA) to FAS mRNA. This has been accomplished by Morris et al. [198] for the goose uropygial gland enzyme. A double-stranded cDNA library was constructed from uropygial gland poly(A$^+$)-RNA. This was recombined into plasmid pBR322 and the recombinant molecules were used to transform E. coli HB101. Colony hybridization with a ^{32}P-labeled cDNA transcribed from partially purified FAS mRNA was used to identify clones containing sequences complementary to FAS mRNA. The identity of these clones was confirmed by hybrid-selected translation. Two plasmids, pFAS$_1$ and pFAS$_3$ selected RNA enriched for FAS mRNA activity. Size of FAS mRNA was determined after electrophoresis of mRNA isolated from the gland followed by Northern analysis with ^{32}P-labeled pFAS$_3$ DNA. It was found that FAS mRNA is 16 kilobases long. Based on a FAS subunit molecular weight of 250 000, it was estimated that FAS mRNA should contain 6.8 kilobases. Thus FAS mRNA contains approximately 9 kilobases more

54

than was required for synthesis of FAS. The function of these additional bases is unknown.

In addition to its use for determining the size of FAS mRNA, the recombinant plasmid, pFAS$_3$ DNA, was used to ascertain the relative FAS mRNA levels in fed and fasting gosling liver by dot-blot hybridization analysis [198]. It was found that 24 h after refeeding, FAS synthesis increased 42-fold, while the abundance of FAS mRNA in total RNA increased 70-fold. Thus, FAS mRNA levels increased in parallel with increased synthesis of FAS in vivo in response to refeeding starved animals.

Thus, it appears that fatty acid synthetase can be regulated by the nutritional state of the animal, by hormonal factors, the development stage and genetic factors. The differences in enzyme activity seen are due to changes in the amount of enzyme and not its intrinsic activity. These changes are in turn controlled by the stimulation of enzyme synthesis or degradation, mediated by the quantity of fatty acid synthetase-mRNA present in the cell.

Acknowledgements

We would like to thank Elizabeth Schroeder for proofreading and Joan Kiliyanski for the typing of this manuscript.

References

1 Lynen, F. (1961) Fed. Proc. 20, 941.
2 Gibson, D.M., Titchener, E.B. and Wakil, S.J. (1958) J. Am. Chem. Soc. 80, 2908.
3 Wakil, S.J. (1958) J. Am. Chem. Soc. 80, 6465.
4 Wakil, S.J. and Ganguly, J. (1959) J. Am. Chem. Soc. 81, 2597.
5 Ganguly, J. (1960) Biochim. Biophys. Acta 40, 110.
6 Alberts, A.W. and Vagelos, P.R. (1961) Fed. proc. 20, 273.
7 Wakil, S.J. and Barnes Jr., E.M. (1971) in: M. Florkin and E.H. Stotz (Eds.), Comprehensive Biochemistry, Vol. 18S, Elsevier, New York, p. 57.
8 Numa, S. and Yamashita, S. (1974) in: B.L. Horecker and E.R. Stadtman (Eds.), Current Topics in Cellular Regulation, Vol. 8, Academic Press, New York, p. 197.
9 Volpe, J.J. and Vagelos, P.R. (1976) Physiol. Rev. 56, 339.
10 Bloch, K. and Vance, D. (1977) Annu. Rev. Biochem. 46, 236.
11 Katiyar, S.S. and Porter, J.W. (1980) Experientia 36, Suppl., 181.
12 Stoops, J.K., Arslanian, M.J., Chalmers Jr., J.H., Joshi, V.C. and Wakil, S.J. (1977) in: E.E. van Tamelen (Ed.), Bioorganic Chemistry, Vol. 1, Academic Press, New York, p. 339.
13 Brindley, D.N., Matsumura, S. and Bloch, K. (1969) Nature (London) 224, 666.
14 Horning, M.G., Martin, D.B., Karmen, A. and Vagelos, P.R. (1961) J. Biol. Chem. 236, 669.
15 Knudsen, J. and Grunnet, I. (1980) Biochem. Biophys. Res. Commun. 95, 1808.
16 Buckner, J.S. and Kolattukudy, P.E. (1976) Biochemistry 15, 1948.
17 Katiyar, S.S., Buedis, A.V. and Porter, J.W. (1974) Arch. Biochem. Biophys. 162, 42.
18 Smith, S. and Abraham, S. (1971) J. Biol. Chem. 246, 2537.
19 Lin, C.Y. and Kumar, S. (1971) J. Biol. Chem. 246, 3284.
20 Kaneda, T. (1973) Can. J. Microbiol. 19, 87.

21 Kaneda, T. (1977) Bacteriol. Rev. 41, 371.

22 Naik, D.N. and Kaneda, T. (1974) Can. J. Microbiol. 20, 1701.

23 Kaneda, T. and Smith, E.J. (1980) Can. J. Microbiol. 26, 893.

24 Seyama, Y., Otsuka, H., Kawaguchi, A. and Yamakawa, T. (1981) J. Biochem. 90, 789.

25 Jacob, J. (1976) in: P.E. Kolattukudy (Ed.), Chemistry and Biochemistry of Natural Waxes, Elsevier, New York, p. 93.

26 Buckner, J.S. and Kolattukudy, P.E. (1975) Biochemistry 14, 1774.

27 Kolattukudy, P.E., Poulose, A.J. and Buckner, J.S. (1981) in: J.M. Lowenstein (Ed.), Methods in Enzymology, Vol. 71, Academic Press, New York, p. 103.

28 Buckner, J.S., Kolattukudy, P.E. and Rogers, L. (1978) Arch. Biochem. Biophys. 186, 152.

29 Frenkel, E.P. and Kitchens, R.L. (1977) Proc. Soc. Exp. Biol. Med. 156, 151.

30 Roncari, D.A.K. and Mack, E.Y.W. (1976) Can. J. Biochem. 54, 923.

31 Buckner, J.S. and Kolattukudy, P.E. (1975) Biochemistry 14, 1768.

32 Yamazaki, T., Seyama, Y., Otsuka, H., Ogawa, H. and Yamakawa, T. (1981) J. Biochem. 89, 683.

33 Turner, W.B. (Ed.) (1971) Fungal Metabolites, Academic Press, New York.

34 Weeks, G. and Wakil, S.J. (1968) J. Biol. Chem. 243, 1180.

35 White III, H.B., Matsukashi, O. and Bloch, K. (1971) J. Biol. Chem. 248, 4751.

36 Knoche, H. and Koths, K.E. (1973) J. Biol. Chem. 248, 3517.

37 Kawaguchi, A., Yoshimura, T., Saito, K., Seyama, Y., Kasama, T., Yamakawa, T. and Okuda, S. (1980) J. Biochem. (Tokyo) 88, 1.

38 Lynen, F. (1980) Eur. J. Biochem. 112, 431.

39 Goldman, P., Alberts, A.W. and Vagelos, P.R. (1961) Biochem. Biophys. Res. Commun. 5, 280.

40 Wood, W.I., Peterson, D.O. and Bloch, K. (1978) J. Biol. Chem. 253, 2650.

41 Smith, S. (1980) J. Dairy Sci. 63, 337.

42 Morrison, W.R. (1970) in: F.D. Gunstone (Ed.), Topics in Lipid Chemistry, Vol. 1, Halsted Press, New York, p. 51.

43 Smith, S., Watts, R. and Dils, R. (1968) J. Lipid Res. 9, 52.

44 Breckenridge, W.C. and Kuksis, A. (1967) J. Lipid Res. 8, 473.

45 Marai, L., Breckenridge, W.C. and Kuksis, A. (1960) Lipids 4, 562.

46 Smith, S. (1973) Arch. Biochem. Biophys. 156, 751.

47 Agradi, E., Libertini, L. and Smith, S. (1976) Biochem. Biophys. Res. Commun. 68, 894.

48 Lin, C.Y. and Smith, S. (1978) J. Biol. Chem. 253, 1954.

49 Libertini, L.J. and Smith, S. (1978) J. Biol. Chem. 253, 1393.

50 Libertini, L.J. and Smith, S. (1979) Arch. Biochem. Biophys. 192, 47.

51 Smith, S. and Libertini, L.J. (1979) Arch. Biochem. Biophys. 196, 88.

52 Smith, S. and Ryan, P. (1979) J. Biol. Chem. 254, 8932.

53 Knudsen, J., Clark, S. and Dils, R. (1975) Biochem. Biophys. Res. Commun. 65, 921.

54 Knudsen, J., Clark, S. and Dils, R. (1976) Biochem. J. 160, 683.

55 Chivers, L., Knudsen, J. and Dils, R. (1977) Biochim. Biophys. Acta 487, 361.

56 Grunnet, I. and Knudsen, J. (1979) Eur. J. Biochem. 95, 497.

57 Grunnet, I. and Knudsen, J. (1978) Biochem. Biophys. Res. Commun. 80, 745.

58 Grunnet, I. and Knudsen, J. (1981) Biochem. Biophys. Res. Commun. 100, 629.

59 Knudsen, J. and Grunnet, I. (1982) Biochem. J. 202, 139.

60 De Renobales, M., Rogers, L. and Kolattukudy, P.E. (1980) Arch. Biochem. Biophys. 205, 464.

61 Rogers, L., Kolattukudy, P.E. and De Renobales, M. (1982) J. Biol. Chem. 257, 880.

62 Linn, T.C. and Srere, P.A. (1980) J. Biol. Chem. 255, 10676.

63 Stern, A., Sedgwick, B. and Smith, S. (1982) J. Biol. Chem. 257, 799.

64 Greenspan, M.D., Birge, C.H., Powell, G., Hancock, W.S. and Vagelos, P.R. (1970) Science 170, 1203.

65 Cronan Jr., J.E., Weinberg, L.J. and Allen, R.G. (1975) J. Biol. Chem. 250, 5835.

66 Barnes Jr., E.M. and Wakil, S.J. (1968) J. Biol. Chem. 243, 2955.

67 Barnes Jr., E.M., Swindell, A.C. and Wakil, S.J. (1970) J. Biol. Chem. 245, 3122.

68 Peterson, D.O. and Bloch, K. (1977) J. Biol. Chem. 252, 5735.
69 Banis, R.J., Peterson, D.O. and Bloch, K. (1977) J. Biol. Chem. 252, 5740.
70 Wood, W.I., Peterson, D.O. and Bloch, K. (1977) J. Biol. Chem. 252, 5745.
71 Kawaguchi, A., Seyama, Y., Sasaki, K., Okuda, S. and Yamakawa, T. (1979) J. Biochem. (Tokyo) 85, 865.
72 Kawaguchi, A., Arai, K., Seyama, Y., Yamakawa, T. and Okuda, S. (1980) J. Biochem. (Tokyo) 88, 303.
73 Nepokroeff, C.M., Lakshamanan, M.R. and Porter, J.W. (1975) in: J.M. Lowenstein (Ed.), Methods in Enzymology, Vol. 35, Academic Press, New York, p. 37.
74 Stoops, J.K., Arslanian, M.J., Oh, Y.H., Aune, K.C., Vanaman, T.C. and Wakil, S.J. (1975) Proc. Natl. Acad. Sci. (U.S.A.) 72, 1940.
75 Stoops, J.K., Ross, P., Arslanian, M.J., Aune, K.C., Wakil, S.J. and Oliver, R.M. (1979) J. Biol. Chem. 254, 7418.
76 Linn, T.C. (1981) Arch. Biochem. Biophys. 209, 613.
77 Smith, S. and Abraham, S. (1975) in: J.M. Lowenstein (Ed.), Methods in Enzymology, Vol. 35, Academic Press, New York, p. 65.
78 Grunnel, I. and Knudsen, J. (1978) Biochem. J. 173, 929.
79 Hardie, D.G. and Cohen, P. (1978) Eur. J. Biochem. 92, 25.
80 Ahmad, F. and Ahmad, P.M. (1981) in: J.M. Lowenstein (Ed.), Methods in Enzymology, Vol. 71, Academic Press, New York, p. 16.
81 Hardie, D.G., Guy, P.S. and Cohen, P. (1981) in: J.M. Lowenstein (Ed.), Methods in Enzymology, Vol. 71, Academic Press, New York, p. 26.
82 Jenik, R.A. and Porter, J.W. (1979) Int. J. Biochem. 10, 609.
83 Jenik, R.A. and Porter, J.W. (1981) in: J.M. Lowenstein (Ed.), Methods in Enzymology, Vol. 71, Academic Press, New York, p. 97.
84 Dils, R. and Carey, E.M. (1975) in: J.M. Lowenstein (Ed.), Methods in Enzymology, Vol. 35, Academic Press, New York, p. 74.
85 Kim, I.C., Unkefer, C.J. and Deal Jr., W.C. (1977) Arch. Biochem. Biophys. 178, 475.
86 Kim, I.C., Neudahl, G. and Deal Jr., W.C. (1981) in: J.M. Lowenstein (Ed.), Methods in Enzymology, Vol. 71, Academic Press, New York, p. 79.
87 Roncari, D.A. (1974) Can. J. Biochem. 52, 221.
88 Roncari, D.A. (1981) in: J.M. Lowenstein (Ed.), Methods in Enzymology, Vol. 71, Academic Press, New York, p. 73.
89 Alberts, A.W., Strauss, A.W., Hennessy, S. and Vagelos, P.R. (1975) Proc. Natl. Acad. Sci. (U.S.A.) 72, 3956.
90 Thompson, B.J., Stern, A. and Smith, S. (1981) Biochim. Biophys. Acta 662, 125.
91 Maitra, S.K. and Kumar, S. (1974) J. Biol. Chem. 249, 1118.
92 Kumar, S. and Dodds, P.F. (1981) in: J.M. Lowenstein (Ed.), Methods in Enzymology, Vol. 71, Academic Press, New York, p. 86.
93 Arslanian, M.J. and Wakil, S.J. (1975) in: J.M. Lowenstein (Ed.), Methods in Enzymology, Vol. 35, Academic Press, New York, p. 59.
94 Stoops, J.K., Arslanian, M.J., Aune, K.C. and Wakil, S.J. (1978) Arch. Biochem. Biophys. 155, 348.
95 Aprahamian, S., Arslanian, M.J. and Stoops, J.K. (1979) Lipids 14, 1015.
96 Muesing, R.A. and Porter, J.W. (1975) in: J.M. Lowenstein (Ed.), Methods in Enzymology, Vol. 35, Academic Press, New York, p. 45.
97 Smith, S. (1973) Arch. Biochem. Biophys. 156, 751.
98 Kumar, S., Srinivasan, K.R. and Asato, N. (1977) Biochim. Biophys. Acta 489, 32.
99 Kumar, S., Muesing, R.A. and Porter, J.W. (1972) J. Biol. Chem. 247, 4749.
100 Katiyar, S.S. and Porter, J.W. (1977) Life Sci. 20, 737.
101 Stoops, J.K. and Wakil, S.J. (1981) J. Biol. Chem. 256, 5128.
102 Bratcher, S.C. and Hsu, R.Y. (1975) Biochim. Biophys. Acta 410, 229.
103 Roncari, D.A., Bradshaw, R.A. and Vagelos, P.R. (1972) J. Biol. Chem. 247, 6324.

104 Qureshi, A.A., Lornitzo, F.A. and Porter, J.W. (1974) Biochem. Biophys. Res. Commun. 60, 158.

105 Roncari, D.A. (1974) J. Biol. Chem. 249, 7035.

106 Bedord, C.J., Kolattukudy, P.E. and Rogers, L. (1978) Arch. Biochem. Biophys. 186, 139.

107 Dileepan, K.N., Lin, C.Y. and Smith, S. (1978) Biochem. J. 175, 199.

108 Smith, S. and Stern, A. (1979) Arch. Biochem. Biophys. 197, 379.

109 Puri, R.N. and Porter, J.W. (1981) Biochem. Biophys. Res. Commun. 100, 1010.

110 Guy, P., Law, S. and Hardie, G. (1978) FEBS Lett. 94, 33.

111 Kumar, S. (1975) J. Biol. Chem. 250, 5150.

112 Kolattukudy, P.E., Buchner, J.S. and Bedord, C.J. (1976) Biochem. Biophys. Res. Commun. 68, 379.

113 Phillips, G.T., Nixon, J.E., Abramovitz, A.S. and Porter, J.W. (1970) Arch. Biochem. Biophys. 138, 357.

114 Joshi, V.C., Plate, C.A. and Wakil, S.J. (1970) J. Biol. Chem. 245, 2857.

115 Kumar, S., Dorsey, J.A., Muesing, R.A. and Porter, J.W. (1970) J. Biol. Chem. 245, 4732.

116 Kumar, S., Opas, E. and Alli, P. (1980) Biochem. Biophys. Res. Commun. 95, 1642.

117 Katiyar, S.S., Pan, D. and Porter, J.W. (1982) Biochem. Biophys. Res. Commun. 104, 517.

118 Stoops, J.K. and Wakil, S.J. (1982) J. Biol. Chem. 257, 3230.

119 Stoops, J.K. and Wakil, S.J. (1982) Biochem. Biophys. Res. Commun. 104, 1018.

120 Brady, R.O., Bradley, R.M. and Trams, E.G. (1960) J. Biol. Chem. 235, 3093.

121 Poulose, A.J. and Kolattukudy, P.E. (1980) Arch. Biochem. Biophys. 199, 457.

122 Poulose, A.J. and Kolattukudy, P.E. (1980) Arch. Biochem. Biophys. 201, 313.

123 Poulose, A.J. and Kolattukudy, P.E. (1981) J. Biol. Chem. 256, 8379.

124 Poulose, A.J., Rogers, L. and Kolattukudy, P.E. (1980) Int. J. Biochem. 12, 591.

125 Prescott, D.J. and Vagelos, P.R. (1968) Adv. Enzymol. 109, 702.

126 Vagelos, P.R., Majerus, P.W., Alberts, A.W., Larrabee, A.R. and Ailhaud, G. (1966) Fed. proc. 25, 1485.

127 Ailhaud, G.P., Vagelos, P.R. and Goldfine, H. (1967) J. Biol. Chem. 242, 4459.

128 Simoni, R.O., Criddle, R.S. and Stumpf, P.K. (1967) J. Biol. Chem. 242, 573.

129 Ahmad, P.M., Stirling, L.A. and Ahmad, F. (1981) J. Gen. Microbiol. 127, 121.

130 Majerus, P.W., Alberts, A.W. and Vagelos, P.R. (1965) Proc. Natl. Acad. Sci. (U.S.A.) 53, 410.

131 Majerus, P.W., Alberts, A.W. and Vagelos, P.R. (1964) Proc. Natl. Acad. Sci. (U.S.A.) 51, 1231.

132 Vanaman, T.C., Wakil, S.J. and Hill, R.J. (1968) J. Biol. Chem. 243, 6420.

133 Alberts, A.W., Majerus, P.W., Talamo, B. and Vagelos, P.R. (1964) Biochemistry 3, 1563.

134 Williamson, I.P. and Wakil, S.J. (1966) J. Biol. Chem. 241, 2326.

135 Ruch, F.E. and Vagelos, P.R. (1973) J. Biol. Chem. 248, 8086.

136 Ruch, F.E. and Vagelos, P.R. (1973) J. Biol. Chem. 248, 8095.

137 Joshi, V.C. and Wakil, S.J. (1971) Arch. Biochem. Biophys. 143, 493.

138 Toomey, R.E. and Wakil, S.J. (1966) J. Biol. Chem. 241, 1159.

139 Greenspan, M.D., Alberts, A.W. and Vagelos, P.R. (1969) J. Biol. Chem. 244, 6477.

140 Prescott, D.J. and Vagelos, P.R. (1970) J. Biol. Chem. 245, 5484.

141 Alberts, A.W., Bell, R.M. and Vagelos, P.R. (1972) J. Biol. Chem. 240, 618.

142 Vagelos, P.R. and Alberts, A.W. (1960) J. Biol. Chem. 235, 2786.

143 Arnstadt, K.I., Schindlbeck, G. and Lynen, F. (1975) Eur. J. Biochem. 55, 561.

144 D'Agnolo, G., Rosenfeld, I.S. and Vagelos, P.R. (1975) J. Biol. Chem. 250, 5289.

145 Garwin, J.L., Klages, A.L. and Cronan Jr., J.E. (1980) J. Biol. Chem. 255, 3263.

146 Garwin, J.L., Klages, A.L. and Cronan Jr., J.E. (1980) J. Biol. Chem. 255, 11949.

147 Numa, S., Matsuhashi, M. and Lynen, F. (1961) Biochem. Z. 334, 203.

148 Korchak, H.M. and Masoro, E.J. (1962) Biochim. Biophys. Acta 58, 353.

149 Allmann, D.W., Hubbard, D.D. and Gibson, D.M. (1965) J. Lipid Res. 6, 63.

150 Gibson, D.M., Hicks, S.E. and Allmann, D.W. (1966) Adv. Enzyme Reg. 4, 239.

151 Diamant, S., Gorin, E. and Shafrir, E. (1972) Eur. J. Biochem. 26, 553.

152 Hill, R., Linazasoro, J.M., Chevallier, F. and Chaikoff, I.I. (1958) J. Biol. Chem. 233, 305.

153 Majerus, P.W. and Vagelos, P.R. (1967) Adv. Lipid Res. 5, 1.

58

154 Wakil, S.J., Pugh, E.L. and Sauer, F. (1964) Proc. Natl. Acad. Sci. (U.S.A.) 52, 106.

155 Burton, D.N., Collins, J.M., Kennan, A.L. and Porter, J.W. (1969) J. Biol. Chem. 244, 4510.

156 Butterworth, P.H.W., Guchhait, R.B., Baum, H., Olson, E.B., Margolis, S.A. and Porter, J.W. (1966) Arch. Biochem. Biophys. 116, 453.

157 Tweto, J. and Larrabee, A.R. (1972) J. Biol. Chem. 247, 4900.

158 Volpe, J.J., Lyles, T.O., Roncari, D.A.K. and Vagelos, P.R. (1973) J. Biol. Chem. 248, 2502.

159 Volpe, J.J. and Vagelos, P.R. (1973) Biochim. Biophys. Acta 326, 293.

160 Chu, L.C., McIntosh, D.J., Hincenbergs, I. and Williams, D. (1969) Biochim. Biophys. Acta 187, 574.

161 Muta, Y. and Gibson, D.M. (1970) Biochem. Biophys. Res. Commun. 28, 9.

162 Flick, P.K., Chen, J. and Vagelos, P.R. (1977) J. Biol. Chem. 252, 4242.

163 Yu, H.L. and Burton, D.N. (1974) Arch. Biochem. Biophys. 161, 297.

164 Gibson, D.M. and Hubbard, D.D. (1960) Biochem. Biophys. Res. Commun. 3, 531.

165 Numa, S., Matsuhashi, M. and Lynen, F. (1961) Biochem. Z. 334, 203.

166 Saggerson, E.D. and Greenbaum, A.L. (1970) Biochem. J. 119, 221.

167 Wieland, O., Neufeld, I., Numa, S. and Lynen, F. (1963) Biochem. Z. 336, 455.

168 Volpe, J.J. and Vagelos, P.R. (1974) Proc. Natl. Acad. Sci. (U.S.A.) 71, 889.

169 Lakshamanan, M.R., Nepokroeff, C.M. and Porter, J.W. (1972) Proc. Natl. Acad. Sci. (U.S.A.) 69, 3516.

170 Volpe, J.J. and Marasa, J.C. (1975) Biochim. Biophys. Acta 380, 454.

171 Goodridge, A.G. (1973) J. Biol. Chem. 248, 1932.

172 Goodridge, A.G. (1973) J. Biol. Chem. 248, 1939.

173 Aprahamian, S., Arslanian, M.J. and Stoops, J.K. (1979) Lipids 14, 1015.

174 Volpe, J.J. and Marasa, J.C. (1976) Biochim. Biophys. Acta 431, 195.

175 Fischer, P.W.F. and Goodridge, A.G. (1978) Arch. Biochem. Biophys. 190 332.

176 Smith, S. and Abraham, S. (1970) Arch. Biochim. Biophys. 136, 112.

177 Volpe, J.J. and Kishimoto, Y. (1972) J. Neurochem. 19, 737.

178 Mellenberger, R.W. and Bauman, D.E. (1974) Biochem. J. 138, 373.

179 Chang, H.C., Seidman, I., Teebor, G. and Lane, M.D. (1967) Biochem. Biophys. Res. Commun. 28, 682.

180 Volpe, J.J. and Marasa, J.C. (1975) Biochim. Biophys. Acta 409, 235.

181 Green, H. and Kehinde, O. (1974) Cell 1, 113.

182 Green, H. and Kehinde, O. (1975) Cell 5, 19.

183 Russell, T.R. and Ho, R.-J. (1976) Proc. Natl. Acad. Sci. (U.S.A.) 73, 4516.

184 Mackall, J.C., Student, A.K., Polakis, S.E. and Lane, M.D. (1976) J. Biol. Chem. 251, 6462.

185 Williams, I.H. and Polakis, S.E. (1977) Biochem. Biophys. Res. Commun. 77, 175.

186 Rubin, C.S., Hirsch, A., Fung, C. and Rosen, O.M. (1978) J. Biol. Chem. 253, 7570.

187 Student, A.K., Hsu, R.Y. and Lane, M.D. (1980) J. Biol. Chem. 255, 4745.

188 Weiss, G.H., Rosen, O.M. and Rubin, C.S. (1980) J. Biol. Chem. 255, 4751.

189 Nepokroeff, C.M., Lau, H.-P. and Porter, J.W. (1979) Int. J. Biochem. 10, 791.

190 Strauss, A.W., Alberts, A.W., Hennessy, S. and Vagelos, P.R. (1975) Proc. Natl. Acad. Sci. (U.S.A.) 72, 4366.

191 Flick, P.K., Chen, J., Alberts, A.W. and Vagelos, P.R. (1978) Proc. Natl. Acad. Sci. (U.S.A.) 75, 730.

192 Lau, H.-P., Nepokroeff, C.M. and Porter, J.W. (1979) Biochem. Biophys. Res. Commun. 89, 264.

193 Adachi, K., Pry, T.A., Nepokroeff, C.M. and Porter, J.W. (1982) Biochim. Biophys. Acta 697, 295.

194 Pry, T.A. and Porter, J.W. (1981) Biochem. Biophys. Res. Commun. 100, 1002.

195 Mattick, J.S., Zehner, Z.E., Calabro, M.A. and Wakil, S.J. (1981) Eur. J. Biochem. 114, 643.

196 Zehner, Z.E., Mattick, J.S., Stuart, R. and Wakil, S.J. (1980) J. Biol. Chem. 255, 9519.

197 Goodridge, A.G., Morris Jr., S.M. and Goldflam, T. (1981) in: J.M. Lowenstein (Ed.), Methods in Enzymology, Vol. 71, Academic Press, New York, p. 139.

198 Morris Jr., S.M., Nilson, J.H., Jenik, R.A., Winberry, L.K., McDevitt, M.A. and Goodridge, A.G. (1982) J. Biol. Chem. 257, 3225.

S. Numa (Ed.) Fatty Acid Metabolism and Its Regulation
© 1984 Elsevier Science Publishers B.V.

CHAPTER 3

Genetics of fatty acid biosynthesis in yeast

ECKHART SCHWEIZER

Institut für Mikrobiologie und Biochemie, Lehrstuhl für Biochemie, Universität Erlangen-Nürnberg, Egerlandstrasse 7, 8520 Erlangen, F.R.G.

1. Introduction

In yeast, as in other eukaryotes, biosynthesis of long-chain fatty acids depends essentially on 4 distinct enzyme systems, i.e. acetyl-CoA carboxylase (ACC), fatty acid synthetase (FAS), desaturase and, in some instances, a malonyl-CoA-independent chain-elongation system. FAS [1] and ACC [2,3] are soluble proteins which have been purified to homogeneity from the yeast cytoplasm. The desaturation [4,5] and elongation systems [6,7], on the other hand, are particulate enzymes associated with the microsomal fraction of the cell. For a long time, both ACC and FAS catalyzing multistep reaction sequences were considered to be classical multienzyme complexes composed of several non-identical and functionally different subunits. Recently, however, this view proved to be wrong when it was demonstrated that in yeast both enzymes were multifunctional proteins combining several different catalytic activities within a single polypeptide chain. Though first indications for this structure came from protein-chemical studies, final proof was obtained from genetic investigations by determining the number of gene loci involved in ACC [8,9] and FAS [10] biosynthesis. For these studies, yeast proved to be an especially well-suited organism: extensive work, especially in Lynen's laboratory, on these two yeast enzymes had characterized them biochemically in extraordinary detail [8,11]. Furthermore, genetic manipulation of yeast is easy and, thus *Saccharomyces cerevisiae* has become the best genetically characterized eukaryote so far [12,13].

The general mechanisms of saturated and unsaturated fatty acid biosynthesis as well as the enzyme systems involved in these processes in many different organisms have been adequately reviewed in the past by other authors [14–23,98]. Therefore, these topics will not be treated systematically in this article. Instead, available data will be presented on the structural organization of catalytic domains on the multifunctional subunits of yeast ACC and FAS. In addition, the functional interplay of different catalytic sites at inter- and intra-molecular levels, the regulation of enzyme activity and the genetic control of their biosynthesis were studied. In this work on multifunctional proteins, genetic methodology proved especially fruitful, providing an experimental approach to questions which could not be answered unequivocally by conventional biochemical or protein-chemical methods.

2. Acetyl-CoA carboxylation

Acetyl-CoA carboxylation (Eqn. 1) represents the first committed step in long-chain fatty acid biosynthesis from acetate.

$$\text{acetyl-CoA} + \text{HCO}_3^- + \text{ATP} \rightarrow \text{malonyl-CoA} + \text{ADP} + \text{P}_i \qquad (1)$$

The overall reaction is composed of 2 distinct partial reactions catalyzed by the biotin carboxylase (Eqn. 2) and transcarboxylase (Eqn. 3) component enzymes.

$$\text{HCO}_3^- + \text{ATP} + \text{biotin enzyme} \rightarrow {}^-\text{O}_2\text{C-biotin enzyme} + \text{ADP} + \text{P}_i \qquad (2)$$

$${}^-\text{O}_2\text{C-biotin enzyme} + \text{acetyl-CoA} \rightarrow \text{malonyl-CoA} + \text{biotin enzyme} \qquad (3)$$

The biotin cofactor is covalently attached to the enzyme protein. Its binding site, the biotin carboxyl carrier protein (BCCP), therefore is the third functional entity of this multicomponent enzyme. A fourth, regulatory, site may be defined in mammalian acetyl-CoA carboxylase. This site is responsible for citrate-induced polymerization and activation of the enzyme [22,24].

Acetyl-CoA carboxylases (ACC), like carboxylases in general, may be attributed to different levels of molecular organization and structural complexity [25]. In most bacteria, the components biotin carboxylase, transcarboxylase and BCCP represent distinct, individual proteins [14,22]. In plant chloroplasts [26–28] and nematodes [29,30], two of them — probably biotin carboxylase and BCCP — are covalently linked to a bifunctional protein. In fungi, higher animals and certain bacterial species, all ACC functions are associated within a single, multifunctional polypeptide chain [8,9,18,31]. Each of the three monofunctional ACC components in bacteria has its own specific quaternary structure. Whether these components are organized, in vivo, into loose aggregates, remains a matter of speculation. The quaternary structure of the bifunctional enzyme is suggested to be $\alpha_2\beta_2$ in chloroplasts [28] and $(\alpha_2\beta_2)_2$ in nematodes [30] and *M. smegmatis* [32]. The trifunctional enzyme of yeast has an α_4 [8] and the tetrafunctional ACC of higher animals an $(\alpha_2)_n$ filamentous [22] structure.

Extensive biochemical studies on yeast ACC have been performed in the laboratories of Lynen and Numa. It was indicated by this work that in 2 different yeast species studied, *Saccharomyces cerevisiae* [8] and *Candida lipolytica* [9], ACC was made up of a single and therefore tri-functional polypeptide chain. Subsequent genetic studies of Roggenkamp et al. [33] and Mishina et al. [34] confirmed these results and provided, in addition, insight into the structural and functional organization of this multi-functional enzyme.

Acetyl-CoA carboxylase-deficient (acc) *Saccharomyces cerevisiae* mutants are obtained, after conventional mutagenesis with UV or ethyl methanesulfonate, with a frequency of 0.5–1×10^{-5}. Enrichment by nystatin treatment [35] in the absence of nutrient fatty acids cannot be achieved with these and other mutants defective in membrane lipid biosynthesis [36]. Acc mutants require appropriately emulsified long-chain (C_{14}–C_{16}) saturated fatty acids for growth. Using odd-chain-length dietary fatty acids it was shown that de novo biosynthesis of even-chain-length fatty acids from acetate is blocked in ACC-deficient yeast cells. On the other hand, fatty acid desaturation and limited elongation of medium-chain-length fatty acids proceed unimpaired [33].

(a) Biotin apocarboxylase ligase mutations

By genetic complementation analysis, Mishina et al. [34] assigned 60 independently isolated *Saccharomyces cerevisiae* acc mutants to 2 unlinked gene loci, acc 1 and acc 2. Both classes of mutants lacked ACC overall activity. 5 out of 57 acc 1 mutants were CRM-negative when challenged with an ACC-specific antiserum, the rest contained enzymatically inactive ACC, the amount and molecular weight of which were essentially the same as in wild-type cells. Biochemical characterization of acc 1 and acc 2 mutants regarding the amount of enzyme-bound biotin, mutational alteration of the two ACC component enzymes and the concomitant inactivation of another yeast carboxylase revealed that only acc 1 mutants represent specific ACC structural gene mutations. ACC 2 mutations, on the other hand, apparently affected a bivalent biotin : apocarboxylase ligase responsible for attaching biotin to 2 different yeast enzymes, acetyl-CoA and pyruvate carboxylase [34]. Consequently, acc 2 mutants contain a biotin-free apo-ACC and are completely defective in ACC overall and both partial activities. At the same time, they also lack pyruvate carboxylase activity. In acc 2 revertants, both carboxylase defects are concomitantly restored, indicating that this double deficiency has not been caused by accidental double mutations. Obviously, the two yeast carboxylases, though being immunologically different, contain structurally similar biotin-binding sites recognizable by the same ligase. This conclusion agrees well with the results of Rylatt and coworkers (see ref. 16) revealing a considerable degree of amino acid sequence homology around enzyme-bound biocytin in several different carboxylases. Furthermore, the immunological resemblance of biotin : apocarboxylase ligases from different sources and their wide substrate specificities as demonstrated by McAllister and Coon [37] lend additional support to this view.

(b) Acetyl-CoA carboxylase mutations

Selected acc 1 mutant acetyl-CoA carboxylases were purified to homogeneity and analyzed for specific ACC component enzyme activities [33,34]. Except for a single mutant (acc 1-167) in which only one partial activity (biotin carboxylase) was specifically inactivated, all other mutants studied were simultaneously affected in both component enzymes, biotin carboxylase and transcarboxylase. As a consequence, ACC overall activity was reduced to 0–8% of the wild-type level (Table 1). More detailed examination of the data contained in Table 1 reveals that in acc 1-4431, acc 1-5083 and acc 1-6463 biotin carboxylase was more seriously affected

TABLE 1

ACC overall and component enzyme activities in purified acc 1-mutant carboxylases

Values indicate percentage of wild-type ACC activities [34].

Strain	Relative enzyme activities (%)		
	Overall acetyl-CoA carboxylase	Biotin carboxylase	Trans-carboxylase
acc 1-4431	4	7	65
acc 1-167	8	3	101
acc 1-5083	1	0	12
acc 1-6463	2	0	12
acc 1-8498	0	0	0
acc 1-2972	4	12	3
acc 1-8785	2	7	1

than transcarboxylase, while in acc 1-2972 and 1-8787 the reverse was true. Thus, the first group of mutants may be considered as biotin carboxylase mutations with concomitantly impaired transcarboxylase activity, while in the latter two mutants a transcarboxylase mutation is accompanied by an additional, partial inactivation of the biotin carboxylase active site. Obviously, both ACC domains have only limited structural autonomy. Thus, a conformational change induced in one of them will usually be conferred on the other. This characteristic is not generally observed in multifunctional proteins. For instance, in yeast fatty acid synthetase (see below, and ref. 38), or in the arom-cluster gene product of *N. crassa* [39,131], protein–protein interactions between heterofunctional domains of the multifunctional polypeptide chain appear to be less pronounced. Therefore, in these systems specific partial enzyme lesions may be induced without obligatory inactivation of other catalytic sites.

(c) Acetyl-CoA carboxylase structure

The results on the genetics of ACC biosynthesis in yeast indicate, in agreement with earlier biochemical findings [8,9] that the ACC apoenzyme is a multifunctional protein, encoded by a single structural gene, acc 1. Conceivably, its constituent active sites represent distinct patches on the surface of the enzyme molecule. This may, or may not, imply that each of them represents an autonomously folded domain containing a contiguous stretch of the polypeptide chain. Apart from conformational interactions, the functional interrelationship between the individual catalytic ACC domains may be visualized in two principally different ways: within the α_4 tetramer, component enzyme interactions may either be restricted to the monomer or two α subunits may cooperate in an α_2 dimeric protomer (Fig. 1). With appropriate acc 1 mutants available, both mechanisms are open to experimental examination.

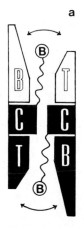 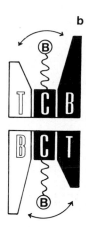

Fig. 1. Hypothetical subunit organization and reaction mechanisms of the ACC α_2 protomer. Arrows indicate intermolecular (a) and intramolecular (b) interaction of catalytic domains. B (open), biotin carboxylase; T, transcarboxylase; C, carboxybiotin carrier protein. White areas indicate mutationally inactivated catalytic domains.

According to the model depicted in Fig. 1, two heterofunctionally defective acc 1 mutants each of them specifically lacking one of the two ACC component enzymes should complement each other if α_2 but not if α were the minimal functional unit in the ACC complex. When Mishina et al. [34] analyzed the various acc 1 mutants available for mutual genetic complementation, it was observed that most heteroallelic diploids contained no functional ACC. This negative complementation is understandable as a result of the biochemical pleiotropy of most acc 1 mutants mentioned above (cf. Table 1). Nevertheless, fatty-acid-independent growth (positive interallelic complementation) was also observed in a number of acc 1 diploids. According to Fig. 2, two acc 1 complementation subgroups (a and b) may be defined in addition to the majority of non-complementing mutants (subgroup c). Subgroups a and b complement each other but not subgroup c. Comparison of biochemical (Table 1) and genetic (Fig. 2) data suggests that subgroup a mutations affected the biotin carboxylase domain while subgroup b comprises transcarboxylase domain mutations. Complementation between subgroups a and b could be explained by the model depicted in Fig. 1b provided the mutant enzymes involved were heterofunctionally defective in only one of the two ACC functions. However, since in most acc 1 mutants both component enzymes are drastically impaired, complementation may rely rather on conformational than on functional interactions between biotin carboxylase and transcarboxylase domains of 2 different α subunits. Therefore restoration of ACC function according to this mechanism cannot be expected for each combination of 2 doubly deficient mutant enzymes. Its occurrence seems to be restricted to acc 1 mutant combinations carrying the primary mutational defect in 2 different catalytic domains. The interallelic complementation patterns then observed were intermediate compared to typical intergenic and intragenic complementation

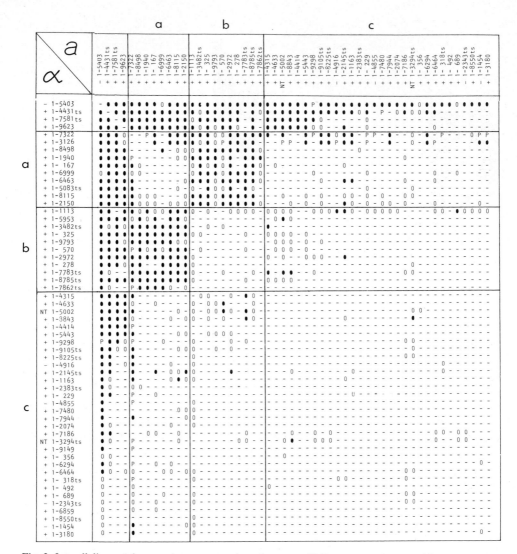

Fig. 2. Interallelic complementation patterns of acc 1 mutants [34]. ts, temperature-sensitive mutants; ●, positive complementation; ○, weak complementation; P, papillae; −, no complementation. + and − symbols preceding the mutant number indicate CRM-positive and -negative character, respectively. NT, not tested.

[40,41]. The double deficiency of acc 1 mutants on one side and heterologous intermolecular interactions between ACC subunits, according to Fig. 1b, on the other may explain these experimental findings. In conclusion, available genetic data suggest that the molecular structure of yeast ACC is $(\alpha_2)_2$. Thus, the catalytic process is likely to consist of intermolecular rather than of intramolecular communi-

cation between biotin carboxylase and transcarboxylase domains. Nevertheless, the conformation of both domains decisively depends on intramolecular protein–protein interactions between them.

3. Saturated fatty acid biosynthesis

(a) Reaction mechanism and FAS enzyme structure

Fatty acid synthetase (FAS) catalyzes, subsequent to acetyl-CoA carboxylation, the biosynthesis of long-chain saturated fatty acids from acetyl-CoA and malonyl-CoA (Eqn. 4).

$$\text{acetyl-CoA} + 7 \text{ malonyl-CoA} + 14 \text{ NADPH} + 14 \text{ H}^+$$

$$\rightarrow \text{palmityl-CoA (palmitate)} + 14 \text{ NADP}^+ + 7 \text{ CO}_2 + 7(8) \text{ CoASH} \qquad (4)$$

This process is one of the basic capacities of living cells. Only very few naturally occurring individuals are known to lack fatty acid synthetase and/or endogenous fatty acid synthesis. In these organisms, straight-chain fatty acids are either replaced, in membrane lipids, by polyisoprenoids, as is observed in Halobacteria [42], or they are exogenously provided by an appropriate host organism. This situation is encountered in certain rumen bacteria [43] or in some parasitic worms [44] and fungi [45].

Depending on the organism, end products of the FAS reaction sequence (Eqn. 4) are either free fatty acids (animals) or their coenzyme A thioesters (bacteria, fungi, etiolated *Euglena gracilis*, see refs. 15 and 11). The overall process is a multistep reaction sequence catalyzed by at least 7 distinct component enzymes [1]. At the start, the priming substrates acetate and malonate are covalently bound to the enzyme. During chain elongation the various reaction intermediates remain covalently linked, as thioesters, to enzyme-bound 4′-phosphopantetheine (acyl carrier protein) [46]. The end products are finally transferred from the enzyme to water and coenzyme A, respectively. Details of the reaction mechanism as well as the characteristics of the various component enzymes involved have been elucidated mainly using the purified yeast [1] and *E. coli* [46] FAS enzymes. The results of these studies, as summarized by Lynen [11], are depicted in Fig. 3.

Fatty acid synthetase has been isolated from a variety of organisms (see ref. 15). Generally, 2 structurally different classes of FAS multienzyme systems are found in nature. Type I fatty acid synthetases constitute high molecular weight ($0.45–2.5 \times 10^6$ dalton) multienzyme complexes. They are found in animals (see ref. 15), fungi [11,47,65] etiolated *Euglena gracilis* [48] and certain bacterial species [18,49]. Type II FAS enzymes on the other hand are represented by a series of distinct and monofunctional enzymes which may, or may not, be organized into loose aggregates, in vivo [50]. These enzymes are found in most bacteria [14] as well as in plant chloroplasts [17].

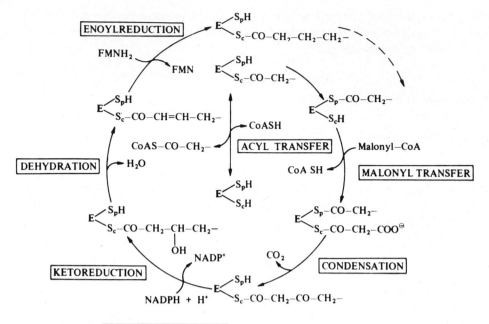

Fig. 3. Reaction sequence catalyzed by yeast FAS [11]. E–S_c, active site of acyl carrier protein; E–S_p, active site of β-ketoacyl synthase. Condensation is synonymous with β-ketoacyl synthesis as used throughout this paper.

As was first demonstrated for yeast FAS the subunit composition of type I FAS complexes is, in spite of their functional complexity, surprisingly simple. By the combination of genetic and biochemical methodology Schweizer et al. [51] proved that yeast FAS contains only 2 non-identical subunits, α and β. Obviously, both subunits are multifunctional proteins of extraordinary functional complexity. This complexity appears to be increased further in animals, etiolated *Euglena gracilis*, *M. smegmatis* and *Corynebacterium diphtheriae* (see refs. 15 and 18) which contain only one type of FAS subunit in an α_n-type ($n = 2$–6) homomultimeric complex.

Biochemically, yeast FAS has been intensively studied by Lynen and coworkers [11]. The enzyme complex was crystallized [52], its component enzymes and the reaction mechanism were characterized in much detail [1]. However, the molecular structure of yeast FAS remained unknown for a long time. Limited proteolytic degradation before, during and even after enzyme purification interfered with the identification and physical characterization of native-size FAS subunits. Only when specific precautions were taken during enzyme purification, i.e. the use of freshly harvested log-phase cells in the presence of a protease inhibitor, were reproducible and stoichiometrically consistent ($\alpha : \beta = 1 : 1$) FAS subunit compositions observed [51,53]. According to Schweizer et al. [51] the molecular weights of α and β are 185 000 and 180 000 dalton, respectively. Probably on the basis of different calibration standards slightly higher values (212 000 and 203 000, respectively) were reported by Stoops et al. [53]. Both subunits may be separated by SDS-polyacrylamide gel electrophoresis. Labeling of enzyme-bound phosphopantetheine [51] with [^{14}C]pantothenic acid as well as alkylation of a specific cysteine residue in the β-ketoacyl synthase active center [54] revealed that both acyl-binding sites are located on subunit α. From the molecular weights of α and β compared with that of the intact complex, the cofactor content of the enzyme (4.5 moles FMN and 5–6 moles pantetheine per mole of enzyme [11]) and the genetic and protein-chemical assignment of FMN and pantetheine to subunits β and α, respectively (see below), it was concluded that yeast FAS has an $\alpha_6 \beta_6$ molecular structure [38].

Studies on the biosynthesis of yeast FAS and on its functional organization at the molecular level have been performed by Schweizer et al. [10,38] using FAS-deficient (fas) *Saccharomyces cerevisiae* mutants. Fas mutants are isolated from ethyl methanesulfonate-treated yeast populations with a frequency of about 5×10^{-4} [55,66]. Selection, growth and supplementation characteristics of fas mutants are identical to those of acc mutants. Genetic complementation studies comprising more than 2000 independently isolated fas mutants revealed the presence of 2 FAS gene loci on the *Saccharomyces cerevisiae* genome. They were designated as fas 1 and fas 2 [56]. Fas 1 has been mapped on chromosome XI [57]. The location of fas 2 which is unlinked to fas 1 still remains to be elucidated.

(b) Biochemical properties of fatty acid synthetase mutants (fas)

Biochemical characterization of selected fas 1 and fas 2 mutants by Schweizer et al. [10] revealed that 3 different FAS functions, i.e. β-ketoacyl synthase, β-ketoacyl reductase and binding of pantetheine (acyl carrier protein function) were associated with fas 2. The remaining 5 FAS activities, i.e. acetyl, malonyl and palmityl transferase, dehydratase and enoyl reductase, were assigned to fas 1. These genetic results were subsequently confirmed, biochemically, by Wieland et al. [58] assaying purified α and β subunits for FAS component activities. As demonstrated by these authors, yeast FAS may be dissociated by reversible acylation with dimethyl maleic anhydride. Subsequently, α and β may be separated on sucrose density gradients. Purified subunit β thus obtained exhibited acetyl and malonyl transferase, dehydratase and enoyl reductase activities. Obviously, these were the same functions as genetically assigned to the gene locus fas 1. Corresponding studies on subunit α were impossible since this component was inactivated when separated from β. In conclusion, it is evident from biochemical as well as genetic data that subunit β of yeast FAS is a pentafunctional peptide while subunit α is trifunctional (Fig. 4).

Biochemically, two distinct and equally large groups of fas mutants may be discriminated [59]. The first group comprises CRM-negative mutants lacking wild-

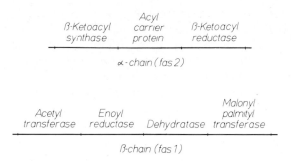

Fig. 4. Allocation of FAS component functions to fas 1 and fas 2. The relative order of domains in each gene is unknown. Thus, the indicated sequence is arbitrary.

type-size FAS protein. FAS overall activity and all partial activities are absent in these mutants. The second, CRM-positive, group produces a mutant FAS complex essentially indistinguishable in size and quantity from that of wild-type cells. In these mutant synthetases usually only one of the FAS component enzymes is specifically inactivated [10]. All other activities remain essentially unaffected no matter whether they are located on the same or on the other FAS subunits. As an exception, acetyl-, malonyl- or palmityl-transferase-deficient fas 1 mutations are often pleiotropic exhibiting double or triple deficiencies in various combinations with each other [10,60]. While acetyl and palmityl transferase defects occur as both specific and as pleiotropic mutations, malonyl transferase is always inactivated together with palmityl transferase. It is concluded from these results that the individual FAS functions represent autonomously folded structural domains of subunits α and β. Obviously, this structural autonomy allows mutational inactivation of most domains without concomitant inactivation of others. On the other hand, occasional loss of two or more acyl transferase activities at the same time suggests that these domains are structurally stabilized by protein–protein interactions between them. Alternatively, strict coupling of malonyl with palmityl transferase inactivation may also be interpreted in terms of partial structural identity of both sites. In this case, both will be affected by the same mutational event.

Active site peptides of acetyl, malonyl and palmityl transferase have been chemically sequenced by Engeser et al. [61] and by Ziegenhorn et al. [62]. In these studies, a homologous sequence of 7 amino acids around the malonyl- and palmityl-binding serine residues of the respective transferases was identified. The amino acid composition of acetyl-binding peptides, however, was different. From these results Engeser et al. [61] proposed overlapping malonyl and palmityl transferase domains around the acyl-binding serine common to both of them. Non-covalent interactions of the malonyl carboxyl group and of the palmitate hydrocarbon chain with appropriately located ionic and hydrophobic centers may be important in controlling the relative rates of chain elongation and termination (see below).

Comparative and more detailed studies on FAS component enzyme activities in a large number of different fas mutants [10] revealed that mutational inactivation of principally any FAS function may be accompanied by allele-specific, positive or negative changes of other FAS activities. These variations, indicating structural interrelationships between both homologous and heterologous FAS subunits are usually only of limited extent. The only pronounced and consistently observed interactions, besides the pleiotropic transferase defects already mentioned, were between enoyl reductase and β-ketoacyl synthase domain on β and α, respectively. Inactivation of enoyl reductase, either by mutation or by removal of FMN [63] enhances β-ketoacyl synthase activity by a factor of 3–8.

The identification of structurally autonomous component enzyme domains on the multifunctional subunits of yeast FAS prompted Lynen and collaborators [11] to fractionate these subunits proteolytically into their constituent active sites. By limited elastase digestion, a 56 000–58 000-dalton fragment was purified which specifically exhibited acetyl transferase activity. The specific activity of this component enzyme was 6 times higher in the fragment than in the intact complex. Other fragments, however, were either enzymatically inactive or they exhibited more than one FAS partial activity. Obviously, the interdomain polypeptide sequences of these functions are not accessible to preferential proteolytic cleavage. Corresponding experiments with mammalian [64] and avian [67] FAS gave similar results. Here, the thioesterase domain was selectively removed from the complex and recovered as a 32 000–35 000-dalton-specific fragment. The question remains open whether the identical behavior of the two different acyl transferases reflects a common evolutionary origin of the respective domains in animal and yeast fatty acid synthetases.

Isolation of individual fas domains is further complicated by the fact that only subunit β but not α retains its native conformation after disintegration of the complex. Isolated subunit α apparently denatures rapidly and refolds into a less compact and slower sedimenting conformation [58]. For this reason, sedimentation of β is faster than that of α in sucrose density gradients although α is larger according to its migration characteristics in SDS-polyacrylamide gels [51]. The stabilization of yeast FAS by subunit association as inferred from these results also became evident in studies on temperature-sensitive fas mutants [68]. Purified ts mutant FAS was fully active when isolated from cells grown at 22°C. Surprisingly, however, it was noted that in vitro the mutant enzyme thus isolated retained its activity even after incubation at non-permissive temperature (35°C) for prolonged periods of time. On the other hand, cells grown at 35°C were fatty acid auxotrophic and contained an inactive FAS complex. This means that the mutated protein is heat labile only before its incorporation into the quaternary structure of the complex. Association obviously stabilizes subunit conformations once adopted at permissive temperature and, thereby, any temperature-induced rearrangement will be prevented.

(c) Interallelic complementation between fas mutants

Interallelic complementation between fas 1 and fas 2 mutants was intensively studied by Schweizer and collaborators [10,38]. About 50% of both types of mutants

70

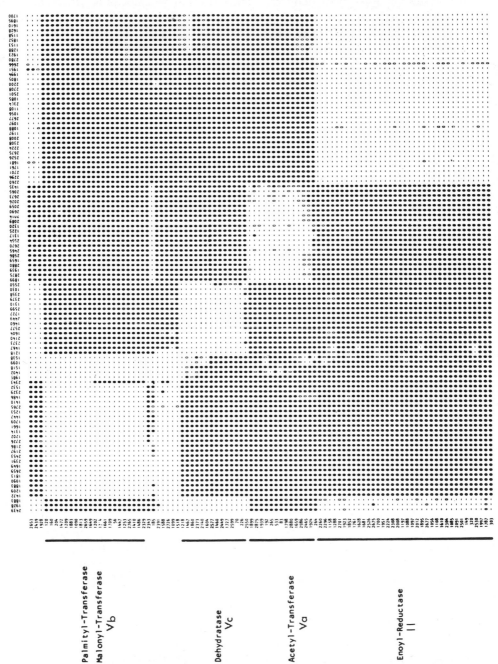

Fig. 5. Interallelic fas 1 complementation patterns. For symbols see Fig. 2. Complementation groups are indicated by roman numbers.

TABLE 2

Fatty acid synthetase overall and component enzyme activities in fas 1 and fas 2 mutants representing different complementation groups [10]

fas mutant	Complementation subgroup	Fatty acid synthetase (%)	Malonyl transferase (%)	Palmityl transferase (%)	Acetyl transferase (%)	β-Ketoacyl synthase (%)	Enzyme bound pantetheine	β-Ketoacyl reductase (%)	Dehydratase (%)	Enoyl reductase (%)
1-246	II	–	205	210	67	350	present	120	500	–
1-1467	Vc	<1	282	198	365	189	present	117	–	77
1-83	Va	2	38	74	–	112	present	100	172	225
1-2329	Vb	<1	125	<1	168	125	present	80	120	34
1-120	Vb	–	–	–	100	–	present	120	100	165
2-15	VI	–	180	100	100	–	present	100	140	100
2-158	VII	–	66	200	40	–	present	25	130	52
2-90	VIII	–	42	220	140	41	present	–	150	220

were strictly non-complementing in heteroallelic crosses. Among the rest, distinct patterns of intragenic complementation were observed. The allelic complementation characteristics of fas 1 mutants, indicating 4 different complementation subgroups are depicted in Fig. 5. According to biochemical studies [10] mutants of the same subgroup have identical component enzyme lesions while different subgroups are characterized by different biochemical defects (Table 2). Corresponding complementation studies performed with fas 2 mutants led to principally the same results [10]. Three interallelic complementation subgroups were defined corresponding to β-ketoacyl synthase, β-ketoacyl reductase and acyl carrier protein deficiencies. Other than fas 1 mutants, however, not only heterofunctionally defective mutants but also a sizeable portion of isofunctionally defective fas 2 mutants complement each other [10].

Available data support the general conclusion that all heterofunctionally defective fas mutants complement each other no matter whether they are allelic or not [10]. On the other hand, complementation between isofunctionally defective fas mutants is only exceptionally observed. This strict correlation between intragenic complementation and functional characteristics of fas mutants suggests that the functional interplay of the α and β domains rather than protein–protein interactions restores enzyme function. As in the case of ACC (cf. Fig. 1) a model may be devised where not the monomers but the dimers α_2 and β_2 are presumed to represent minimal functional entities of yeast FAS. According to this model, dimers of 2 appropriately oriented, heterofunctionally defective subunits contain one double-defective and one wild-type-like subsite combination (Fig. 6). Thus, restoration of FAS activity in diploids of 2 heterofunctionally defective allelic fas mutants should be a predictable characteristic in all appropriate crosses. By this criterion the model is in full agreement with the experimental data. Different lines of experimental evidence led Stoops and Wakil [69–71] to similar conclusions regarding the molecular structure of yeast and animal FAS. They found that the bifunctional thiol reagents 5,5′-dithiobis(2-nitrobenzoic acid) and 1,3-dibromo-2-propanone produced intermolecular and not intramolecular cross-links between enzyme-bound phosphopantetheine

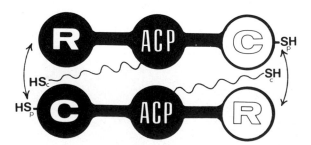

Fig. 6. Intermolecular cooperation of heterofunctional domains in FAS α_2 protomers. R, β-ketoacyl reductase; C, ketoacyl synthase (condensation reaction); ACP, acyl carrier protein; $-SH_p$, active site of β-ketoacyl synthase; $-SH_c$, active site of acyl carrier protein; open circles, mutationally inactivated domains.

and the reactive cysteine of the β-ketoacyl synthase domain. Thus, covalently linked α_2 dimers were produced in agreement with the relative orientation of the two SH groups as schematically depicted in Fig. 6.

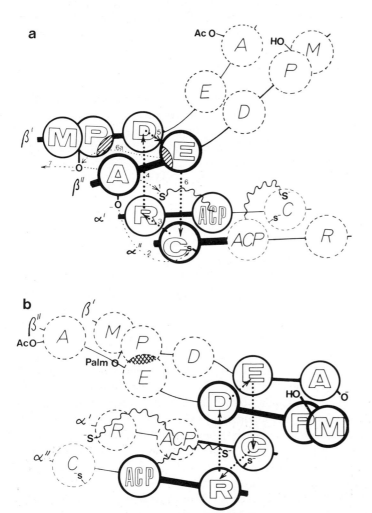

Fig. 7. Model of the intermolecular FAS reaction mechanism in the $\alpha_2\beta_2$ protomer. A, acetyl transferase; E, enoyl reductase; D, dehydratase; P, palmityl transferase; M, malonyl transferase; C, β-ketoacyl synthase; R, β-ketoacyl reductase; ACP, acyl carrier protein. Dotted lines and arrows delineate the route taken by intermediates when sequentially processed on different FAS domains. Numbers indicate the reaction sequence. Catalytically active domains, at a specific moment, are marked by bold lines. Shaded areas on E and P domains potentially interact by hydrophobic attraction in the presence of palmitate (b). On the protomer depicted in (a) fatty acyl chain elongation occurs in one half of the $\alpha_2\beta_2$ protomer. In (b) chain termination is induced by hydrophobic interaction between E-bound palmitate and P. Subsequently, palmitate is transferred to its O-ester binding site on P. Inactivation of the left half of $\alpha_2\beta_2$ simultaneously activates its right half (b).

The model proposed for α_2 interaction in yeast FAS implies that acetyl- and malonyl-binding sites which are located on different but not on the same α subunit cooperate in the β-ketoacyl synthase reaction. Corresponding mechanisms may be operating in the functional interplay of the other FAS component enzymes. Thus, intermolecular rather than intramolecular interactions are presumed for the α domains of β-ketoacyl synthase and β-ketoacyl reductase as well as for the β domains of dehydratase and enoyl reductase. α/β interactions are necessary for acetyl, malonyl and probably also palmityl transacylation. A hypothetical scheme of the reaction steps catalyzed by one of the three protomers $\alpha_2\beta_2$ of yeast FAS is depicted in Fig. 7. In this scheme intermediates of a single reaction cycle are shuffled around between subunits α', α'', β' and β''. Palmitate synthesized at the end of the reaction sequence on the β'' enoyl reductase domain induces, by hydrophobic interaction with palmityl transferase on β', a conformational alteration in β'/β'' (Fig. 7b). Thereby, palmitate transfer to palmityl transferase (reaction 6a) and, consequently, to coenzyme A (reaction 7) are facilitated. At the same time, palmityl transacylation to β-ketoacyl synthase (reaction 6) and its subsequent elongation are blocked. Apart from this local alteration of β'/β'', presumably also the overall orientation of α_2 and β_2 changes relative to each other. By the palmitate-induced β'/β'' interaction the cooperation of α_2 and β_2 may be interrupted at one end of the protomer and, at the same time, initiated at the other (Fig. 7b). Thus, only one set of reactive sites in $\alpha_2\beta_2$ will be active at a specific moment. This assumption takes earlier findings on half-of-the-sites reactivity [88] of yeast FAS into consideration. Interference of reactions 2 and 6 in Fig. 7, i.e. restart of fatty acid synthesis at the expense of chain elongation, is avoided in yeast FAS. This control may be achieved if acetyl transferase reacts with acetyl CoA preferably in that state of β where the surrounding domains are inactive.

As already mentioned, restoration of FAS function is occasionally observed between isofunctionally defective fas 2 mutants. This phenomenon is considered to reflect "classical" interallelic complementation due to protein–protein interactions between homologous subunits of an oligomer [40,41,72]. Both patterns of fas 2 complementation are superimposed on each other. Therefore, the fas 2 complementation map is considerably more complex than that of fas 1. The frequencies and patterns of interallelic complementation between isofunctional fas 2 mutants correspond to those reported for other, monofunctional fungal genes [40]. Since this type of complementation is only observed between fas 2 and not between fas 1 mutants, homologous interactions between α subunits appear to prevail considerably over those between β subunits. The hypothetical model of yeast FAS derived by Wieland et al. [73] from immunological and electron microscopic data essentially agrees with these genetic conclusions. The concentration of subunits in the central part of the molecule may facilitate α/α interactions compared with those between α and β subunits. However, the model may have to be refined to account also for the formation of β_2 functional protomers.

Since association of at least 2 homologous FAS subunits is a prerequisite for interallelic complementation [72] no complementation will be observed either if at least 1 of the 2 subunits is missing or if it has lost the ability to associate with another subunit of its kind. Thus, nonsense and deletion mutants as well as missense mutations causing proteolytic instability of the mutant subunit are expected to be non-complementing in interallelic crosses [59]. In fact, about half of the fas mutants studied by Schweizer et al. [10] exhibit non-complementing characteristics. As expected, all non-complementing fas mutants, so far studied, drastically differ from wild type regarding the amount and protein chemical characteristics of the mutant FAS contained in them. Immunologically, most non-complementing fas mutants are CRM negative when challenged with an antiserum prepared against the native wild-type FAS [59]. In some mutants, a weak and temporary immunological response is observed during early log-phase growth. Probing cell homogenates of non-complementing fas mutants with antisera prepared against SDS denatured purified subunits α and β indicated that either both or only the mutated subunit were missing (B. Schuh, unpublished data). Thus, these mutants apparently contain either incompletely associated FAS complexes or only one of the two FAS subunits. In both cases the FAS protein synthesized is likely to be proteolytically unstable. In early log-phase cultures of some mutants the short-lived intermediates may be identified due to their higher steady-state concentrations under these conditions. As indicated by hybridization of mRNA with specific fas 1 and fas 2 DNA probes, fas 1 and fas 2 transcription rates appear not to be affected in non-complementing mutants (C. Postius, unpublished data). Proteolytic instability of unassociated subunits may be physiologically meaningful even in wild-type cells. It allows the two FAS subunits to be synthesized at proper stoichiometry although fas 1 and fas 2 are unlinked and possibly read at different rates.

(d) In vitro complementation between fas mutant synthetases

Recently, Wieland et al. [58] have shown that yeast FAS may be reversibly dissociated into subunits α and β by acylation with dimethyl maleic anhydride. Upon subsequent deacylation, subunits α and β reassemble to the native-size complex, exhibiting full FAS activity again. This technique was used by Werkmeister et al. [74] for in vitro complementation of appropriate pairs of mutant FAS proteins. These combinations included iso- and heterofunctionally defective enzymes representing allelic as well as non-allelic mutations. The hybrid synthetases thus prepared exhibited full overall FAS activity. Component enzyme activities of the hybrids were usually the average of those measured in the constituting mutant enzymes. As far as this was examined, in vitro and in vivo complementation patterns were identical. When the same dissociation/reassociation protocol was applied to an aged wild-type FAS preparation, a considerable increase of FAS-specific activity was observed in the reconstituted enzyme. Obviously, contaminating denatured subunits were excluded from reassociation and thereby selectively removed from the enzyme complex.

(e) Incorporation of 4'-phosphopantetheine into apo-FAS

Among pantetheine-deficient fas 2 mutants, interallelic complementation has been observed in a few cases, in vivo [75]. In vitro, the corresponding pantetheine-free FAS apoenzymes have been hybridized to a mixed apoenzyme which should be capable of accepting phosphopantetheine. Thereby, it would become activated to holo-FAS. By incubation with coenzyme A in the presence of a partially purified yeast cell extract Werkmeister et al. [76] succeeded in activating the in vitro prepared apoenzymes to holo-FAS of low specific activity. It remains to be studied further whether by these experiments a physiologically significant coenzyme A:apo-FAS phosphopantetheine transferase has been identified. In *E. coli* a corresponding activity was found transferring part of coenzyme A onto the bacterial apo-acyl carrier protein [77]. The apo-FAS of yeast thus prepared in vitro may be useful in further studies on the mechanism of holo-FAS biosynthesis in yeast.

4. Unsaturated fatty acid biosynthesis

In yeast, monounsaturated fatty acids are synthesized by aerobic desaturation of the corresponding saturated fatty acids (Eqn. 5).

$$\text{stearyl-CoA} + NAD(P)H + H^+ + O_2 \rightarrow \text{oleyl-CoA} + NAD(P)^+ + 2\,H_2O \quad (5)$$

No polyunsaturating enzymes have been identified in *Saccharomyces cerevisiae* [78]. As in other eukaryotes the yeast desaturase is a multienzymic mixed function oxidase containing at least 3 different functional components, i.e. NADH cytochrome *b* oxidoreductase (flavoprotein), cytochrome b_5 and the O_2-dependent desaturase proper [5,79,81,89]. Difficulties in purification and stabilization of the microsome-associated enzyme system so far prevented a detailed characterization of its molecular properties and reaction mechanism.

Although biochemical genetic studies on fatty acid desaturation in yeast have not been performed systematically, oleic-acid-requiring (ole) mutants have been known for a long time. They were the first lipid-requiring yeast mutants isolated [82]. Available ole mutants represent 4 different gene loci [83,84], only one of them coding for the acyl-CoA desaturase proper (ole 1) [83]. Stearate desaturation was shown to be absent in ole 1 cells and Δ^9-*cis*-monounsaturated fatty acids of 12–18 carbon atoms chain length may be used as growth supplements. On the other hand, ole 2, 3 and 4 mutants are defective in porphyrin and, consequently, in cytochrome b_5 biosynthesis [84]. These mutants are phenotypically pleiotropic being simultaneously oleate and ergosterol requiring as well as respiratory deficient. For this reason they have also been designated as olerg [85] or as porphyrin (por)-deficient mutations [86]. More detailed biochemical studies, especially on ole 1 mutants and, possibly, the characterization of additional ole loci may provide further insight into function and molecular structure of yeast desaturase.

5. Regulation of fatty acid biosynthesis in yeast

(a) Feedback inhibition of ACC and FAS

In yeast, as in other organisms, biosynthesis of long-chain fatty acids is efficiently blocked by long-chain acyl-CoA derivates [15,22–24,80,87]. The inhibition increases with the length of the acyl chain [87,94] and affects both the specific activities and cellular concentrations of ACC [90,93] and FAS [80,87]. By studies using acyl-CoA synthetase-deficient Candida lipolytica [91] and Saccharomyces cerevisiae [90,92] mutants Numa and coworkers demonstrated that acyl-coenzyme A thioesters rather than free fatty acids were responsible for ACC repression [90,93]. Long-chain acyl-CoA derivatives are known to inhibit, unspecifically, a variety of different enzymes [15,95]. Nevertheless, in contrast to these instances, their effect on ACC and FAS is considered to reflect specific feedback regulation rather than unspecific detergent effects. Both enzymes are inactivated well below the critical micellar concentration [104] of the inhibitor. Though ACC is usually inhibited at lower palmityl-CoA concentrations than FAS, this is not true for all organisms [18,15]. In some instances the palmityl-CoA-binding capacity of ACC is higher than that of all other cellular enzymes studied [101].

At low concentrations palmityl-CoA competitively interferes with malonate binding to yeast FAS [80,97]. Correspondingly, malonyl-CoA counteracts the inhibition of FAS by palmityl-CoA. The identity of malonyl- and palmityl-binding sites on yeast FAS [61] explains this competition. On the other hand, higher concentrations of palmityl-CoA dissociate the yeast FAS enzyme complex [99]. Similar results have been reported for M. smegmatis and pigeon liver FAS [100]. At low palmityl-CoA concentration, animal ACC forms an equimolar enzyme–inhibitor complex which prevents citrate-induced polymerization [96]. At higher molar ratios (palmityl-CoA/enzyme $\geqslant 20$) dissociation of ACC into the monomeric subunits is observed. In overall fatty acid biosynthesis from acetate both ACC or FAS may be rate-limiting, depending on the organism [18]. In yeast the comparatively higher sensitivity of ACC towards palmityl-CoA suggests that this enzyme rather than FAS is rate-limiting [101]. Furthermore, it was demonstrated by Sumper and Träuble that in vitro the rate of fatty acid synthesis from acetyl-CoA using a combination of ACC and FAS may be stimulated by replacing ACC and acetyl-CoA by malonyl-CoA [102].

Due to the inhibition of FAS by long-chain acyl-CoA derivatives the end products of bacterial and yeast FAS have to be relased from the enzyme surface otherwise the synthetic process will come to a standstill [18,102]. In vitro, this type of product inhibition is relieved in the presence of lecithin liposomes, bovine serum albumin or certain polysaccharides. The capacity of these compounds to serve as fatty acyl-CoA acceptors is well established [103]. In vivo, either the same or corresponding lipid-binding substances may have to fulfil this function.

(b) Regulation of enzyme synthesis

Depending on the yeast strain studied, external fatty acids reduce cellular levels of ACC and FAS to varying degrees. According to enzymological and immunological criteria, both enzymes are absent in *Candida lipolytica* [91,87] grown on long-chain fatty acids as a carbon source. In *Saccharomyces cerevisiae* cells which were grown on glucose in the presence of fatty acids, enzyme repression is less drastic [87,90]. Other than Candida, Saccharomyces is unable to use fatty acids as a carbon source. Thus, the different extent of ACC and FAS repression in both yeasts appears to be qualitatively related to their different capacities of growth on exogenous fatty acids. In vitro translation rates of ACC mRNA preparations isolated from Candida after growth in the presence or absence of fatty acids, suggest that repression of this enzyme operates at the transcriptional level [105].

(c) Control of FAS component enzyme activities

Conceivably, cellular levels of ACC and FAS may also be controlled by the equilibrium between the respective apo- and holoenzymes. Limited variations of apo-/holoenzyme ratios have been observed in animal systems depending on nutritional or hormonal conditions [106–108, 113]. However, nothing is known, so far, as to whether apo-/holoenzyme interconversion is a significant control mechanism in yeast fatty acid synthesis. There are a number of control mechanisms specifically observed in animal fatty acid biosynthesis but not in yeast. Among these are certain dietary and hormonal effects [20,107,109], cell differentiation characteristics [111,115], citrate-induced ACC activation [110], cAMP-dependent enzyme phosphorylation [112] and enhancement of medium- [114] or branched-chain [116] fatty acid biosynthesis. On the other hand, there are several other physiological parameters known which influence the activities and product patterns of fatty acid synthetase, quite generally. For instance, FAS product patterns are shifted towards lower-chain-length fatty acids by increased acetyl-CoA vs. malonyl-CoA molar ratios [117]. This shift may be explained by the competition of acetyl-CoA and enzyme-bound intermediates for the active site of β-ketoacyl synthase. Furthermore, free coenzyme A exerts both a stimulating [11,118] and inhibitory effect (E. Schweizer, unpublished data) on FAS, depending on its concentration. At low concentrations, as experimentally produced by a coenzyme A-consuming system, stimulation prevails. This stimulation is observed not only with yeast FAS [11] but also with the animal enzyme which synthesizes free fatty acids rather than acyl-CoA ester as end products. Therefore, the role of coenzyme A as an acceptor for enzyme-bound palmitate in the terminal transacylase reaction cannot be the only explanation of CoA-dependent stimulation of FAS activity. In addition, either allosteric interaction or the temporary formation of so far unidentified acyl-CoA intermediates may have to be presumed [119,120]. At higher concentrations, on the other hand, coenzyme A interferes with acetyl and malonyl enzyme formation and thus reduces FAS overall activity.

Apart from external conditions, the chain length determination of the end products of fatty acid synthesis is an intrinsic property of each FAS. According to the elegant model of Sumper et al. [117] the chain length of intermediates bound to yeast FAS influences, in opposite directions, the turnover rates of β-ketoacyl synthase and fatty acyl transferase. Both component enzymes compete for the saturated acyl-FAS intermediates. Therefore, the probability of enzyme-bound fatty acids being released from the enzyme rather than elongated further will increase with their chain length. Similar variations in the relative activities of other FAS component enzymes during the chain elongation process are unknown, though likely. Among the more than 30 discrete reaction steps catalyzed by yeast FAS when synthesizing palmityl-CoA from acetyl-CoA and malonyl-CoA the rate-limiting step may change in each elongation cycle. Therefore, kinetic data obtained for individual FAS component enzymes by the use of model substrates are only of questionable value for the physiological process.

(d) Control of yeast fatty acid composition

Apart from the rate of fatty acid synthesis the composition of membrane lipids in yeast and other microorganisms is also subject to regulatory processes. This control probably serves to maintain the optimal membrane fluidity at varying external conditions [121]. At different growth temperatures, for instance, homeostasis of membrane fluidity may be achieved by changing the relative amounts of extra-long [18], medium-chain-length, branched [122] or unsaturated fatty acids synthesized. *S. cerevisiae* lipids contain essentially no extra-long, branched or polyunsaturated fatty acids [110,133]. In this organism, the proportion of palmitate vs. stearate increases with increasing temperature [124]. In addition, an inverse relationship between temperature and the extent of fatty acid desaturation is observed [124]. This may be due either to the higher oxygen tension at low temperature or to the known temperature-dependent inactivation of acyl CoA desaturases [89]. In Candida, the induction of a second desaturase activity at low temperature has been reported [125] and probably serves the same effect.

6. Concluding remarks

The study of appropriate mutants may often help in characterizing the specific contribution of an enzyme to a complex metabolic sequence. In animals, 3 different enzyme systems cooperate in the biosynthesis of long-chain saturated fatty acids. Besides the soluble, malonyl-CoA-dependent FAS responsible for de novo fatty acid formation a mitochondrial, malonyl-CoA-independent elongation system and a malonyl-CoA-dependent microsomal fatty acid elongation system have been described [15,126]. In *Saccharomyces cerevisiae,* the isolation of acc and fas mutants together with the use of mitochondria-free rho⁻ mutants clearly demonstrated that (i) there is no malonyl-CoA-independent de novo fatty acid synthesis, (ii) malonyl-

CoA-independent chain elongation is not located in the mitochondria [127], and (iii) malonyl-CoA-dependent chain elongation is irrelevant in yeast, if present at all [127]. So far, no elongation-deficient yeast mutants are available. Chain length modification of FAS reaction products may be necessary under certain physiological conditions such as elevated temperature or high acetyl/malonyl-CoA ratios. Nevertheless, a vital role of this enzyme system in yeast remains to be elucidated.

The multifunctional character of ACC and FAS subunits in yeast is evident from the biochemical and interallelic complementation characteristics of acc and fas mutants. While the ACC subunit structure seems to be similar in yeast and higher animals, the molecular structure of yeast FAS is obviously of intermediate complexity compared to the bacterial type II and animal type I synthetase. Comparison of different type I synthetase structures at the DNA level may reveal homologies reflecting evolutionary and/or functionally indispensable correlations, if there are any. From taxonomic data, the evolution of multifunctional enzymes due to their selective advantage over multienzyme complexes or non-aggregated systems cannot be deduced, generally [11,15,21,128,129]. Furthermore, the catalytic efficiency of multifunctional enzymes when compared to that of multienzyme complexes is probably not superior, either. On the other hand, the kinetics and economy of enzyme biosynthesis are certainly favored by fusing several structural genes into a unique cluster gene. Subunit association will thus be replaced by protein folding and a 1 : 1 stoichiometry of active sites is achieved without elaborate control mechanisms or wasteful overproduction of any component. An appropriate topological organization of component enzymes on the multifunctional protein chain may direct the formation of a functionally most efficient and spatially compact enzyme architecture. Being part of a multifunctional protein, each catalytic domain probably requires less protein mass than an independent enzyme.

From the biochemical and genetic characterization of 2 yeast multienzyme systems, ACC and FAS, it became clear that the individual functional sites in a multifunctional protein may be both autonomous or structurally interdependent domains. In this definition autonomy implies that mutational inactivation of a specific component enzyme does not simultaneously affect others. In spite of the phenotypic differences between acc and fas mutations regarding the pleiotropy of mutational lesions both multienzyme complexes have probably the same basic structure, i.e. they are both oligomers of dimeric protomers. This was inferred from the specific interallelic complementation characteristics of acc 1, fas 1 and fas 2 mutants. Other multifunctional enzymes may be organized similarly. For instance, cross-linking studies of Stoops and Wakil [130] suggest that in animal FAS, like in yeast, the acetyl- and malonyl-binding sites of β-ketoacyl synthase originate from two rather than from the same subunit. In multifunctional enzymes, intramolecular distances between functionally related domains located on the same subunit may be longer than intermolecular ones between two neighboring subunits. Therefore, the oligomeric structure of all known multifunctional enzymes may be intrinsically related to their reaction mechanisms.

References

1 Lynen, F. (1969) Methods Enzymol. 14, 17–39.
2 Sumper, M. (1981) Methods Enzymol. 71, 34–36.
3 Mishina, M., Kamiryo, T. and Numa, S. (1981) Methods Enzymol. 71, 37–43.
4 Bloomfield, D.K. and Bloch, K. (1960) J. Biol. Chem. 235, 337–345.
5 Schultz, J. and Lynen, F. (1971) Eur. J. Biochem. 21, 48–54.
6 Stoops, J.K. and Wakil, S.J. (1981) J. Biol. Chem. 256, 8364–8370.
7 Orme, T.W., McIntyre, J., Lynen, F., Kühn, L. and Schweizer, E. (1972) Eur. J. Biochem. 24, 407–415.
8 Sumper, M. and Riepertinger, C. (1972) Eur. J. Biochem. 29, 237–248.
9 Mishina, M., Kamiryo, T., Tanaka, A., Fukui, S. and Numa, S. (1976) Eur. J. Biochem. 71, 295–300.
10 Schweizer, E., Werkmeister, K. and Jain, K. (1978) Mol. Cell. Biochem. 21, 95–107.
11 Lynen, F. (1980) Eur. J. Biochem. 112, 431–442.
12 Mortimer, R.K. and Hawthorne, D.C. (1966) Annu. Rev. Microbiol. 20, 151–168.
13 Mortimer, R.K. and Schild, D. (1980) Microbiol. Rev. 44, 519–571.
14 Volpe, J.J. and Vagelos, P.R. (1973) Annu. Rev. Biochem. 42, 21–60.
15 Bloch, K. and Vance, D. (1977) Annu. Rev. Biochem. 46, 263–298.
16 Wood, H.G. and Barden, R.E. (1977) Annu. Rev. Biochem. 46, 385–413.
17 Stumpf, R.K. (1977) Int. Rev. Biochem. 14, 215–237.
18 Bloch, K. (1977) Adv. Enzymol. 46, 1–84.
19 Jeffcoat, R. (1979) Essays Biochem. 15, 1–35.
20 Hardie, D.G. (1980) in: P. Cohen (Ed.), Molecular Aspects of Cellular Regulation, Vol. 1, Elsevier, Amsterdam, pp. 33–62.
21 Lynen, F. (1972) in: J. Ganguly and R.M.S. Smellie (Eds.), Current Trends in the Biochemistry of Lipids, Academic Press, New York, pp. 5–26.
22 Laue, M.D., Moss, J. and Polakis, S.E. (1974) Curr. Topics Cell. Regul. 8, 139–195.
23 Vagelos, P.R. (1971) Curr. Topics Cell. Regul. 4, 119–166.
24 Numa, S., Bortz, W.M. and Lynen, F. (1965) Adv. Enzyme Regul. 3, 407–423.
25 Obermayer, M. and Lynen, F. (1976) TIBS 1, 169–171.
26 Nielsen, N.C. (1981) Methods Enzymol. 71, 44–54.
27 Ernst-Fonberg, M.L. and Wolpert, J.S. (1981) Methods Enzymol. 71, 60–72.
28 Egin-Bühler, B., Loyal, R. and Ebel, J. (1980) Arch. Biochem. Biophys. 203, 90–100.
29 Meyer, H. and Meyer, F. (1981) Methods Enzymol. 71, 55–59.
30 Meyer, H., Nevaldine, B. and Meyer, F. (1978) Biochemistry 17, 1822–1827.
31 Tanabe, T., Nakanishi, S., Hashimoto, T., Ogiwara, H., Nikowa, J.I. and Numa, S. (1981) Methods Enzymol. 71, 5–15.
32 Erfle, J.D. (1973) Biochim. Biophys. Acta 316, 143–155.
33 Roggenkamp, R., Numa, S. and Schweizer, E. (1980) Proc. Natl. Acad. Sci. (U.S.A.) 77, 1814–1817.
34 Mishina, M., Roggenkamp, R. and Schweizer, E. (1980) Eur. J. Biochem. 111, 79–87.
35 Snow, R. (1966) Nature (London) 211, 206–207.
36 Henry, S.A. (1973) J. Bacteriol. 116, 1293–1303.
37 McAllister, H.C. and Coon, M.J. (1966) J. Biol. Chem. 241, 2855–2861.
38 Schweizer, E. (1980) in: H. Bisswanger and E. Schmincke-Ott (Eds.), Multifunctional Proteins, Wiley, New York, pp. 197–215.
39 Giles, N.H., Case, M.E., Partridge, C.W.H. and Ahmed, S.I. (1967) Proc. Natl. Acad. Sci. (U.S.A.) 58, 1453–1460.
40 Fincham, J.R.S. (1977) Carlsberg Res. Commun. 42, 421–430.
41 Schlesinger, M.J. and Levinthal, C. (1965) Annu. Rev. Microbiol. 19, 267–284.
42 Oesterhelt, D. (1976) Progr. Mol. Subcell. Biol. 4, 133–166.
43 Hazlewood, G. and Dawson, R.M.C. (1979) J. Gen. Microbiol. 112, 15–27.
44 Meyer, F., Meyer, H. and Bueding, E. (1970) Biochim. Biophys. Acta 210, 257–266.

82

45 Shifrine, M. and Marr, A.G. (1963) J. Gen. Microbiol. 32, 263–270.
46 Vagelos, P.R., Alberts, A.W. and Majerus, P.W. (1969) Methods Enzymol. 14, 39–43.
47 Elovson, J. (1975) J. Bacteriol. 124, 524–533.
48 Goldberg, I. and Bloch, K. (1972) J. Biol. Chem. 247, 7349–7357.
49 Knoche, H.W. and Koths, K.E. (1973) J. Biol. Chem. 248, 3517–3519.
50 Van den Bosch, H., Williamson, J.R. and Vagelos, P.R. (1970) Nature (London) 228, 338–341.
51 Schweizer, E., Kniep, B., Castorph, H. and Holzner, U. (1973) Eur. J. Biochem. 39, 353–362.
52 Oesterhelt, D., Bauer, H. and Lynen, F. (1969) Proc. Natl. Acad. Sci. (U.S.A.) 63, 1377–1382.
53 Stoops, J.K., Awad, E.S., Arslanian, M.J., Gunsberg, S. and Wakil, S.J. (1978) J. Biol. Chem. 253, 4464–4475.
54 Kresze, G.B., Oesterhelt, D., Lynen, F., Castorph, H. and Schweizer, E. (1976) Biochem. Biophys. Res. Commun. 69, 893–899.
55 Schweizer, E. and Bolling, H. (1970) Proc. Natl. Acad. Sci. (U.S.A.) 67, 660–666.
56 Kühn, L., Castorph, H. and Schweizer, E. (1972) Eur. J. Biochem. 24, 492–497.
57 Burkl, G., Castorph, H. and Schweizer, E. (1972) Mol. Gen. Genet. 119, 315–322.
58 Wieland, F., Renner, L., Verfürth, C. and Lynen, F. (1979) Eur. J. Biochem. 94, 189–197.
59 Dietlein, G. and Schweizer, E. (1975) Eur. J. Biochem. 58, 177–184.
60 Knobling, A., Schiffmann, D., Sickinger, H.D. and Schweizer, E. (1975) Eur. J. Biochem. 56, 359–367.
61 Engeser, H., Hübner, K., Straub, J. and Lynen, F. (1979) Eur. J. Biochem. 101, 413–422.
62 Ziegenhorn, J., Niedermeyer, R., Nüssler, C. and Lynen, F. (1972) Eur. J. Biochem. 30, 285–300.
63 Werkmeister, K., Johnston, R.B. and Schweizer, E. (1981) Eur. J. Biochem. 116, 303–309.
64 Smith, S., Agradi, E., Libertini, L. and Dileepan, K.N. (1976) Proc. Natl. Acad. Sci. (U.S.A.) 73, 1184–1188.
65 Packter, N.M. and Alan, A. (1978) Biochem. Soc. Trans. 6, 195–197.
66 Henry, S. and Fogel, S. (1971) Mol. Gen. Genet. 113, 1–19.
67 Rogers, L., Kolattukudy, P.E. and deRenobales, M. (1982) J. Biol. Chem. 257, 880–886.
68 Knobling, A. and Schweizer, E. (1975) Eur. J. Biochem. 59, 415–421.
69 Stoops, J.K. and Wakil, S.J. (1982) Biochem. Biophys. Res. Commun. 104, 1018–1024.
70 Stoops, J.K. and Wakil, S.J. (1981) J. Biol. Chem. 256, 8364–8370.
71 Stoops, J.K. and Wakil, S.J. (1981) J. Biol. Chem. 256, 5128–5133.
72 Crick, F.H.C. and Orgel, L.E. (1964) J. Mol. Biol. 8, 161–165.
73 Wieland, F., Siess, E.A., Renner, L., Verfürth, C. and Lynen, F. (1978) Proc. Natl. Acad. Sci. (U.S.A.) 75, 5792–5796.
74 Werkmeister, K., Johnston, R.B. and Schweizer, E. (1981) Eur. J. Biochem. 116, 303–309.
75 Schweizer, E. (1977) Naturwissenschaften 64, 366–370.
76 Werkmeister, K., Wieland, F. and Schweizer, E. (1980) Biochem. Biophys. Res. Commun. 96, 483–490.
77 Elovson, J. and Vagelos, P.R. (1968) J. Biol. Chem. 243, 3603–3611.
78 Silbert, D.F. (1975) Annu. Rev. Biochem. 44, 315–339.
79 Ohba, M., Sato, R., Yoshida, Y., Bieglmayer, C. and Ruis, H. (1979) Biochim. Biophys. Acta 572, 352–362.
80 Lust, G. and Lynen, F. (1968) Eur. J. Biochem. 7, 68–72.
81 Bloomfield, D.K. and Bloch, K. (1960) J. Biol. Chem. 235, 337–345.
82 Resnick, M.A. and Mortimer, R.K. (1966) J. Bacteriol. 92, 597–600.
83 Keith, A.D., Resnick, M.R. and Haley, A.B. (1969) J. Bacteriol. 98, 415–420.
84 Bard, M., Woods, R.A. and Haslam, J.M. (1974) Biochem. Biophys. Res. Commun. 56, 324–330.
85 Karst, F. and Lacrote, F. (1973) Biochem. Biophys. Res. Commun. 52, 741–747.
86 Plischke, M.E., von Borstel, R.C., Mortimer, R.K. and Cohn, W.E. (1976) in: G.D. Fasman (Ed.), Handbook of Biochemistry and Molecular Biology: Nucleic Acid Section, Vol. 2, CRC Press, Cleveland, OH, pp. 767–832.
87 Meyer, K.H. and Schweizer, E. (1976) Eur. J. Biochem. 65, 317–324.
88 Oesterhelt, D., Bauer, H., Kresze, G.B., Steber, L. and Lynen, F. (1977) Eur. J. Biochem. 79, 173–180.

89 Fulco, A.J. (1974) Annu. Rev. Biochem. 43, 215–241.
90 Kamiryo, T., Parthasarathy, S. and Numa, S. (1976) Proc. Natl. Acad. Sci. (U.S.A.) 73, 386–390.
91 Mishina, M., Kamiryo, T., Tanaka, A., Fukui, S. and Numa, S. (1976) Eur. J. Biochem. 71, 301–308.
92 Kamiryo, T. and Numa, S. (1973) FEBS Lett. 38, 29–32.
93 Kamiryo, T., Nishikawa, Y., Mishina, M., Terao, M. and Numa, S. (1979) Proc. Natl. Acad. Sci. (U.S.A.) 4390–4394.
94 Nikawa, J., Tanabe, T., Ogiwara, H., Shiba, T. and Numa, S. (1979) FEBS Lett. 102, 223–226.
95 Wieland, O., Weiss, L., Eger-Neufeldt, J., Teinzer, A. and Westmann, B. (1965) Klin. Wochenschr. 43, 645–654.
96 Ogiwara, H., Tanabe, T., Nikawa, J. and Numa, S. (1978) Eur. J. Biochem. 89, 33–41.
97 Engeser, H., Hübner, K., Straub, J. and Lynen, F. (1979) Eur. J. Biochem. 101, 407–412.
98 Harwood, J.L. (1979) Progr. Lipid Res. 18, 55–86.
99 Willecke, K. and Lynen, F. (1969) Progr. Biochem. Pharmacol. 5, 91–98.
100 Dorsey, J.A. and Porter, J.W. (1968) J. Biol. Chemie 243, 3512–3516.
101 Sumper, M. (1974) Eur. J. Biochem. 49, 469–475.
102 Sumper, M. and Träuble, H. (1973) FEBS Lett. 30, 29–34.
103 Tanford, C. (1980) in: The Hydrophobic Effect: Formation of Micelles and Biological Membranes, Wiley, New York, pp. 155–157.
104 Zahler, W.L., Barden, R.E. and Cleland, W.W. (1968) Biochim. Biophys. Acta 164, 1–11.
105 Horikawa, S., Kamiryo, T., Nakarishi, S. and Numa, S. (1980) Eur. J. Biochem. 104, 191–198.
106 Stoops, J.K., Arslanian, M.J., Aune, K.C. and Wakil, S.J. (1978) Arch. Biochem. Biophys. 188, 348–359.
107 Mason, J.V. and Donaldson, W.E. (1972) J. Nutr. 102, 667–672.
108 Das, D.K. (1980) Arch. Biochem. Biophys. 203, 25–36.
109 Lane, M.D. and Mooney, R.A. (1981) Curr. Top. Cell. Regul. 18, 221–242.
110 Welch, J.W. and Burlingame, A.L. (1973) J. Bacteriol. 115, 464–466.
111 Ahmad, P.M., Russell, T.R. and Ahmad, F. (1979) Biochem. J. 182, 509–514.
112 Qureshi, A.A., Jenik, R.A., Kim, M., Lornitzo, F.A. and Porter, J.W. (1975) Biochem. Biophys. Res. Commun. 66, 344–351.
113 Vagelos, P.R. (1974) Biochem. Lipids 4, 99–140.
114 Grunnet, J. and Knudsen, J. (1979) Eur. J. Biochem. 95, 497–502.
115 Student, A.K., Hsu, R.Y. and Lane, M.D. (1980) J. Biol. Chem. 255, 4745–4750.
116 Kim, Y.S. and Kolattukudy, P.E. (1978) Arch. Biochem. Biophys. 190, 585–597.
117 Sumper, M., Oesterhelt, D., Riepertinger, C. and Lynen, F. (1969) Eur. J. Biochem. 10, 377–387.
118 Linn, T.C. and Srere, P.A. (1980) J. Biol. Chem. 255, 10676–10680.
119 Poulose, A.J. and Kolattukudy, P.E. (1982) Int. J. Biochem. 14, 445–448.
120 Stern, A., Sedgwick, B. and Smith, S. (1982) J. Biol. Chem. 257, 799–803.
121 McElhaney, R.N. (1976) in: M.R. Heinrich (Ed.), Extreme Environments: Mechanisms of Microbial Adaption, Academic Press, New York, pp. 255–281.
122 Kaneda, T. (1977) Bacteriol. Rev. 41, 391–418.
123 Nurminen, T., Kouttinen, K. and Suomalainen, H. (1975) Chem. Phys. Lipids 14, 15–32.
124 Okuyama, H., Saito, M., Joshi, V.C., Gunsberg, S. and Wakil, S.J. (1979) J. Biol. Chem. 254, 12281–12284.
125 Kates, M. and Paradis, M. (1973) Can. J. Biochem. 51, 184–197.
126 Murad, S. and Kishimoto, Y. (1978) Arch. Biochem. Biophys. 185, 300–306.
127 Schweizer, E., Meyer, K.H., Schweizer, M. and Fischer, W. (1978) in: R. Diels and J. Knudsen (Eds.), Regulation of Fatty Acid and Glycerolipid Metabolism, FEBS Proc., Vol. 46, Pergamon Press, Oxford, pp. 11–19.
128 Kirschner, K. and Bisswanger, H. (1976) Annu. Rev. Biochem. 45, 143–166.
129 Stark, G. (1977) TIBS 2, 64–66.
130 Stoops, J.K. and Wakil, S.J. (1981) J. Biol. Chem. 256, 5128–5133.
131 Gaertner, F.H. and Cole, K.W. (1977) Biochem. Biophys. Res. Commun. 75, 259–264.

S. Numa (Ed.) Fatty Acid Metabolism and Its Regulation
© *1984 Elsevier Science Publishers B.V.*

CHAPTER 4

The regulation of desaturation and elongation of fatty acids in mammals

R. JEFFCOAT and A.T. JAMES

Biosciences Division, Unilever Research, Colworth House, Sharnbrook, Bedford MK44 1LQ, Great Britain

This chapter will discuss the control of desaturases and elongases as influenced by dietary and hormonal changes and will thus complement and up-date previous reviews on this subject [1–3]. In particular it will focus on the control of these enzymes in terms of the overall control of lipid synthesis with special emphasis on those conditions prevailing in the liver. References to other desaturase systems will be made for comparison only. Although it is well recognized that cytoplasmic enzymes, notably acetyl-CoA carboxylase and fatty acid synthetase play key roles in controlling the synthesis of fatty acids in the liver, relatively little attention has been given to those enzymes responsible for the further elongation and desaturation of de novo synthesised fatty acids. Particular attention will be made to the influence of dietary carbohydrate and fat on the activity of the desaturases and the effect this has on the amount and type of triacylglycerol secreted by the liver.

1. Introduction

The success of any living system depends upon its ability to adapt to its environment, i.e. to be able to use the available raw materials to synthesise those components which are essential to life. In times of plenty, excess available raw materials can be stored in animals as glycogen or as lipid in the form of tri-acylglycerols. Since fatty acids are also required for phospholipid biosynthesis, the essential lipids of cellular membranes, a balance has to be maintained between (a) the storage of fatty acids as triacylglycerols and (b) the synthesis of phospholipids as essential membrane components. Furthermore the fatty acids required for these lipids can be derived either from a dietary source or from de novo synthesis. (Table 1 gives a list of the more common fatty acids with their trivial names and double-bond positions.) In general saturated and monounsaturated fatty acids can be derived from either source but polyunsaturated fatty acids (i.e. those with two or more double bonds) can only be derived from dietary linoleic or α-linolenic acids which in turn have been derived directly or indirectly from a plant source. Since these fatty acids cannot be synthesised by animal tissue they are often referred to as essential fatty acids. Chronic deficiencies of these fatty acids from the diet lead, in experimental animals, to the classic symptoms first described by Burr and Burr [4] of decreased growth rate, development of scaly paws, skin and tail, and fatty liver.

The biosynthesis of fatty acids may therefore be considered as a complex series of integrated reactions in which substrates compete for available enzymes which in turn are controlled by many factors. (The key enzymes concerned with the de novo synthesis of fatty acids, i.e. the conversion of acetate to fatty acids are acetyl-CoA carboxylase (EC 6.4.1.2) and fatty acid synthetase and will not be considered further as they have been described in full detail in Chapters 1 and 2.) The metabolic fate of either dietary or de novo synthesised fatty acids will therefore depend upon the balance of a series of enzymic reactions as follows: chain elongation, retroconversion, desaturation, incorporation into complex lipid and β-oxidation. The product of each of the above reactions then becomes a potential substrate for one of the other pathways shown in Fig. 1. The preferred route of any particular fatty acid will thus depend not only upon the structure of the fatty acid in relation to the specificity of each of the participating enzymes, but also on dietary factors which are capable of influencing metabolism by: (a) influencing the level of specific enzymes by increasing/decreasing the rate of breakdown/synthesis of enzyme protein; (b) controlling enzyme activities by end-product inhibition; (c) influencing fatty acid pool sizes and composition and thus affecting reactions competing for common enzymes, e.g. the competition of oleate and linoleate for the Δ^6-desaturase giving rise to 6,9-18:2 and

TABLE 1

Shorthand notation

The number immediately before the colon (:) refers to the number of carbon atoms in the fatty acid chain, while the number after the colon refers to the number of double bonds; thus 16:1 indicates a fatty acid of 16 carbon atoms with 1 double bond. The letter c indicates that the double bond is in the *cis* configuration, and the number before the letter c refers to the position of that double bond; thus 9c indicates a *cis* double bond between carbons 9 and 10.

Trivial name	Shorthand notation	Systematic name
Palmitate	16:0	*n*-Hexadecanoic acid
Palmitoleate	9c-16:1	*cis*-9-Hexadecanoic acid
	17:0	*n*-Heptadecanoic acid
Stearate	18:0	*n*-Octadecanoic acid
Oleate	9c-18:1	*cis*-9-Octadecanoic acid
cis-Vaccenate	11c-18:1	*cis*-11-Octadecanoic acid
Linoleate	6c,9c-18:2	*cis,cis*-6,9-Octadecadienoic acid
	9c,12c-18:2	*cis,cis*-9,12-Octadecadienoic acid
γ-Linolenate	6c,9c,12c-18:3	*all-cis*-6,9,12-Octadecatrienoic acid
α-Linolenate	9c,12c,15c-18:3	*all-cis*-9,12,15-Octadecatrienoic acid
Arachidonate	5c,8c,11c,14c-20:4	*all-cis*-5,8,11,14-Eicosatetraenoic acid

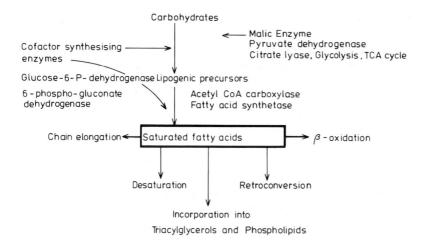

Fig. 1. Synthesis and metabolic fate of fatty acids.

6,9,12-18 : 3 respectively; (d) changing hormone levels/sensitivity.

An example of the effects of enzyme specificity and rates of reaction is shown in Fig. 2 describing the metabolism of palmitic acid, the preferred end-product of fatty acid synthetase. Potentially each substrate competes for desaturation, elongation or transfer into triacylglycerol, where it is effectively removed from further modification. However, Bernert and Sprecher [5] have demonstrated that the rates of elongation are considerably greater than those of desaturation. Furthermore Jeffcoat et al. [6] have confirmed the earlier observations of Gurr et al. [7] that the preferred chain length of the substrate for the Δ^9-desaturation is stearoyl-CoA. A consequence of this is that the major fatty acids found in de novo synthesised lipids are stearic acid, oleic acid and palmitic acid.

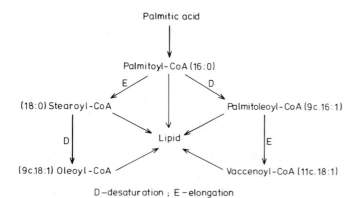

Fig. 2. Metabolic fate of palmitic acid. Taken from Jeffcoat, R. (1979) Essays in Biochemistry, Vol. 15, Academic Press, London, pp. 1–36.

Although the chemical composition of fatty acids has been known for a very long time, the biochemical synthesis of saturated fatty acids has only been recently described by Lynen [8]. However, of equal intrigue to the biochemist and nutritionist has been the question of interconversion of fatty acids and in particular the detailed mechanism of enzymic desaturation.

2. The biochemistry of desaturation

(a) Characterisation of the enzyme

Although recent studies have been focussed on mammalian liver, early studies were carried out by Nagai and Bloch [9]. Using *Euglena gracilis* they were able to show that extracts of this organism could convert stearic acid into oleic acid by a reaction that required both reduced pyridine nucleotide and molecular oxygen. The subsequent fractionation of these extracts resulted in the first evidence that the desaturase was not a single enzyme but was composed of at least 3 individual proteins: an NADPH oxidase, a non-haem iron sulphur protein, ferredoxin and the desaturase. The very unstable nature of the latter protein $t_{1/2}$ 10 h prevented further detailed studies but nonetheless laid the foundation for the biochemical understanding of mammalian oxidative desaturation. Furthermore it identified a separate mechanism of desaturation to that described for anaerobic desaturation by microorganisms. The major difference here is that under anaerobic conditions, bacteria do not desaturate the preformed fatty acids but rather introduce the *cis* double bond during the synthesis of the fatty acid [10] in the following way:

3–*cis* double bond   2–*trans* double bond

(b) Characterisation of the substrate

After the early studies of Nagai and Bloch [9], work on the oxidative desaturation was focussed on mammalian systems and it was soon established that the true substrates for these reactions were not the free fatty acids but the coenzyme-A esters. Further studies by Raju and Reiser [11] demonstrated that incorporation of saturated fatty acids into triacylglycerols prevented the desaturation and indeed established that the true substrates for mammalian desaturases were the coenzyme-A esters. This has been confirmed several times since [6,12,13] and the only exception is the

---

* The key enzyme involved in this isomerisation is 3-hydroxydecanoyl thiolester dehydrase.

observation of Pugh and Kates [14]. They have demonstrated that the Δ^5-desaturase of rat liver (see later) can act both on the coenzyme-A or phospholipid form of eicosatrienoic acid (8c,11c,14c-20:3) to form arachidonic acid (5c,8c,11c,14c-20:4). This is the only example of a complex lipid acting as a substrate for oxidative desaturation apart from those described for polyenoic acid biosynthesis in plants. In lower plants the conversion of oleic acid (9c-18:1) to linoleic acid (9c,12c-18:2) as its phosphatidyl choline derivative was first reported in *Chlorella vulgaris*. Similar conversions have also been reported for higher plants by Stymme and Appelquist [15], Slack et al. [16] and Murphy and Stumpf [17].

3. The enzymology of desaturation

(a) Mechanism of enzyme activity

Desaturation of preformed fatty acids serves two major functions related to their physiological role [18]: (1) the desaturation of saturated fatty acids catalysed by the Δ^9-desaturase to form monounsaturated fatty acids with sufficiently reduced melting points to allow them to be further metabolised and transported via the blood stream [3] and (2) the desaturation of unsaturated fatty acids to form polyunsaturated fatty acids derived from oleic, linoleic and α-linolenic acids to provide suitable precursors of phospholipids to maintain the physiological state of membranes (Fig. 3). Those

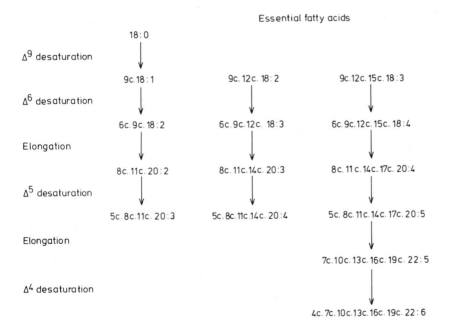

Fig. 3. Unsaturated fatty acid biosynthesis.

fatty acids derived from linoleic and α-linolenic acid also provide the precursors of prostaglandin, prostacyclin, thromboxone and leucotriene biosynthesis [19].

Initial studies were focussed on the Δ^9-desaturase and were pioneered by the work of James and his colleagues [1] who set out to establish the detailed substrate specificity in relation to the enzyme-active centre and to understand the mechanism by which the enzyme selectively removes 2 hydrogens from the saturated methylene chain of stearic acid to produce cis Δ^9-octadecanoic acid (oleic acid) [20]. Those experiments fall into 3 groups: (1) Studies designed to determine which 2 of the possible 4 hydrogens were removed during desaturation. It was demonstrated using deuterium-labelled stearic acid that only the D-hydrogens were removed from carbon atoms 9 and 10 and in a concerted reaction. It was, therefore, suggested that as a result of the substrate interacting with the enzyme, the linear steroyl-CoA was twisted about carbon atoms 9–10 to take on a "pseudo-oleic acid" conformation with the D-hydrogens on the same side of the molecule.

H▷ C9 ◁H⦁   H▷ C ◁H⦁   H∖   ∕
                                         C
⦁H∼ C10 ∼H   H▷ C ◁H⦁   ‖
                                         C
                                       ∕   ∖
                                     H

This appears to be a common feature of desaturation as it has also been shown to be true for the synthesis of linoleic acid by *Chlorella vulgaris* [20]. (2) Further studies in which monosubstituted methyl derivatives of C-10 to C-18 fatty acid were tested as substrates for the Δ^9-desaturase, indicated that the stearoyl-CoA fitted into a narrow cleft in the enzyme since those molecules which had been substituted in carbons 5–15 failed to be a substrate [21]. Similar results have been obtained by Do and Sprecher [22] for the Δ^5-desaturase. (3) Furthermore, when the enzyme was incubated with a range of substrates from C-10 to C-19 saturated fatty acids, the product was always a *cis*-Δ^9-monounsaturated fatty acid indicating that in the case of the Δ^9-desaturase the position of the double bond is always determined relative to the carboxyl group. Attempts to further elucidate the mechanism of desaturation was focussed on the purification of the enzyme — most of the work being carried out using rat-liver or hen-liver, microsomal preparations.

(b) Fractionation of the Δ^9-desaturase complex

Due to the early work of Bloch (see [23] for a review) it was demonstrated that the true substrates for the enzymes were coenzyme-A esters and that the enzyme itself was bound to the microsomal membranes. Once this latter point had been established the question was asked, 'What is the function of the membrane lipid?' Jones et al. [24] removed the microsomal lipid by solvent extraction and with it the enzyme activity — the latter was restored only after the total lipid fraction had been added back. Safford et al. [25] attempted to answer the question by a different approach. Lyophilised hen-liver microsomes were extracted with a range of water in acetone

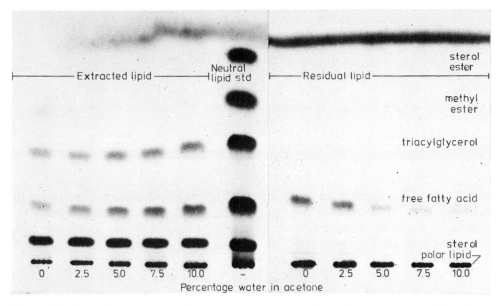

Fig. 4. Thin-layer chromatography of acetone/water extracts of hen-liver microsomes. Taken from Safford, R., Jeffcoat, R. and James, A.T. (1975) Biochim. Biophys. Acta 409, 86–96.

solutions (maximum 10% (v/v) water in acetone). The results shown in Fig. 4 indicated that all the neutral lipid and 44% of the phospholipid could be removed without significant loss of enzyme activity and therefore contrary to earlier observations, only phospholipid was required for enzyme activity. This was supported by the latter work of Strittmatter et al. [12] and Prasad and Joshi [13].

Attempts to purify the protein were made either by "solubilisation" in high salt or by using surface active reagents such as sodium deoxycholate and/or Triton X-100. Gurr and Robinson [26] using hen-liver microsomes 'solubilised' the desaturase in 1 M potassium phosphate buffer pH 8.0 followed by partial purification on Sepharose 6B.

Undoubtedly the most significant initial breakthrough in our understanding of the desaturase enzyme came from the initial studies of Holloway [27] working with hen-liver microsomes and Shimakata et al. [28] working with rat-liver microsomes. Their approach had been to totally solubilise the microsomal protein in detergent followed by traditional protein chemical methods. Shimakata et al. [28] used a mixture of 1% (w/v) sodium deoxycholate and 1% (v/v) Triton X-100 followed by ammonium sulphate fractionation and chromatography on DEAE-cellulose. Although this method resulted in considerable loss of enzyme activity, they did succeed in demonstrating at the same time as Holloway, that the mammalian desaturase is composed of 3 proteins, NADH-cytochrome b_5 reductase (EC 1.6.2.2), cytochrome b_5 and the desaturase protein which was shown to be the cyanide-sensitive component of the desaturase complex. It was thus demonstrated that the desaturation of stearoyl CoA was catalysed by a complex of 3 proteins, two of which constituted a mini-electron transport chain shown below:

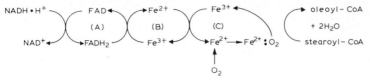

(A) NADH–cytochrome b_5 reductase
(B) cytochrome b_5
(C) desaturase

The actual arrangement of the 3 proteins and their orientation with respect to each other in the membrane has largely been studied by Strittmatter and his colleagues. From the detailed protein chemistry carried out by this group it is now clear that both NADH–cytochrome b_5 reductase and cytochrome b_5 consist of 2 domains — a globular hydrophilic region exposed to the cytoplasm and anchored to the microsomal membrane via a hydrophobic tail (see diagrammatic representation in Fig. 5). Purification of these proteins using detergent-isolation methods [28–30] resulted in protein which readily aggregated when the detergent was removed and which showed a higher molecular weight when compared with protein solubilised by controlled digestion of the membranes with trypsin. Furthermore Rogers and Strittmatter [31] demonstrated that the removal of the lipid fraction from rabbit-liver microsomes by treatment with sodium deoxycholate in conjunction with gel filtration on Bio-gel P.30 followed by gel filtration on Sephadex G25 to remove the detergent resulted in loss of NADH–cytochrome b_5 reductase activity but had little effect on the activity when an artificial electron acceptor (potassium ferricyanide) was used. When the sonicated isolated lipid fraction was added back to the lipid-depleted microsomes, full activity was restored. From these results it was clear that removal of the lipid did not affect the enzyme activity since the enzyme was still capable of reducing potassium ferricyanide. The most likely function of the lipid is therefore to act as a medium to anchor the proteins in the correct orientation with respect to each other, since in its absence, the proteins clump together.

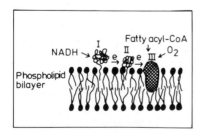

Fig. 5. Schematic representation of desaturase complex. I, NADH-cytochrome b_5 reductase; II, cytochrome b_5; III, stearoyl-CoA desaturase. Taken from Jeffcoat, R. (1979) Essays in Biochemistry, Vol. 15, Academic Press, London, pp. 1–36.

Similarly the desaturase is also embedded in the membrane but since it is not removed by low concentrations of detergent (sodium deoxycholate and Nonidet P-40) which solubilise the electron-transport proteins, it would appear to have a greater affinity for the membrane lipids. Further support for this hypothesis came from a more detailed analysis of the purified protein which was achieved in the following way. Jeffcoat et al. [6] adopted an approach of solubilising the desaturase protein from the microsomal membrane using increasing concentrations of the non-ionic detergent Nonidet P-40. Strittmatter et al. [12] adopted a similar approach using sodium deoxycholate followed by Triton X-100 and polyethylene glycol and produced the first homogeneous preparation of a desaturase. Comparisons of the amino acid composition of the hydrophilic and hydrophobic domains of cytochrome b_5 and detergent-isolated desaturase indicated to Jeffcoat et al. [6] that the hydrophobicity of the desaturase, as determined by the rules of Capaldi and Vanderkooi [32], was very similar to that of the hydrophobic tail of the cytochrome b_5 molecule. However, since the active centre of the desaturase must be accessible to electrons from cytochrome b_5 which is exposed to the cytoplasm, it follows that most of the desaturase is located in the membrane with only a small part exposed to the cytoplasm [6].

The Δ^9-desaturase has now been purified to homogeneity from hen-liver microsomes by Prasad and Joshi [13] and has been shown to have similar properties to that described by others for the rat-liver enzyme. Thus at least within the animal/avian kingdom the Δ^9-desaturase appears to have similar properties. However such generalities cannot be extended to other living systems since McKeon and Stumpf [33] have shown for sunflower that the Δ^9-desaturase is absolutely specific with respect to chain length and the form of the ester. The enzyme is cytoplasmic and acts only on stearoyl-acyl carrier protein. In bacterial systems the oxidative desaturation occurs via the coenzyme-A derivative, while in yeast the ACP derivative is the preferred substrate.

4. The physiological role of Δ^6- and Δ^5-desaturases

(a) The enzymology of Δ^6- and Δ^5-desaturases

In contrast to the Δ^9-desaturase, the Δ^6- and Δ^5-desaturases (and maybe the Δ^4-desaturase) are solely responsible for the conversion of essential polyunsaturated fatty acids into fatty acids as components of membrane phospholipids or precursors of prostaglandins. Thus the types of reaction they catalyse may be summarised as follows:

$$18:2 \xrightarrow{\Delta^6} 18:3 \xrightarrow{E} 20:3 \xrightarrow{\Delta^5} 20:4$$

| 9c,12c | 6c,9c,12c | 8c,11c,14c | 5c,8c,11c,14c |
| Linoleic acid | γ-Linolenic acid | Eicosatrienoic acid | Arachidonic acid |

$$18:3 \quad \overset{\Delta^6}{\to} \quad 18:4 \quad \overset{E}{\to} \quad 20:4 \quad \overset{\Delta^5}{\to} \quad 20:5$$

9c,12c,15c	6c,9c,12c,15c	8c,11c,14c,17c	5c,8c,11c,14c,17c
α-Linolenic			
acid			

In some species, notably the cat, the Δ^6-desaturase is absent [34,35] and the nutritional implications of this has been discussed by Hassam et al. [35].

The Δ^6-desaturase acting on linoleic acid and α-linolenic acid are one and the same enzyme although Brenner and Peluffo [36] have shown that the preferred substrate is the trienoic acid 9c,12c,15c-18:3. Thus where both acids are ingested there is competition for the two substrates — however in the Western diet the dominant pathway will be the linoleic acid one while in those populations, e.g. Eskimos, eating a predominantly fish oil diet, the α-linolenic acid pathway will dominate. Under those circumstances where neither fatty acid is present (i.e. EFA deficiency) then the substrates for the Δ^6- and Δ^5-desaturases are as follows:

$$18:0 \quad \underset{\Delta^9}{\to} \quad 18:1 \quad \overset{\Delta^6}{\to} \quad 18:2 \quad \overset{E}{\to} \quad 20:2 \quad \overset{\Delta^5}{\to} \quad 20:3$$

	9c	6c,9c	8c,11c	5c,8c,11c
Stearic	Oleic			
acid	acid			

In this case an unusual eicosatrienoic acid (5c,8c,11c-20:3) which is different to the one produced by the Δ^6-desaturase acting on linoleic acid (8c,11c,14c-20:3) is formed. Normally this triene is not produced since linoleic acid is the preferred substrate over oleic acid. However under conditions of essential fatty acid deficiency the unusual triene accumulates and the ratio of 20:4/20:3 in the blood (and in particular the red blood cell membrane) is used as a clinical diagnostic tool of essential fatty acid deficiency.

(b) The biochemistry of Δ^6- and Δ^5-desaturases

The role of the desaturases falls very clearly into 2 categories — the Δ^9-desaturase as has been described is primarily responsible for the conversion of saturated fatty acids into monounsaturated fatty acids which thus facilitates their transport as very-low-density lipoproteins via the blood stream to the adipose tissue to act as a carbon and energy store. The Δ^6- and Δ^5-desaturases act primarily on unsaturated fatty acids (although exceptions have been reported; Cook and Spence [37]) and in conjunction with elongases (see later) give rise to the parent fatty acids in prostaglandin biosynthesis and also the polyunsaturated fatty acids found in membrane phospholipids. In spite of the important role of these lipids the characterisation of the Δ^6-desaturase has lagged far behind that of the Δ^9-desaturase and as yet nothing is known about the Δ^5-desaturase protein complex.

Once it had been established that the Δ^9-desaturase required cytochrome b_5 as an electron donor, similar investigations were focussed upon the Δ^6-desaturase. Evidence for such an involvement came from the work of Lee et al. [38] and Okayasu et al. [39] who used an immunochemical approach. They were able to demonstrate that rat-liver microsomes lost their capacity to desaturate either linoleic acid or oleoyl-CoA when incubated with rabbit anti-cytochrome b_5 IgG. Incubation of the microsomes with IgG from non-immunised rabbits had no effect. These observations clearly indicated that although it had been established that the Δ^9- and Δ^6-desaturases were separate and distinct proteins they did share a common electron-transport protein.

The exact nature of the cytochrome b_5 interaction with the desaturases is not really known. Is the cytochrome b_5 free to move about in the lipid bi-layer of the microsomal membrane making only transitory interactions with the cytochrome b_5 reductase and Δ^6-desaturase/Δ^9-desaturase or does each desaturase exist as a complex bound to its own electron-transport proteins? Some evidence for the close affinity of cytochrome b_5 and the Δ^6-desaturase protein came from the studies of Okayasu et al. [40] who used an affinity approach to purify rat-liver microsomal Δ^6-desaturase. Rat-liver microsomes were solubilised in 2% (w/v) Triton X-100 and the Δ^6-desaturase partially purified using DEAE-cellulose and CM-Sephadex. The final purification was achieved using affinity chromatography on a cytochrome b_5–Sepharose column which yielded a homogeneous non-haem iron-containing protein of molecular weight 60 000 as judged by SDS-polyacrylamide gel electrophoresis. The reconstituted Δ^6-desaturase activity could be achieved only by the addition of cytochrome b_5, NADH–cytochrome b_5 reductase, the Δ^6-desaturase

```
NADH ──▶ cytochrome b₅                                      linoleoyl – CoA
          reductase                                          (        + O₂
                      ╲▶ cytochrome b₅ ──▶ Δ⁶ – desaturase  (
NADPH ──▶ cytochrome P-450                                   linolenyl – CoA
          reductase
```

(Okayasu, T., Nagao, M., Ishibashi, T. and Imai, Y. (1981) Arch. Biochem. Biophys. 206, 21–28)

TABLE 2

Comparison of Δ^9- and Δ^6-desaturases

	Δ^9-r	Δ^9-c	Δ^6-r	Δ^5-r
Microsomal	+	+	+	+
Cytochrome b_5	+	+	+	NK
Cytochrome b_5 reductase	+	+	+	NK
Mol. wt.	53 K	33.6 K	66 K	NK
Non-haem Fe	+	+	+	NK
Inhibition by: KCN	+	+	+	NK
Bathophenanthroline				
sulphonate	+	NK	+	NK
PCMBS	+	+	+	NK
Polarity index	62%	NK	49%	NK

r, rat liver; c, chicken liver; PCMBS, p-chloromercuribenzene sulphonate; NK, not known.

protein, NADH and lipid or detergent. Enoch and Strittmatter [41] reported that the Δ^9-desaturase could also be reconstituted by NADPH–cytochrome P-450 reductase but Okayasu reported that this protein only restored 60% of the Δ^6-desaturase activity measured in the presence of NADH–cytochrome b_5 reductase.

Our current knowledge of desaturases is summarised in Table 2.

5. Evidence for other desaturases

(a) Δ^8-Desaturase

It is now generally believed that in the liver, the presence of a Δ^9-, Δ^6- and Δ^5-desaturase can account for all the unsaturated fatty acids that occur from metabolism. However in specialised tissue such as the testes of the rat, Albert and Coniglio [42] have provided convincing evidence that this tissue contains a Δ^8-desaturase and have demonstrated similar conversions in human testes [43]. Incubation of rat testes with $[1\text{-}^{14}C]\text{-}11:14\,20:2$ showed significant conversion into $8,11,14\text{-}20:3$ under conditions which rule out the possibility of β-oxidation or retroconversion to $9,12\text{-}18:2$ followed by Δ^6-desaturation and chain elongation. The biochemical significance of the Δ^8-desaturase is not known but may reflect the relatively high activity of elongases in the testes coupled with a low-specificity Δ^9-desaturase. This speculation still has to be supported by experimental evidence.

	18:2 (9,12)	18:2 (9,12)	
	↓ Elongation	↓ Δ^6-desaturation	
	20:2 (11,14)	18:3 (6,9,12)	
TESTES	↓ Δ^8-desaturation	↓ Elongation	LIVER
	20:3 (8,11,14)	20:3 (8,11,14)	
	↓ Δ^5-desaturation	↓ Δ^5-desaturation	
	20:4 (5,8,11,14)	20:4 (5,8,11,14)	

(b) Δ^4-Desaturase

A characteristic of fish-liver oils is the presence of long-chain polyunsaturated fatty acids as shown in Fig. 3 and characterised by such fatty acids as $22:5$.

The presence of Δ^6- and Δ^5-desaturases with the appropriate elongases can account for all but the final steps, i.e. feeding $22:4(7,10,13,16)$ failed to produce $22:5(4,7,10,13,16)$ but resulted in the formation of arachidonic acid [44]. However, injection of $[1\text{-}^{14}C]20:3(7,10,13)$ did result in a small conversion into $20:4(4,7,10,13)$ [45] and may therefore reflect tight specificity for certain chain-length fatty acids.

These studies have been carried out with rat microsomal preparations. For more clear-cut results it might be necessary to use tissues which are known to synthesise high levels of these polyunsaturated fatty acids.

6. General properties of desaturases

(a) Specificity

It has already been stated that the substrate for all mammalian desaturases with one exception [14] is the fatty acyl-CoA ester and that for the Δ^9-desaturase the preferred substrate is stearoyl-CoA. Work on this area has been carried out with a wide range of systems, using free fatty acids, coenzyme-A esters, with/without carrier proteins such as bovine serum albumin but in general the conclusions are the same, even between species as shown in the composite Fig. 6 comparing the specificity of rat-liver and avian-liver Δ^9-desaturase. The results shown here agree

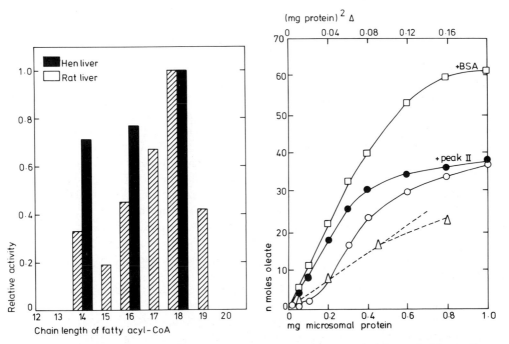

Fig. 6. Specificity of Δ^9-desaturase from rat liver and hen liver. Data was taken from ref. 6 for rat liver and from ref. 13 for hen liver.

Fig. 7. Enzymic desaturation of stearoyl-CoA in the absence ($\bigcirc$) and presence ($\square$, $\bullet$) of carrier proteins. $\bigcirc$, control; $\square$, with bovine serum albumin; $\bullet$, with ligandin. Taken from Jeffcoat, R., Brawn, P.R. and James, A.T. (1976) Biochim. Biophys. Acta 431, 33–44.

with those reported earlier using crude preparations and free fatty acids reported by Gurr et al. [7]. The results of Prasad and Joshi [13] would however indicate that hen-liver preparations showing apparently 2 peaks of Δ^9-desaturase activity [7] is unlikely to be due to 2 Δ^9-desaturases since antisera to the purified stearoyl-CoA desaturase also inhibited dodecanoyl-CoA, myristoyl-CoA, palmitoyl-CoA as well as stearoyl-CoA desaturation.

In the case of Δ^6-desaturation, it has already been stated that the preferred substrates are α-linolenic > linoleic > oleic acid although all are desaturated in the 6-position (Fig. 3). Whereas both Δ^9- and Δ^6-desaturases have clearly defined substrate preferences, this cannot be stated with certainty for the Δ^5-desaturase where the major discernible effect is a dependence on chain length for Δ8c, Δ9t, Δ8c:11c, Δ11c:14c or Δ8c:11c:14c acids. All studies carried out on the Δ^5-desaturation of fatty acids have made use of crude extracts which contain lipids which can act as potential substrates for the enzyme. Results should therefore be interpreted with caution until more purified systems are available for experimental confirmation. The list of potential substrates (both natural and unnatural) for desaturation is vast and has been comprehensively reviewed by James [1] and Sprecher and James [2].

(b) Role of cytoplasmic proteins

The substrate of the hepatic Δ^9-desaturase is derived from de novo synthesised fatty acid, dietary lipid or albumin-bound fatty acids from the adipose tissue. Considering hepatic fatty acid biosynthesis, the question can be asked: 'How are the free fatty acids — the known products of mammalian fatty acid synthetase — directed from their site of synthesis in the cytoplasm to the membranes for further elongation (see later), desaturation and/or incorporation into triacylglycerols?' Three possibilities exist: (i) the product of fatty acid synthesis is released from the complex and diffuses through the cytoplasm, (ii) the complex associates with membranes and loads its product on the next enzyme in the membrane or (iii) specific carrier molecules such as those described by Knoche et al. [46], direct the fatty acids to the appropriate organelles, e.g. mitochondria,, microsomes, etc. The possibility that binding proteins are involved in the desaturation of stearoyl-CoA came from Jeffcoat et al. [6] and linoleoyl-CoA from the studies of Catala et al. [47] and Jeffcoat et al. [48,49].

From work on the Δ^9-desaturase, Jeffcoat et al. [48] demonstrated that the non-linear relationship between enzyme activity and microsomal protein concentration could be alleviated either by the addition of bovine serum albumin or fatty-acid-binding protein which was similar to, if not identical with, a ligandin fraction described by Litwack et al. [50] (Fig. 7). Since in purified systems [6,12,40] full desaturase activity could be restored without the additions of these proteins, they are clearly not obligatory, but may be involved in modulating activity by organisation of the enzyme complex in the membrane [51]. In crude preparations, and perhaps in vivo, their function may be to bind fatty acyl-CoA derivatives in a controlled way such that their subsequent metabolism is optimised. For example, Jeffcoat et al. [6] demonstrated that in the presence of optimum concentrations of bovine serum albumin, the rate of hydrolysis of stearoyl-CoA was halved and the rate of desaturation increased. Similar effects of soluble proteins from developing rat brain on the hydrolysis of fatty acyl-CoAs have also been described by Brophy and Vance [52]. The stimulation of the Δ^6- and Δ^5-desaturase by catalase is not understood but may play a protective role in those tissues where there is low desaturase activity and high superoxide dismutase activity [53]. Its role in influencing the Δ^9-desaturase however is far from clear [54], but has also been implicated in linoleate desaturase in linseed cotyledons by Browse and Slack [55].

(c) Metal ions

As well as requiring cytochrome b_5, cytochrome b_5 reductase, lipid, reduced pyridine nucleotides, molecular oxygen and maybe fatty-acid-binding proteins, desaturases also seem to be influenced by metal ions in vivo although in the purified system the requirement for these is restricted to the non-haem iron of the desaturase [12,13] and the haem ion of the cytochromes. However work by Thompson et al. [56] has demonstrated that pigs fed a copper-deficient diet have a higher stearate/oleate ratio in the outer subcutaneous fat and perirenal fat depots when compared with pigs fed a copper-supplemented diet. Similar changes in rat-microsomal Δ^9-desaturase were also observed when rats were injected intraperitoneally with copper sulphate, i.e. higher desaturase activity after injection [57].

By way of contrast, it has been shown (Jeffcoat, unpublished data) that incubations of rat-liver microsomes with the iron chelator, bathophenanthroline sulphonate caused 80% inhibition of stearoyl-CoA desaturase whereas the copper chelator, diethyldithiocarbamate had no effect. In chicks, Sreekrishna and Joshi [58] demonstrated that copper and copper complexes of tyrosine, histidine, and lysine inhibited stearoyl-CoA desaturase in microsomal and purified enzyme systems. They postulated that the effect might be explained by the copper chelates acting as superoxide scavengers.

Other reports of the effect of metal ions on desaturation have been cited but as yet it is unclear whether or not this is a direct effect upon the desaturases. For example, zinc has a stimulatory effect on hepatic Δ^9- and Δ^6-desaturation [59–61] and selenium while stimulating Δ^6-desaturation has an unknown effect on the Δ^9-desaturation [62,63]. In testes, zinc deficiency increases Δ^9-desaturation and decreases Δ^6- and Δ^5-desaturation.

7. Elongation of fatty acids

It has been established that fatty acid biosynthesis (Chapter 2, this volume) occurs via a complex of enzymes, collectively known as the fatty acid synthetase. These reactions involve the condensation of acetyl-CoA and malonyl-CoA units which have been transferred to the complex via the appropriate transferases. The action of the condensing enzyme is followed by reduction, dehydration and a second reduction. The process is repeated with the C-2 units derived from malonyl-CoA until a 16-carbon acyl chain is formed. At this point the fatty acid, palmitic acid, is released from the complex via the action of palmitic acid thioesterase. The fate of the palmitic acid is thus usually conversion to its coenzyme-A ester followed by further elongation by the action of mitochondrial or microsomal elongases which in essence consist of all the enzymes of the fatty acid synthetase complex described above, but are membrane bound and use acetyl-CoA and malonyl-CoA respectively. The actual nature of the elongase system is still unclear due to the difficulty of purification of membrane-bound enzymes but indirect studies based on enzymology would suggest that the complex is made up of individual enzyme proteins each with its own distinct catalytic activity [65] (Fig. 8).

Although the overall elongation of fatty acids by chain elongation is analogous to fatty synthesis, Keyes et al. [66] have implicated cytochrome b_5 based on (a) the increased rate of reoxidation of liver microsomal cytochrome b_5, following reduction by NADH in the presence of malonyl-CoA and ATP and (b) a 60% inhibition of incorporation of malonyl-CoA into microsomal fatty acids by anti-cytochrome b_5 IgG. It has been concluded by the authors that it is most probable that cytochrome b_5 can transfer electrons from NADH to the reductases acting upon the β-ketoacyl-CoA and the $trans$-α-β-unsaturated acyl-CoA [67] (Fig. 8).

The early observations of Abraham et al. [68] first drew attention to the possibility of the microsomal elongation system when they demonstrated that

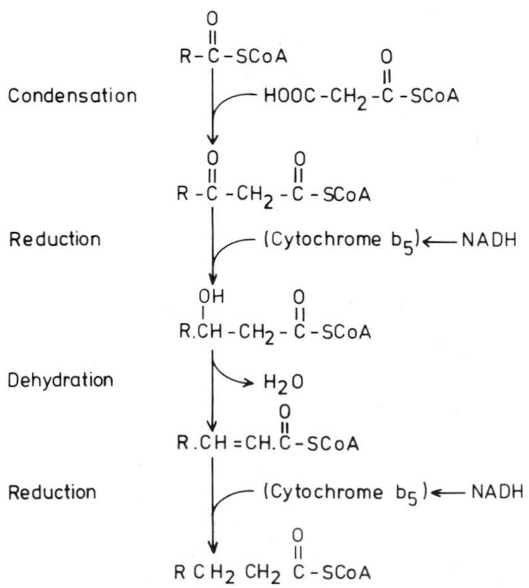

Fig. 8. Generalised scheme for chain elongation.

incubations including microsomes, NADPH, cytosol and [^{14}C]malonyl-CoA resulted in significant synthesis of long-chain fatty acids. However, it was the work of Nugteren [69] and Stoffel and Ach [70] which underlined the significance of the observations. Nugteren [69] demonstrated that in the following conversion of myristic acid to palmitic acid, the overall reaction was limited by the condensation of acyl-CoA and malonyl-CoA.

$$R-\overset{\overset{O}{\|}}{C}-SCoA \;+\; \underset{\underset{\underset{O}{\|}}{C-SCoA}}{\overset{\overset{COOH}{/}}{CH_2}} \;\longrightarrow\; R-\overset{\overset{O}{\|}}{C}-CH_2-\overset{\overset{O}{\|}}{C}-SCoA$$

THis was followed by a reduction, dehydration and a second reduction to yield $R \cdot CH_2CH_2CH_2 \cdot SCoA$ in an analogous way to fatty acid synthetase as outlined previously. More recent studies by Bernert and Sprecher [71] have shown by direct measurement that the rate of condensation of malonyl-CoA and palmitoyl-CoA equals the overall rate of chain elongation. The substrate for these elongation reactions was shown by Nugteren [69] to be the acyl-CoA derivatives since the need for the presence of CoA and ATP was obviated by the use of fatty acyl-CoA derivatives.

Although most studies have been carried out with rat-liver preparation, Cook [72] has studied chain elongation in the brain where polyunsaturated fatty acids are major components of the membrane phospholipids. Substrate specificity studies on 3–4-week-old rats indicated that the preferred substrates were 6,9,12-18 : 3 (100%) > 16 : 0 (75%) > 5,8,11,14-20 : 4 (57%) > 9,12,15-18 : 3 (30%) > 9,12-18 : 2 (10%) > 8,11,14-20 : 3 (6%).

The enzymology of chain elongation has lagged behind that of conventional fatty acid synthesis largely as a result of the fact that the elongases are membrane-bound and hence difficult to isolate and characterise. In an attempt to understand the partial reactions of elongation Bernert and Sprecher [73] studied the effects of bovine serum albumin on the condensation reaction in relation to the overall elongation. When albumin was included in the incubations in a 2 : 1 molar ratio (acyl-CoA : albumin), both the condensation and α,β-enoyl-CoA reductase reactions were elevated, but the dehydrase reaction was unaffected [73]. The major conclusions of the authors [73] was that bovine serum albumin can influence the partial reactions in the microsomal chain elongation of palmitate to stearate in different ways. The three most likely modes of operation suggested by the authors [73] are (1) to limit the availability of the acyl-CoA for the hydrolysis by thiol esterases, (2) to bind the substrate in such a way that the free acyl-CoA is below the critical micelle concentration and (3) to substitute for in vivo binding proteins which are capable of binding fatty acids and their coenzyme-A esters and thus prevent inhibition of lipid-metabolising enzymes.

Complete purification of all the enzymes of the elongase complex has not yet been achieved but Bernert and Sprecher [73] successfully solubilised and partially purified the β-hydroxyacyl-CoA dehydrase. Under conditions of solubilisation using 0.5% sodium deoxycholate, neither the condensation nor the enoyl-CoA reductase activation could be solubilised. The 90-fold purified dehydrase was capable of acting upon a range of even numbered acyl-CoAs with chain lengths of 14–20 carbons — V_{max} varied little, but as the chain length increased so did the K_m.

From these purification studies it was interesting to note that the condensation and reductase activities although not solubilised were irreversibly inhibited by the deoxycholate. In the light of these data it was suggested by the authors that the inhibition of these two enzymes by their substrates and the protection by bovine serum albumin reflects the detergent-like properties of the acyl-CoA substrates. The partially purified dehydrase did not require any added lipid but it is possible that the solubilisation step, salt precipitation and ion-exchange chromatography had not removed some tightly bound essential lipid.

In contrast to the condensation and reductase enzymes, the requirement of the dehydrase for a micellar substrate, raised the possibility [73] of an additional regulatory step in elongation. It was suggested that since the condensation is the regulatory step in the overall elongation, several enzymes might contribute to a common pool of substrate for the dehydrase; the pool thus providing substrates as micelles of long-chain fatty acids with lower critical micelle concentrations.

8. The control of lipogenesis by desaturation and elongation

(a) Dietary control

Lipids not only form the basis of membranes in the form of phospholipids but also act as a valuable store of energy. It is therefore perhaps not surprising that numerous control systems have evolved to influence the fate of fatty acid precursors and the fatty acids themselves. Lipids can be derived from dietary sources and this is a prerequisite for the essential fatty acids, or from de novo synthesis from such raw materials as carbohydrates (Fig. 9). Although it is apparent that many enzymes are involved in lipid synthesis [74,75], this review will be restricted to the control of desaturases and elongases.

The early studies of Yudkin's group [76] demonstrated that rats fed high concentrations of sucrose or fructose showed elevated levels of fatty acid synthetase. Similar effects were observed with acetyl-CoA carboxylase and these effects could be augmented by pre-starving the animals before feeding the high-carbohydrate diet. Jeffcoat and James [78] have also demonstrated that starving and refeeding rats in the way described, not only enhanced fatty acid synthetase, but also stearoyl-CoA desaturase. It thus appeared that key enzymes involved in lipid synthesis show co-ordinately induced activity when provided with lipogenic substrates in this way. This was further confirmed by Gibson et al. [74] who have also demonstrated similar effects with malic enzymes (EC 1.1.1.40), citrate lyase (EC 4.1.3.6), glucose-6-P dehydrogenase (EC 1.1.1.49) and 6-phosphogluconate dehydrogenase (EC 4.2.1.12) which provide substrates and co-factors for lipogenesis.

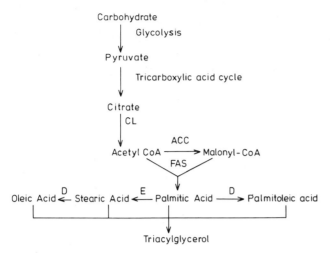

Fig. 9. Biosynthesis of triacylglycerol. CL, citrate lyase; ACC, acetyl-CoA carboxylase; FAS, fatty acid synthetase; D, desaturase; E, elongase.

It is to be anticipated that when animals are challenged with levels of dietary carbohydrate over and above their immediate requirements, there will be an increase in the activity of those enzymes responsible for the conversion of carbohydrate into storage lipid. Conversely it might be expected that diets rich in the products of lipid synthesis would result in a decrease in lipogenesis. Inkpen et al. [79] demonstrated that the change from a hydrogenated coconut diet to a safflower oil diet resulted in decreased activity of rat-liver stearoyl-CoA desaturase. Further, Jeffcoat and James [78] have shown that whereas all dietary fatty acids inhibit to some extent fatty acid synthetase and stearoyl-CoA desaturase activity, the most potent inhibitor was the polyunsaturated fatty acid, linoleic acid — an observation which has also been made by others for fatty acid synthetase [80]. Since saturated fatty acids and monounsaturated fatty acids were not the most effective inhibitors of synthesis and desaturation respectively, it suggested that the action of polyunsaturated fatty acids is by a mechanism other than end-product inhibition. Furthermore, Jeffcoat and James [81] have demonstrated a close interrelationship between fatty acid synthesis and desaturation in terms of the control by sucrose and polyunsaturated fatty acid [82].

Although much work has been carried out on the control of fatty acid synthesis by fatty acid synthetase and acetyl-CoA carboxylase, the involvement of stearoyl-CoA desaturase now raises the question as to which enzyme controls overall fatty acid synthesis. In the past, control has been divided into short term and long term with the general consensus of opinion that fatty acid synthetase controls the latter and acetyl-CoA carboxylase the former. Since fatty acid synthesis and Δ^9-desaturation appear to be influenced by common factors, the question can be asked — what role does the Δ^9-desaturase play in influencing the total lipid synthesis in the liver? The first indication of the relative importance of synthesis and desaturation came from

104

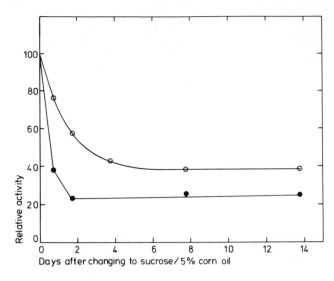

Fig. 10. Effect of dietary polyunsaturated fatty acids on fatty acid synthetase (○) and stearoyl-CoA desaturase (●). Taken and modified from Jeffcoat, R. and James, A.T. (1978) FEBS Lett. 85, 114–118.

studies of Jeffcoat and James [81] who demonstrated that whilst groups of weanling rats were fed a high-carbohydrate fat-free diet for 2 weeks, and the expected elevated levels of fatty acid synthetase and stearoyl-CoA desaturase activities were achieved, when the animals were switched to the same diet supplemented with 5% (w/w) corn oil containing 60% (w/w) linoleic acid, then both enzyme activities decayed, with a half-life of 2–3 days for fatty acid synthetase and < 12 h for the stearoyl-CoA desaturase (Fig. 10). This observation clearly identified that the nutritional control of hepatic lipid synthesis cannot be by the action of linoleic acid on fatty acid synthesis but rather via its action on desaturation since the time course of its action fell within the diurnal feeding pattern of the rat [83,84]. The general trend in the response of the two enzymes is of the same order of magnitude as the reported half-life for the fatty acid synthetase ∼ 72 h [80] and stearoyl-CoA desaturase ∼ 3–4 h [84] and it is thus tempting to identify the polyunsaturated fatty acid effect with a control of enzyme levels. So far this has only been studied for the synthetase (Flick et al. [80]; Alberts, this volume) and similar studies for the desaturase have been awaiting the purification of the desaturase and the availability of antibodies, which have been hampered by the difficulty in purifying the enzyme.

The observation that stearoyl-CoA desaturase responds 3–4 times more quickly than fatty acid synthetase to changes in dietary linoleic acid only compares the enzyme activities under optimum conditions of available substrate and enzyme. The question as to whether or not this relates to the in vivo situation is still a real one. Jeffcoat et al. [82] went some way to answering this question with the use of isolated hepatocytes from animals nutritionally manipulated.

Using rats which had been starved for 24 h and then refed a fat-free/high-

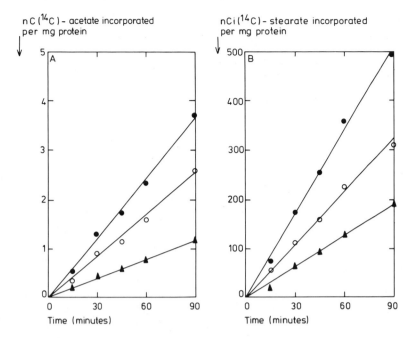

Fig. 11. Incorporation of acetate (A) and stearate (B) in saturated (○), monounsaturated (▲) and total fatty acids (●). Taken from Jeffcoat, R., Roberts, P.A., Ormesher, J.A. and James, A.T. (1979) Eur. J. Biochem. 101, 439–445.

carbohydrate diet, hepatocytes were isolated and incubated with [2-^{14}C]acetate. Analysis of the lipid fractions indicated a time-dependent formation of fatty acids with the rate of formation of saturated fatty acids being approximately 2.5 times that of monounsaturated fatty acids (Fig. 11). This indicates that in the formation of monounsaturated fatty acids from acetate, the rate-limiting step is the desaturation of the saturated fatty acids.

However the end-product of lipid biosynthesis in the liver is triacylglycerol in the form of very-low-density lipoprotein. How does the activity of stearoyl-CoA relate to this overall synthesis? Jeffcoat et al. [82] studied the rate of triacylglycerol biosynthesis from stearic acid using hepatocytes derived from rats fed (a) a diet containing 20% (w/w) sucrose and (b) a diet containing 20% (w/w) sucrose and 5% (w/w) corn oil. It was shown from these studies that the effect of corn oil was to suppress triacylglycerol production by 54% accompanied by a decrease in stearoyl-CoA desaturase activity by 55%. Since it was also demonstrated that the incorporation of oleic acid into the triacylglycerol fraction was 3 times as fast as the incorporation of stearic acid, it was concluded that desaturation of fatty acids plays an important role in the overall synthesis of lipid by the liver. These observations are further supported by other workers who have also shown a more rapid metabolism of unsaturated fatty acid than stearic acid [85,86] and the correlation in perfused liver experiments between fatty acid synthesis and lipoprotein secretion [87]. The view therefore that stearoyl-CoA desaturase plays a key role in lipid synthesis can be summarised as follows:

(1) Diurnal variation of stearoyl-CoA desaturase (Δ^9) coincides with the food intake.

(2) Desaturation responds rapidly to dietary polyunsaturated fatty acid.

(3) The half-life of the Δ^9-desaturase is 3–4 h.

(4) Desaturation is the rate-limiting step in the sequence from acetate to oleic acid.

(5) Oleic acid is incorporated 3 times as quickly as stearic acid into tri-acylglycerols.

(6) Chain elongation of preformed fatty acids is generally faster than desaturation.

Since the main reason for the induction of liver lipogenesis is the conversion of dietary carbohydrate into storage lipid, it is interesting to consider the fate of dietary carbohydrates when ingested in the presence of linoleic acid in the form of triacylglycerols — in this situation the carbohydrate stimulates lipogenesis and the polyunsaturated fatty acid suppresses it. Studies by Jeffcoat et al. [88] demonstrated that the long-term effects (20 weeks) of feeding either sucrose or sucrose supplemented with corn oil did result in sustained differences in the levels of fatty acid synthetase and stearoyl-CoA desaturase and that these differences were independent of the sex of the animals (Fig. 12). The consequences of this were not striking but can be summarised as follows: changing the diets from a starch-based one (A) to one with 20% (w/w) sucrose (B), or 20% (w/w) sucrose and 4% (w/w) corn oil (C) or 4% (w/w) tallow (D) resulted in an increase in body weight and a decrease in body fat as shown in Fig. 13 in spite of the fact that food intakes varied by no more than $\pm 1\%$ between dietary groups. The metabolic fate of the sucrose in the presence of dietary linoleic acid thus still remains an unsolved problem. If sucrose stimulates

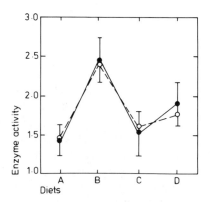

Fig. 12. The change in hepatic fatty acid synthesis (●) and stearoyl-CoA desaturase (○) after 20 weeks feeding starch (A), sucrose (B), sucrose plus corn oil (C) and sucrose plus tallow (D). Taken from Jeffcoat, R., Roberts, P.A. and James, A.T. (1979) Eur. J. Biochem. 101, 447–453.

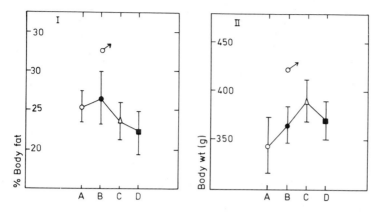

Fig. 13. Changes in body fat (I) and body weight (II) as a result of feeding diets described in Fig. 12. Taken from Jeffcoat, R., Roberts, P.A. and James, A.T. (1979) Eur. J. Biochem. 101, 447–453.

hepatic lipogenesis and dietary linoleic acid represses lipogenesis, then when both are ingested together since sucrose is normally converted into fat in the liver, the normal metabolic pathway is blocked. From the results of Jeffcoat et al. [88] it would appear that sucrose is neither directed to glycogen nor fatty acid synthesis directed to the adipose tissue. It is clear that generalities can be misleading since Jeffcoat et al. [82] have shown that when rats are feed ad libitum sucrose and corn oil, linoleic acid does override the inductive effect of the sucrose, but when the animals are starved for 24 h prior to feeding, then both fatty acid synthetase and Δ^9-desaturase are induced in the usual way. Furthermore Loriette and Lapous [89] and Waterman et al. [90] have shown that unlike hepatic lipogenesis, lard containing only 7% (w/w) linoleic acid is a better inhibitor of adipose tissue lipogenesis than is sunflower oil containing 67% (w/w) linoleic acid. it is thus apparent that when considering the overall control of lipogenesis, several factors must be taken into consideration: (1) The species — in the hen the major site of lipid synthesis is the liver, while in the pig, the adipose tissue is the major site [90]. (2) The carbohydrate in the diet — fructose stimulates hepatic lipogenesis but represses adipose tissue lipogenesis [91] whereas in mouse [92] and man [93] glucose is preferentially converted to lipid in the adipose tissue [94]. (3) The lipid in the diet — saturated fat inhibits fatty acid synthesis whereas polyunsaturated fat controls the enzyme levels. (4) The feeding regime — starved/refed, continuous or continuous plus intubation. (5) Previous nutritional history of the animal. In view of the complexity of the control systems, it is often still not possible to predict with certainty the overall lipogenic state of the animal in question.

(b) Hormonal control

Although it has been clearly demonstrated that specific components in the diet can significantly affect key lipid-synthesising enzymes, it is still not clear how these effects are brought about. One possibility is through the endocrine system with one or more hormones controlling metabolic activity.

(i) Desaturation

Although much work has been carried out with the effects of individual hormones on specific desaturases and elongases [95–103], the overall control of these enzymes by hormones is still a confusing picture [3]. As a result of the close association of carbohydrate and lipid metabolism, it is perhaps not surprising that much of the hormonal study has been focussed upon the action of insulin and glucagon in the liver and adipose tissue [104].

When studying the effects of hormones, two questions need answering: (1) Does the hormone exert its effect on enzyme activity or on the level of enzyme protein? (2) Is the effect a direct influence by the hormone on the enzyme system in question or an indirect effect acting through other hormones or immediates? The answers to these questions have been attempted by inducing (artificially) a stressed state in the animal (starving or chronically inducing diabetes) and then attempting to reverse the effects using hormonal treatment. For example, Mercuri et al. [105] demonstrated that the diabetic state induced by intravenous injection of streptozotoxin caused a reduction in the Δ^9-desaturase activity which could be reversed by feeding fructose, glycerol or saturated fatty acids. It was concluded that the fructose and saturated fatty acids by-passed the insulin-sensitive glucose metabolic steps, while glycerol removed the products of desaturation as triacylglycerols. It would appear from these observations that under these conditions insulin has an indirect effect on desaturation by controlling glucose metabolism and the flux of carbohydrate intermediates into lipid metabolic pools. By way of contrast to these results, Salmon and Hems

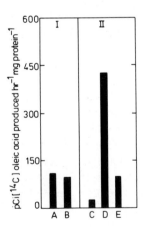

Fig. 14. Effect of insulin on oleic acid production in isolated hepatocytes. A and B: stearoyl-CoA desaturase activity measured at zero time in the presence and absence of insulin respectively. C, D and E: stearoyl-CoA desaturase activity after 48 h incubation without insulin (C), with insulin (D) and with insulin and cycloheximide (E). Taken from Jeffcoat, R., Roberts, P.A., Ormesher, J.A. and James, A.T. (1979) Eur. J. Biochem. 101, 439–445.

[106] have demonstrated indirectly that in short-term perfusion studies, insulin affects desaturase activity. During a 3-h perfusion they demonstrated that in the absence of insulin the ratio of saturated to unsaturated fatty acid increased. More recent studies by Jeffcoat et al. [82] have shown that insulin can directly influence the level of desaturase protein. In a series of experiments, hepatocytes were prepared from rats fed a laboratory chow diet and incubated for 48 h (C) with insulin, (D) without insulin and (E) with insulin and cycloheximide (Fig. 14). In the absence of insulin the Δ^9-desaturase activity dropped by 75%, while in the presence of insulin the enzyme activity increased by 4.5-fold. Finally, when hepatocytes were incubated with insulin and cycloheximide there was neither an increase nor a decrease in enzyme activity. Thus it was concluded that insulin not only controls the synthesis of new enzyme but also stabilises existing enzyme by a mechanism which is as yet not understood. Finally, confirmation of these results awaits the direct measurement of enzyme levels with specific antibodies raised against the enzyme protein.

(ii) Elongation

In contrast to the relatively large amount of work carried out on the hormonal control of individual desaturases, little work has been directed towards a study of the effect of hormones on elongation of fatty acids either by mitochondrial or microsomal elongases. From the work of Fass et al. [107] and Landriscina et al. [108,109] it was demonstrated that chain elongation was largely unaffected by the action of thyroxine but that starving [110] or the administration of hypolipidaemic drugs [111] did depress the activity of microsomal chain elongation. Those results would indicate that elongation is clearly under a different set of controls than that which influences fatty acid synthetases and desaturation.

9. Conclusions

The object of this review has been to assess the control of fatty acid metabolism with particular reference to desaturation and elongation of preformed fatty acids. It is now apparent that in order to appreciate the complexity of the control systems, the individual enzymic steps must be evaluated in terms of the overall lipid-synthe-sising process. Clearly the physiological state of the animal and the nature of the diet will affect the relative importance of individual enzymes in controlling the overall metabolism. In this review, attention has been focussed on the effect of carbohydrate and polyunsaturated fatty acid on desaturation since it has already been reported that these dietary components can significantly influence fatty acid biosynthesis by influencing fatty acid synthetase and acetyl-CoA carboxylase. From studies on the desaturation of the products of fatty acid synthetase, it would now appear that, under conditions of high-carbohydrate intake, what is true qualitatively for the control of fatty acid synthetase is also true for the Δ^9-desaturase. However, when the rates of the effects of polyunsaturated fatty acid on the synthetase and desaturase are compared, it can be demonstrated that not only does the desaturase respond at least 4 times as quickly as does the synthetase, but that there is a decreased secretion of triacylglycerol and the composition reflects the availability of less oleic acid [3,82]. This implies that dietary polyunsaturated fatty acid controls desaturation of saturated fatty acid and in so doing controls fatty acid synthesis and triacylglycerol secretion by the liver when animals are subjected to high-carbohydrate intake [3]. However, many interesting questions remain, the not least of which relates to the understanding of the mode of action of linoleic acid at the molecular level. Is linoleic acid the important dietary species or is it a metabolite of this fatty acid? Using eicosa-5,8,11,14-tetraynoic acid, which inhibits the conversion of linoleate to arachidonate, Abraham et al. [112] were able to alleviate linoleate-induced inhibition of fatty acid and cholesterol synthesis. From these observations it appears that linoleic acid is the active dietary component controlling lipid metabolism. Its mode of action will, however, have to await the studies on the effect of polyunsaturated fatty acid on the level/activity of the Δ^9-desaturase which will be greatly aided by the work on fatty acid synthetase and the availability of specific Δ^9-desaturase antibodies.

References

1 James, A.T. (1977) Advances in Experimental Medicine and Biology, Vol. 83, Plenum New York, pp. 51–74.
2 Sprecher, H. and James, A.T. (1979) Geometrical and Positional Fatty Acid Isomers, Champaign, American Oil Chemists Press, pp. 303–338.
3 Jeffcoat, R. (1979) Essays in Biochemistry, Vol. 15, Academic Press, London, pp. 1–36.
4 Burr, G.O. and Burr, M.M. (1929) J. Biol. Chem. 82, 345–367.
5 Bernert Jr., J.T. and Sprecher, H. (1975) Biochim. Biophys. Acta 398, 354–363.
6 Jeffcoat, R., Brawn, P.R., Safford, R. and James, A.T. (1977) Biochem. J. 161, 431–437.
7 Gurr, M.I., Robinson, M.P., James, A.T., Morris, L.J. and Howling, D. (1972) Biochim. Biophys. Acta 280, 415–421.
8 Lynen, F. (1980) Eur. J. Biochem. 112, 431–442.
9 Nagai, J. and Bloch, K. (1968) J. Biol. Chem. 243, 4626–4633.
10 Kass, L.R., Brock, D.J.H. and Bloch, K. (1967) J. Biol. Chem. 242, 4418–4431.
11 Raju, P.K. and Reiser, R. (1967) J. Biol. Chem. 242, 379–384.
12 Strittmatter, P., Spatz, L., Corcoran, D., Rogers, M.J., Setlow, B. and Redline, R. (1974) Proc. Natl. Acad. Sci. (U.S.A.) 71, 4565–4569.
13 Prasad, M.R. and Joshi, V.C. (1979) J. Biol. Chem. 254, 6362–6369.
14 Pugh, E.L. and Kates, M. (1977) J. Biol. Chem. 252, 68–73.
15 Stymme, S. and Appelquist, L.A. (1978) Eur. J. Biochem. 90, 223–229.
16 Slack, C.R., Roughan, P.G. and Browse, J. (1979) Biochem. J. 179, 649–656.
17 Murphy, D.J. and Stumpf, P.K. (1980) Plant Physiol. 66, 666–671.
18 Jeffcoat, R. (1977) Biochem. Soc. Trans. 5, 811–818.
19 Bergstrom, S. (1981) Progr. Lipid Res. 20, 7–12.
20 Morris, L.J. (1970) Biochem J. 118, 681–693.
21 Brett, D., Howling, D., Morris, L.J. and James, A.T. (1971) Arch. Biochem. Biophys. 143, 535–547.
22 Do, U.H. and Sprecher, H. (1975) Arch. Biochem. Biophys. 171, 597–603.
23 Gurr, M.I. (1974) MTP International Review of Science, Biochemistry of Lipids, Vol. 4, Butterworth, London, pp. 181–235.
24 Jones, P.D., Holloway, P.W., Peluffo, R.O. and Wakil, S.J. (1969) J. Biol. Chem. 244, 744–754.
25 Safford, R., Jeffcoat, R. and James, A.T. (1975) Biochim. Biophys. Acta 409, 86–96.

26 Gurr, M.I. and Robinson, M.P. (1970) Eur. J. Biochem. 15, 335–341.
27 Holloway, P.W. (1971) Biochemistry 10, 1556–1560.
28 Shimakata, T., Mihara, K. and Sato, R. (1972) J. Biochem. (Tokyo) 72, 1163–1174.
29 Spatz, L. and Strittmatter, P. (1971) Proc. Natl. Acad. Sci. (U.S.A.) 68, 1042–1046.
30 Spatz, L. and Strittmatter, P. (1973) J. Biol. Chem. 248, 793–799.
31 Rogers, M.J. and Strittmatter, P. (1973) J. Biol. Chem. 248, 800–806.
32 Capaldi, R.A. and Vanderkooi, G. (1972) Proc. Natl. Acad. Sci. (U.S.A.) 69, 930–932.
33 McKeon, T. and Stumpf, P.K. (1981) Methods Enzymol. 71, 275–281.
34 Rivers, J.P.W., Hassam, A.G., Crawford, M.A. and Brombell, M.R. (1976) Fed. Eur. Biochem. Soc. 67, 269–70.
35 Hassam, A.G., Rivers, J.P.W. and Crawford, M.A. (1977) Nutr. Metab. 21, 321–328.
36 Brenner, R.R. and Peluffo, R.O. (1966) J. Biol. Chem. 241, 5213–5219.
37 Cook, H.W. and Spence, M.W. (1974) Biochim. Biophys. Acta 369, 129–141.
38 Lee, T.C., Baker, R.C., Stephens, N. and Snyder, F. (1977) Biochim. Biophys. Acta 489, 25–31.
39 Okayasu, T., Ono, T., Shinojima, K. and Imai, Y. (1977) Lipids 12, 267–271.
40 Okayasu, T., Nagao, M., Ishibashi, T. and Imai, Y. (1981) Arch. Biochem. Biophys. 206, 21–28.
41 Enoch, H.G. and Strittmatter, P. (1979) J. Biol. Chem. 254, 8976–8981.
42 Albert, D.H. and Coniglio, J.G. (1977) Biochim. Biophys. Acta 489, 390–396.
43 Albert, D.H., Rhamy, R.K. and Coniglio, J.G. (1979) Lipids 14, 498–500.
44 Sprecher, H. (1967) Biochim. Biophys. Acta 144, 296–304.
45 Budny, J. and Sprecher, H. (1971) Biochim. Biophys. Acta 239, 190–207.
46 Knoche, H., Esders, T.W., Koths, K. and Bloch, K. (1973) J. Biol. Chem. 248, 2317–2322.
47 Catala, A., Nervi, A.M. and Brenner, R.R. (1975) J. Biol. Chem. 250, 7481–7484.
48 Jeffcoat, R., Brawn, P.R. and James, A.T. (1976) Biochim. Biophys. Acta 431, 33–44.
49 Jeffcoat, R., Dunton, A. and James, A.T. (1978) Biochim. Biophys. Acta 528, 28–35.
50 Litwack, G., Ketterer, B. and Arias, I.M. (1971) Nature (London) 234, 466–467.
51 Jones, D.P. and Gaylor, J.L. (1979) Biochem. J. 183, 405–415.
52 Brophy, P.J. and Vance, D.E. (1976) Biochem. J. 160, 247–251.
53 Okayasu, T., Kameda, K., Ono, T. and Imai, Y. (1977) Biochim. Biophys. Acta 489, 397–402.
54 Baker, R.C., Wykle, R.L., Lockmiller, J.C. and Snyder, F. (1976) Arch. Biochem. Biophys. 177, 299–306.
55 Browse, J.A. and Slack, C.R. (1981) FEBS Lett. 131, 111–114.
56 Thompson, E.H., Allen, C.E. and Meade, R.J. (1973) J. Anim. Sci. 36, 868–873.
57 Wahle, K.W.J. and Davies, N.T. (1975) Br. J. Nutr. 34, 105–112.
58 Sreekrishna, K. and Joshi, V.C. (1980) Biochim. Biophys. Acta 619, 267–273.
59 Clejan, S., Maddaiah, V.T., Castromagana, M. and Collip, P.J. (1981) Lipids 16, 454–460.
60 Huang, Y.S., Cunnane, S.C., Horrobin, D.F. and Davignon, J. (1982) Atherosclerosis 41, 193–207.
61 Cunnane, S.C. and Wahle, K.W.J. (1981) Lipids 16, 771–774.
62 Fischer, W.C. and Whanger, P.D. (1977) J. Nutr. 107, 1493–1501.
63 Fischer, W.C. and Whanger, P.D. (1977) J. Nutr. Sci. Vitam. 23, 273–280
64 Clejan, S., Castromagana, M., Collip, P.J., Jonas, E. and Maddaiah, V.T. (1982) Lipids 17, 129–135.
65 Bernert Jr., J.T. and Sprecher, H. (1979) Biochim. Biophys. Acta 573, 436–442.
66 Keyes, S.R., Alfano, J.A., Jansson, I. and Cinti, D.L. (1979) J. Biol. Chem. 254, 7778–7784.
67 Keyes, S.R. and Cinti, D.L. (1980) J. Biol. Chem. 255, 11357–11364.
68 Abraham, S., Chaikoss, I.L., Bortz, W.M., Klein, H.P. and Den, H. (1961) Nature (London) 192, 1287–1288.
69 Nugteren, D.H. (1965) Biochim. Biophys. Acta 106, 280–290.
70 Stoffel, W. and Ach, K.L. (1964) Z. Physiol. Chem. 337, 123–132.
71 Bernert Jr., J.T. and Sprecher, H. (1978) Biochim. Biophys. Acta 531, 44–55.
72 Cook, H.W. (1982) Arch. Biochem. Biophys. 214, 695–704.
73 Bernert Jr., J.T. and Sprecher, H. (1977) J. Biol. Chem. 252, 6736–6744.
74 Gibson, D.M., Lyons, R.T., Scott, D.F. and Muto, Y. (1972) Adv. Enzyme Regul. 10, 187–204.
75 Denton, R.M. and Halestrap, A.P. (1979) Essays in Biochemistry, Vol. 15, Academic Press, London, pp. 37–77.

76 Bruckdorfer, K.R., Khan, I.H. and Yudkin, J. (1972) Biochem. J. 129, 439–446.

77 Volpe, J.J. and Vagelos, P.R. (1976) Physiol. Rev. 56, 339–417.

78 Jeffcoat, R. and James, A.T. (1977) Lipids 12, 469–474.

74 Inkpen, C.A., Harris, R.A. and Quackenbush, F.W. (1969) J. Lipid Res. 10, 277–282.

80 Flick, P.K., Chen, J. and Vagelos, P.R. (1977) J. Biol. Chem. 252, 4242–4249.

81 Jeffcoat, R. and James, A.T. (1978) FEBS Lett. 85, 114–118.

82 Jeffcoat, R., Roberts, P.A., Ormesher, J. and James, A.T. (1979) Eur. J. Biochem. 101, 439–445.

83 Actis Dato, S.M., Catala, A. and Brenner, R.R. (1973) Lipids 8, 1–6.

84 Oshino, N. and Sato, R. (1972) Arch. Biochem. Biophys. 149, 369–377.

85 Goodridge, A.G. (1973) J. Biol. Chem. 248, 4318–4326.

86 Sundler, R., Akesson, B. and Nilsson, A. (1974) J. Biol. Chem. 249, 5102–5107.

87 Windmueller, H.G. and Spaeth, A.E. (1967) Arch. Biochem. Biophys. 122, 362–369.

88 Jeffcoat, R., Roberts, P.A. and James, A.T. (1979) Eur. J. Biochem. 101, 447–453.

89 Loriette, C. and Lapous, D. (1976) Experientia 3, 881–882.

90 Waterman, R.A., Romsos, D.R., Tsai, A.C., Miller, E.R. and Leveille, G.A. (1975) Proc. Soc. Exp. Biol. Med. 150, 347–351.

91 Romsos, D.R. and Leveille, G.A. (1974) Biochim. Biophys. Acta 360, 1–11.

92 Hems, D.A., Rath, E.A. and Verrinder, T.R. (1975) Biochem. J. 150, 167–173.

93 Baker, N., Learn, D.B. and Bruckdorfer, K.R. (1978) J. Lipid Res. 19, 879–893.

94 Chinayon, S. and Goldrick, R.B. (1978) Aust. J. Exp. Biol. 56, 421–425.

95 Gellhorn, A. and Benjamin, W. (1964) Biochim. Biophys. Acta 84, 167–175.

96 Mercuri, O., Peluffo, R.O. and Brenner, R.R. (1966) Biochim. Biophys. Acta 116, 408–411.

97 Mercuri, O., Peluffo, R.O. and Brenner, R.R. (1967) Lipids 2, 284–285.

98 Castuma, J.C., Catala, A. and Brenner, R.R. (1972) J. Lipid Res. 13, 783–789.

99 Brenner, R.R. (1972) Mol. Cell. Biochem. 3, 41–52.

100 De Gomez Dumm, I.N.T., de Alaniz, M.J.T. and Brenner, R.R. (1975) J. Lipid Res. 16, 264–268.

101 De Gomez Dumm, I.N.T., de Alaniz, M.J.T. and Brenner, R.R. (1976) J. Lipid Res. 17, 616–621.

102 Fass, F.H., Carter, W.J. and Wynn, J.O. (1977) Arch. Biochem. Biophys. 182, 71–81.

103 De Gomez Dumm, I.N.T., de Alaniz, M.J.T. and Brenner, R.R. (1976) Lipids 11, 833–836.

104 Enser, M. (1979) Biochem. J. 180, 551–558.

105 Mercuri, O., Peluffo, R.O. and de Tomas, M.E. (1974) Biochim. Biophys. Acta 369, 264–268.

106 Salmon, D.M. and Hems, D.A. (1975) Biochem. Soc. Trans. 3, 510–512.

107 Fass, F.H., Carter, W.J. and Wynn, J. (1972) Endocrinology 91, 1481–1492.

108 Landriscina, C., Gnoni, G.V. and Quagliariello, E. (1976) Eur. J. Biochem. 71, 135–143.

109 Gnoni, G.V., Landriscina, C. and Quagliariello, E. (1978) FEBS Lett. 94, 179–182.

110 Donaldson, W.E., WH-Peeters, E.M. and Scholte, H.R. (1970) Biochim. Biophys. Acta 202, 35–42.

111 Landriscina, C., Ruggiero, F.M., Gnoni, G.V. and Quagliariello, E. (1977) Biochem. Pharmacol. 26, 1401–1404.

112 Abraham, S., McGarth, H. and Rao, G.A. (1977) Lipids 12, 446–449.

S. Numa (Ed.) Fatty Acid Metabolism and Its Regulation
© *1984 Elsevier Science Publishers B.V.*

CHAPTER 5

Fatty acid oxidation and its regulation

JON BREMER and HARALD OSMUNDSEN *

Institute of Medical Biochemistry, University of Oslo, P.O. Box 1112, Blindern, Oslo 3, Norway

1. Introduction

In the mammalian organism fatty acids fulfil the two major roles as integral components of membrane lipids, and as the body's major energy store in the form of triacylglycerol. Oxidation of fatty acids is the mechanism by which the body can utilize the relatively large amounts of energy contained in fatty acids. This process is strictly regulated by the energy requirement of body tissues.

Our knowledge of the mechanisms of fatty acid oxidation started to develop around the turn of the last century when Geelmuyden [1] showed that ketone bodies are formed from fatty acids and when Knoop [2] formulated his ingenious theory of β-oxidation. However, nearly 50 years had to pass before the details of fatty acid oxidation and its cellular organization could be worked out. The discovery of coenzyme A, and its function as a carrier of activated fatty acids, in the early 1950s [3] led to the isolation and characterization of the individual mitochondrial enzymes involved in fatty acid β-oxidation [4]. Development of methods for tissue fractionation, leading to isolation of subcellular fractions of mitochondria and of other organelles [5] made studies on the subcellular organization of fatty acid metabolism possible. Finally, the discoveries in 1955 of the acetylation of carnitine [6] and of carnitine as a cofactor in fatty acid oxidation [7] led to the demonstration of carnitine as a carrier of activated fatty acids across the mitochondrial membrane. This has been an important basis for further studies of organization and regulation of fatty acid oxidation.

2. Compartmentation of fatty acid metabolism

In all tissues we can distinguish between 3 main functional cellular compartments as regards oxidation of fatty acids: (1) the extramitochondrial compartment, includ-

* Present address: Department of Biochemistry, Norwegian College of Veterinary Medicine, Oslo (Norway).

ing the endoplasmic reticulum, the cytosol, and the outer mitochondrial membrane, (2) the peroxisomes, and (3) the mitochondrial matrix. The peroxisomal membrane and the inner mitochondrial membrane represent the borderlines between these compartments.

The metabolic function of the different compartments varies depending on the fatty acid chain length (Fig. 1).

(a) Long-chain fatty acids

Long-chain fatty acids (chain length C_{12-24}), taken up by the cell, are rapidly activated to acyl-CoA esters in the extramitochondrial compartment by long-chain acyl-CoA synthase(s):

$$Fatty\ acid + ATP + CoA \rightleftharpoons acyl\text{-}CoA + AMP + PP_i$$

After activation, the fatty acid group can be incorporated into phospholipids and triacylglycerol, or it can be oxidized in the mitochondria. The fatty acid can also undergo desaturation, chain elongation, chain shortening and saturation. Desaturation and chain elongation take place in the endoplasmic reticulum. Chain shortening takes place by partial β-oxidation in the peroxisomes. This is particularly important for the longer fatty acids (C_{22}–C_{24}) [8] (Section 5.b). The quantitatively less important ω-oxidation of fatty acids, which occurs prior to activation, takes place in

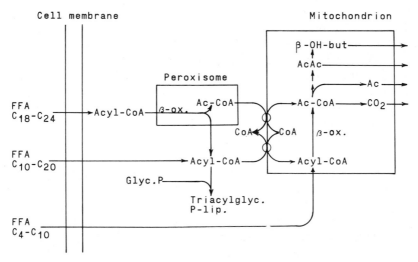

Fig. 1. Compartmentation of fatty acid metabolism in liver. Abbreviations: FFA, free fatty acids; Glyc.P, glycero-3-phosphate; P-lip, phospholipids; Ac-CoA, acetyl-CoA; AcAc, acetoacetate; β-ox., β-oxidation. The circles across the mitochondrial membrane represent the carnitine-dependent transport of acetyl and long-chain acyl groups from extramitochondrial to intramitochondrial CoA (see Fig. 2). In this scheme it is assumed that acetyl-CoA formed in the peroxisomes is transported into the mitochondria via this carnitine-dependent mechanism.

the extramitochondrial compartment (Section 7). In the mitochondria, the fatty acids are broken down by β-oxidation to acetyl-CoA, which is converted to CO_2 and water in the citric acid cycle. In the liver mitochondria acetyl-CoA can also be converted to ketone bodies (Section 4.e). α-Oxidation of fatty acids also takes place in the mitochondria (Section 6).

It is important to recognize that acyl-CoA esters cannot penetrate the inner mitochondrial membrane. Hence, the need for carnitine to carry the activated fatty acid across this membrane (Section 4.a). The regulatory mechanisms of long-chain fatty acid metabolism seem to be localized mainly in the extramitochondrial compartment, and in the inner mitochondrial membrane.

(b) Short-chain fatty acids

The metabolism of short-chain fatty acids (C_{4-10}) is different from the long-chain fatty acids in that their activation to acyl-CoA by specific acyl-COA synthetases takes place in the mitochondrial matrix. The short-chain fatty acids therefore bypass the extramitochondrial processes and the carnitine-dependent transfer mechanism. Their metabolism consequently appears to be subjected to little regulation [9]. Once a short-chain fatty acid is taken up by a cell it is automatically oxidized to acetyl-CoA, irrespective of the physiological situation in the cell.

3. Fatty acid activation

Fatty acids are activated by a number of different acyl-CoA synthases. The physiologically most important characteristics of these enzymes are their fatty acid chain-length specificities, and their cellular localization. The overlapping of their chain-length specificities and their tissue distribution are such that any saturated or unsaturated fatty acids of chain lengths from C_2 to C_{22} or more can be activated in all animal tissues, although with differing rates [10,11]. These enzymes also activate long-chain dicarboxylic acids, branched-chain fatty acids, and carboxylic acids with other unusual groups. However, it should be noted that there are separate, specific enzymes for the activation of bile acids [12] and probably also for some aromatic carboxylic acids like salicylic acid [13].

Corresponding to the acyl-CoA synthases, a series of acyl-CoA hydrolases with variable chain-length specificities exist. But these enzymes have been less well characterized [14,15]. The function of the hydrolases, which convert the acyl-CoA thioesters back to free fatty acids, are probably to ensure that free CoA is always available for the cellular metabolism.

(a) Short- and medium-chain acyl-CoA synthases

(i) Acetyl-CoA synthase (EC 6.2.1.1)
Acetyl-CoA synthase has been isolated in crystalline form from heart mitochondria

[16,17]. It activates acetate with a K_m of approximately 1 mM. The enzyme also activates propionate, but with a lower rate and a higher K_m ($\sim$ 5 mM) [13]. In heart, skeletal muscle and kidney the enzyme is found only in the mitochondrial matrix. It permits activation of acetate to acetyl-CoA, which can then be oxidized in the citric acid cycle. In adipose tissue and in mammary gland it is found both in the mitochondria and in the extramitochondrial cytosol. In the liver the acetyl-CoA synthase is found only in the cytosol, while it is absent from the mitochondria [11]. The extramitochondrial localization in liver, adipose tissue and mammary gland reflects the utilization of acetate for the biosynthesis of long-chain fatty acids in these tissues.

The acetyl-CoA synthase and other short-chain acyl-CoA synthases are particularly important in ruminant animals where large amounts of acetate and other short carboxylic acids are formed by microorganisms in the rumen [18]. Free acetate is also formed in the liver, from ethanol by the alcohol and acetaldehyde dehydrogenases, and from fatty acids via β-oxidation and acetyl-CoA hydrolase under ketotic conditions in which both acetate and ketone bodies are end-products of fatty acid oxidation [19]. The absence of acetyl-CoA synthase from liver mitochondria and its presence in the mitochondria (and in the cytosol) of other tissues, explain why acetate is transported from the liver, and taken up and oxidized (or incorporated into fatty acid) in other tissues.

(ii) Propionyl-CoA synthase (EC 6.2.1.?)

Propionyl-CoA synthase has been purified from the matrix of liver mitochondria. It seems to be absent from other animal tissues where propionate is activated by the acetyl- and butyryl-CoA synthases [20,21]. Its localization and function can be seen in connection with the liver as the main organ for gluconeogenesis for which propionate is an important precursor, particularly in ruminants where propionate is formed in large amounts by microorganisms in the rumen [18].

(iii) Butyryl-CoA synthase (EC 6.2.1.?)

Butyryl-CoA synthase has been isolated from heart mitochondria [22]. It shows its highest activity with butyrate ($K_m \sim$ 1.5 mM), but it is active also with propionate and with carboxylic acids with chain lengths up to 7 carbons. It is found exclusively in the matrix of the mitochondria of heart and probably other extrahepatic tissues, but it has not been found in the liver.

(iv) Medium-chain acyl-CoA synthase (EC 6.2.1.2)

Medium-chain acyl-CoA synthase has been isolated from liver mitochondria [23]. This enzyme is distinctly different from the butyryl-CoA synthase of the heart. It has its highest reation rate with heptanoate, while its lowest K_m (0.15 mM) is obtained with octanoate as substrate. The enzyme is active with fatty acids of chain lengths from C_4 to C_{12}. The matrix of liver mitochondria also contains a second enzyme activating medium-chain-length fatty acids [20,25]. However, this enzyme is more active with benzoate, and also activates salicylate. Its specific function therefore is probably in the formation of glycine conjugates of aromatic carboxylic acids [24].

(b) Long-chain acyl-CoA synthase(s)

(i) Cellular localization

The long-chain acyl-CoA synthase (EC 6.2.1.3) originally found by Kornberg and Pricer [26] in liver microsomes, has since been established to be present also in the outer membrane of mitochondria [27,28] and in liver peroxisomes [29,30]. About 7% of the total long-chain acyl-CoA synthase activity of normal rat liver is found in the peroxisomes, and the remainder is about equally distributed between mitochondria and endoplasmic reticulum. Hence the different sites of fatty acid metabolism can activate free fatty acids as required by local demands (phospholipid and tri-acylglycerol synthesis in the endoplasmic reticulum, chain shortening in the peroxisomes, and (lyso)phosphatidic acid and acylcarnitine formation in the mitochondria). It is not known with certainty whether these separate acyl-CoA synthase activities result in separate pools of long-chain acyl-CoA in the cell. This is a possibility since it has been established that the yeast *Candida lipolytica* has two different long-chain acyl-CoA synthases, one which feeds fatty acids into cellular lipids and one which activates fatty acids for oxidation [31].

A slow activation of long-chain fatty acids can also take place in the matrix of the mitochondria. However, this activity is most likely due to a low, but detectable activity of the medium-chain acyl-CoA synthase with long-chain fatty acids as substrate [10,32].

(ii) Properties

The long-chain acyl-CoA synthases are firmly membrane-bound, and detergents have to be used in their purification. There is no general agreement about the properties of the long-chain acyl-CoA synthase(s). Maes and Bar-Tana [33] and Philip and Parson [34] have isolated microsomal and mitochondrial synthases with different peptides. However, Tanaka et al. [35] who have obtained the highest relative specific activities from their enzyme preparations, found the microsomal and the mitochondrial long-chain acyl-CoA synthases of rat liver to be identical, with the same molecular weight.

Kornberg and Pricer [26] found fatty acids of chain lengths C_{10}–C_{18} to be activated at approximately equal rates in microsomes, while shorter and longer fatty acids are activated at decreasing rates. A similar chain length specificity has been found for the purified microsomal and mitochondrial enzymes [34,35]. A somewhat different specificity has been found in fatty-acid-depleted rat-liver microsomes [36], where a distinct chain length optimum at C_{12} was found. Introduction of double bonds into long-chain fatty acids increases the activation rate.

In the intact cell its activity is probably regulated mainly by the availability of free fatty acids and CoA, and by product inhibition by acyl-CoA [37].

(c) Reaction mechanism of acyl-CoA synthases

The activation of acetate and of butyrate by the heart acetyl-CoA and butyryl-CoA synthases has been found to proceed in two steps [38,39]:

$$\text{Carboxylic acid} + \text{ATP Mg}^{2+} \quad \rightleftharpoons \quad \text{acyl-AMP} + \text{PP}_i$$

$$\text{Acyl-AMP} + \text{CoA} \quad \rightleftharpoons \quad \text{acyl-CoA} + \text{AMP}$$

The overall reaction is freely reversible, but in the tissues the reactions are driven to the right by pyrophosphatase and by the rephosphorylation of AMP. The acyl-AMP is bound to the enzyme and has only been isolated from experiments with substrate amounts of acetyl-CoA synthase or medium-chain acyl-CoA synthase [40]. However, it is doubtful that acyl-AMP exists as a physiological enzyme-bound intermediate in the activation of long-chain fatty acids [34,41,42]. Intermediary enzyme complexes were formed when enzyme was incubated with ATP and fatty acid, but acyl-AMP could not be identified. It has been suggested therefore that acyl-AMP is formed as a side-product or that it is formed only by "unphysiological" or conformationally changed forms of the medium-chain or long-chain acyl-CoA synthases.

(d) Acyl-CoA synthase (GDP-forming)

Besides the ATP-dependent acyl-CoA synthases a GTP-dependent acyl-CoA synthase (EC 6.2.1.?) has been found in the mitochondria of liver and other tissues [43]. It catalyzes the activation of fatty acids of widely different chain lengths in a reaction analogous to that of the succinate thiokinase:

$$\text{RCOOH} + \text{GTP} + \text{CoA} \quad \rightleftharpoons \quad \text{Acyl-CoA} + \text{GDP} + \text{P}_i$$

The enzyme requires phosphopantetheine as a cofactor suggesting that acylpantetheine may be an enzyme-bound intermediate [44]. Since the enzyme is localized in the mitochondrial matrix, it should permit carnitine-independent oxidation of long-chain fatty acids. However, the physiological significance of the enzyme is uncertain. It has a low activity compared with the ATP-dependent acyl-CoA synthases [45,46], and careful studies seem to show that it does not permit any significant carnitine-independent fatty acid oxidation [47].

4. Mitochondrial oxidation of fatty acids

(a) The function of carnitine

CoA esters of fatty acids are poorly oxidized by isolated, intact mitochondria, while they are well oxidized in the presence of carnitine [48]. Carnitine esters are rapidly oxidized [48,49], and simultaneously the mitochondrial pool of CoA is acylated [50]. These observations are explained by the presence of carnitine acyl transferases [51] and of a (acyl)carnitine translocase [52,53] in the inner membrane of the mitochondria. The carnitine acyltransferases catalyse the freely reversible reaction [6]:

$$\text{acyl-CoA} + \text{carnitine} \ \rightleftharpoons \ \text{acylcarnitine} + \text{CoA}$$

and the translocase makes the membrane permeable to carnitine and carnitine esters (Fig. 2).

Thus, the *O*-ester bond of acylcarnitine is unique in having a free energy similar to the thioester bond of acyl-CoA. The reversibility of the carnitine ester formation and the permeability of the mitochondria to carnitine esters also explain that acetylcarnitine is formed by isolated mitochondria oxidizing pyruvate [54,55]. Studies on isolated mitochondria have shown that each carnitine acyltransferase in the inner membrane is divided into two pools, functionally linked by the carnitine translocase. An outer transferase on the outer surface is accessible to cytosolic acyl-CoA, and an inner, latent pool on the inner surface is accessible to the separate CoA pool of the mitochondrial matrix [50,56]. The outer transferase can be selectively solubilized with digitonin. After removal of this outer transferase the mitochondria can still oxidize carnitine esters, but not CoA esters in the presence of carnitine [57]. The outer transferase shows the lower activity and is rate-limiting in the transfer of activated fatty acids into the mitochondria. It is likely that the outer and the inner carnitine acyltransferases are identical [58,59].

From chain-length specificity studies it has been suggested that 3 different carnitine acyltransferases exist, one carnitine acetyl, one carnitine octanoyl and one carnitine palmitoyl transferase with overlapping chain-length specificities [60–62]. However, in careful studies only 2 different carnitine acyltransferases could be isolated from heart mitochondria, one carnitine acetyltransferase, and one carnitine long-chain acyltransferase [63]. It is possible that the apparent presence of a separate octanoyltransferase may be attributed to different assay conditions and effects of the membrane environment on the chain-length specificity of the transferase [58,59].

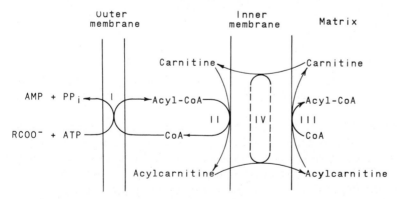

Fig. 2. Carnitine-dependent transport of acyl groups across the inner mitochondrial membrane. I, long-chain acyl-CoA synthase of the outer mitochondrial membrane; II, outer carnitine acyltransferase; III, inner carnitine acyltransferase; IV, carnitine translocase; PP_i, pyrophosphate.

Originally the carnitine acyltransferases were found only in the mitochondria [51], but more recently both carnitine acetyl transferase and carnitine octanoyltransferase have been found in the peroxisomes [64,67]. The carnitine acyltransferases in the peroxisomes may have a function in the transfer of acetyl and shortened fatty acid groups to the mitochondria after their chain shortening by partial β-oxidation in the peroxisomes [68] (see Section 5.b).

(i) Carnitine acetyltransferase (EC 2.3.1.7)

Carnitine acetyltransferase has been prepared in crystalline form from pigeon breast muscle [69]. It shows its highest activity with acetyl- and propionyl-CoA ($K_m \approx 0.4$ mM for both), but it also reacts, with declining rates, with acyl-CoA esters with chain lengths up to C_{10}.

The enzyme is inhibited by long-chain acyl-CoA esters. The enzyme forms a ternary complex with its substrates [70,71]. The enzyme is present in the mitochondria of all tissues with the highest activities in heart and testis, while the activity in the liver varies. It is relatively low in rat liver, while it is high in sheep and ox liver [72,73].

The carnitine acetyltransferase is also active with branched-chain acyl-CoA esters, and branched-chain acylcarnitines have been found in heart and other tissues oxidizing the α-ketoacids of branched-chain amino acids [74,75].

(ii) Carnitine palmitoyltransferase (EC 2.3.1.21)

Carnitine palmitoyltransferase has been purified from calf liver [61] and from ox heart [76]. The calf liver enzyme was found to be a dimer with a subunit molecular weight of 75 000. The beef heart enzyme was found to be a polymer with subunits of 67 000.

A peculiar feature of the carnitine palmitoyltransferase is that palmitoyl-CoA, beside being a substrate, also behaves as a competitive inhibitor to carnitine, the second substrate. This property of the enzyme can also be demonstrated in intact mitochondria [77,78]. The apparent K_m for carnitine is therefore strongly dependent on the palmitoyl-CoA concentration used. The K_i for palmitoyl-CoA against carnitine was found to be even lower than its K_m as substrate in the reaction. The physiological significance of this property of the enzyme may be to prevent excessively high acylcarnitine/carnitine ratios in the cell and "flooding" of the mitochondrial matrix with long-chain acyl-CoA under conditions with a rapid influx of fatty acids.

Both long-chain acyl-CoA and long-chain acylcarnitines are amphipatic compounds with low critical micellar concentrations and with the ability to bind to proteins and membrane surfaces. Hence the kinetic properties of the enzyme vary with the conditions, and are strongly influenced by detergents, presumably because of mixed micelle formation [63,79]. With purified or partially purified enzyme the following K_m values have been reported: palmitoyl-CoA, 10–30 μM; carnitine, 0.25–0.45 mM; CoA, 10–50 μM; palmitoylcarnitine, 40–140 μM.

The properties of the carnitine palmitoyltransferase are influenced by its environment in the mitochondrial membrane. The outer transferase in the membrane is inhibited by malonyl-CoA [80] while solubilized transferase is unaffected by malonyl-CoA. The inhibition of malonyl-CoA is probably an important regulatory mechanism in the oxidation of fatty acids. The inner transferase seems to lose appreciable activity on solubilization [59,81]. The carnitine palmitoyltransferase most probably forms a ternary complex with its substrates, and has a similar reaction mechanism as the carnitine acetyltransferase [77].

(iii) Carnitine translocase

Carnitine translocase catalyses a 1 : 1 exchange of carnitine and acylcarnitines across the inner mitochondrial membrane [82–84]. The translocase apparently also catalyses a slow unidirectional transport of carnitine [82,85]. The K_m for external carnitine is around 0.5–1.5 mM when measured close to 0°C, and much lower for acylcarnitines [86]. The K_m decreases with the chain length of the fatty acid [87]. The exchange rate also depends on the intramitochondrial concentration of carnitine. The exchange is 5–10 times faster with the (−)-carnitine isomer than with the (+) isomer (in contrast to the active transport of carnitine across the liver cell membrane which shows little or no stereospecificity [88]).

The K_m for carnitine exchange in the mitochondria is in the same range as the concentration of carnitine in the tissues, and the lower K_m for acylcarnitines indicates that the acylcarnitines are preferentially transported into the mitochondria. At 37°C the exchange capacity probably exceeds the capacity of the mitochondria to oxidize fatty acids by a wide margin. However, at low tissue concentrations of acylcarnitines the translocase may be rate-limiting for fatty acid oxidation, and the intramitochondrial acyl-CoA concentration may be kept low by a significant difference in the extra- and intra-mitochondrial acylcarnitine/carnitine ratios. A specific carnitine translocase protein has not been isolated.

(b) β-Oxidation enzymes of the mitochondria

When fatty acids have been converted to acyl-CoA esters in the matrix of the mitochondria, either by the carnitine-dependent transfer through the inner membrane of the mitochondria (long-chain fatty acids), or by the acyl-CoA synthases of the matrix (short-chain fatty acids), they are normally β-oxidized quantitatively to acetyl-CoA by the β-oxidation enzymes which are all present in the matrix [89].

The main reaction sequence of Fig. 3 shows how 4 consecutive enzyme reactions complete one β-oxidation cycle of saturated fatty acids, producing one acetyl-CoA and an acyl-CoA ester shortened by 2 carbons. The shortened acyl-CoA ester is then repeatedly β-oxidized until it has been completely converted to acetyl-CoA units. One β-oxidation cycle requires participation of the following enzymes: (a) acyl-CoA dehydrogenase; (b) enoyl-CoA hydratase (crotonase); (c) β-hydroxyacyl-CoA dehydrogenase; and (d) acyl-CoA:acetyl-CoA acyltransferase (thiolase).

(i) Acyl-CoA dehydrogenases

Three different acyl-CoA dehydrogenases (EC 1.3.99.2 and EC 1.3.99.3) with

122

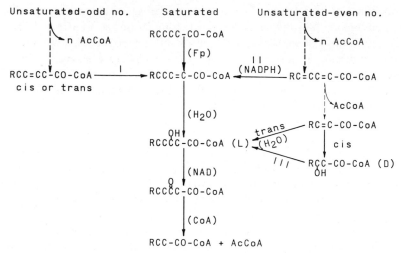

Fig. 3. Catabolism of saturated and unsaturated fatty acids. Abbreviations: AcCoA, acetyl-CoA; Fp, flavoprotein (acyl-CoA dehydrogenases); I, Δ^3,Δ^2-enoyl-CoA isomerase, converting *cis*- or *trans*-Δ^3-enoyl-CoA to Δ^2-*trans*-enoyl-CoA; II, 2,4-dienoyl-CoA reductase, converting 2,4-dienoyl-CoA to 2-enoyl-CoA with NADPH; III, β-hydroxyacyl-CoA epimerase, converting D-(−)-β-hydroxyacyl-CoA to L-(+)-β-hydroxyacyl-CoA.

different and overlapping chain length specificities have been isolated from the mitochondria of animal tissues (Fig. 4) [90–93]. All the enzymes are tetramers with similar molecular weights and similar amino acid compositions [92].

The acyl-CoA dehydrogenases have firmly bound FAD as prosthetic groups which are reduced to $FADH_2$ at the same time as the acyl-CoA is converted to a *trans*-2-enoyl-CoA. The reduced enzyme is reoxidized by a second flavoprotein, the electron-transfer flavoprotein [94]. From this, the electrons are fed into the mitochondrial electron-transport chain at the level of coenzyme-Q–cytochrome *b* [95]. In accordance with this path of electron flow, the oxidative phosphorylation linked to the acyl-CoA dehydrogenases has been shown to have a P/O ratio of 2 [96].

The acyl-CoA dehydrogenases have a strong affinity for their substrates ($K_s = 1–2$ μM) and for their enoyl-CoA reaction products [97]. The enzymes therefore show strong product inhibitions. They are also strongly inhibited by β-ketoacyl-CoA esters, a later intermediate in the β-oxidation sequence [93]. Both substrate and β-ketoacyl-CoA form charge-transfer complexes with the enzymes [98]. The inhibition by products, and by later β-oxidation intermediates, probably decreases the likelihood of accumulation of β-oxidation intermediates in the mitochondria.

(ii) Enoyl-CoA hydratases (crotonases)

Two enoyl-CoA hydratases have been isolated from pig-heart mitochondria, one short-chain crotonase (EC 4.2.1.17) and one long-chain crotonase [99–100]. The enzymes add water to the double bond by a stereospecific mechanism. The reaction

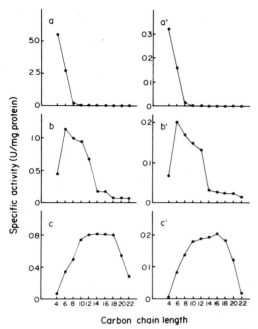

Fig. 4. Fatty acid chain length specificity of the three mitochondrial acyl-CoA dehydrogenases. a, short-chain acyl-CoA dehydrogenase; b, medium-chain acyl-CoA dehydrogenase; c, long-chain acyl-CoA dehydrogenase. The assays were performed with electron-transfer protein as electron acceptor (a, b, c) or with phenazine methosulphate as artificial electron acceptor (a', b', c'). (Reproduced from ref. 92 with the permission of the authors and of J. Biochem.) The figure shows why C_{22} fatty acids are poorly oxidized by mitochondria and why chain shortening of C_{22} fatty acids in peroxisomes facilitates their oxidation (see also Fig. 7).

is freely reversible. *trans*-2-Enoyl-CoA, the product of the acyl-CoA dehydrogenase reaction, is converted to the L-(+)-β-hydroxyacyl-CoA while *cis*-2-enoyl esters are converted to D-(−)-β-hydroxyacyl-CoA [101]. This stereospecificity is important in the oxidation of unsaturated fatty acids which usually contain *cis* double bonds. The short-chain crotonase reacts only poorly with 2,4-dienoyl-CoA esters [102,103], formed during oxidation of some unsaturated fatty acids (see Section 4.c).

The long-chain crotonase has a broad chain-length specificity [100]. The K_m is relatively independent of chain length (25 μM). The short-chain crotonase also reacts with branched-chain enoyl-CoA esters indicating that the enzyme is active in the breakdown of branched-chain amino acids and other compounds [99].

(iii) L-(+)-β-Hydroxyacyl-CoA dehydrogenases

The mitochondria contain 2 β-hydroxyacyl-CoA dehydrogenases (EC 1.1.1.35) with overlapping chain-length specificities. A short-chain dehydrogenase is found in the mitochondrial matrix, while a long-chain dehydrogenase is associated with the inner mitochondrial membrane [104]. The short-chain dehydrogenase has been purified [105]. The enzymes react with NAD and with the L-(+) isomer of β-hydroxyacyl-CoA, while it is completely inactive with the D-(−) isomer (the hydration reaction product of *cis*-enoyl-CoA).

(iv) Acetyl-CoA acyltransferases (thiolases)

Two different thiolases (EC 2.3.1.9 and EC 2.3.1.16) have been isolated from animal mitochondria [106] catalysing the reaction:

$$\beta\text{-ketoacyl-CoA} + \text{CoA} \quad \rightleftharpoons \quad \text{acyl-CoA} + \text{acetyl-CoA}$$

The reaction is strongly displaced to the right ($K_{eqv} = 10^5$ with acetoacetyl-CoA as substrate). One of the thiolases is capable of using β-ketoacyl-CoA esters of widely differing carbon-chain lengths as substrates. The other is specific for acetoacetyl-CoA [106]. These enzymes are active in fatty acid β-oxidation and ketogenesis. A third thiolase is localized in the cytosol and is specific for acetoacetyl-CoA. The function of the cytosolic enzyme [13] is to generate acetoacetyl-CoA for cholesterol biosynthesis [106]. All thiolases have been found to be tetramers with similar molecular weights [107].

The mitochondrial acetoacetyl-CoA thiolase has a K_m of approximately 10 μM for acetoacetyl-CoA and 80 μM for acetyl-CoA in the reverse reaction. The general thiolase reaction shows decreasing K_m with increasing chain length of the β-keto-acyl-CoA (2 μM with β-ketodecanoyl-CoA) [106–108]. The low K_m along with the displacement of the equilibrium toward cleavage of the β-ketoacids, will prevent accumulation of β-oxidation intermediates. An acetylated enzyme has been shown to be intermediate in the thiolase reaction [105,109].

(c) Oxidation of unsaturated fatty acids

Most natural unsaturated fatty acids contain *cis* double bonds. In polyun-saturated fatty acids the double bonds are spaced out with an interval of 3 carbons, i.e. the double bonds are alternately even and odd numbered. Therefore, when unsaturated fatty acids are β-oxidized, sooner or later Δ^3-*cis*-enoyl-CoA or Δ^2-*trans*-Δ^4-*cis*-dienoyl-CoA esters will appear as intermediates (Fig. 3). However, crotonase does not react with a double bond in the 3-position, and poorly with 2,4-dienoyl-CoA, presumably because of the resonance between the conjugated Δ^2 and Δ^4 double bonds. Also, if a Δ^2-*cis*-enoyl-CoA is formed, crotonase will catalyse the formation of the wrong optical isomer of β-hydroxyacyl-CoA which cannot be oxidized by the β-hydroxyacyl-CoA dehydrogenase in the mitochondria. However, the β-oxidation of unsaturated fatty acids is still possible due to 3 auxiliary mitochondrial enzymes, which transform these intermediates to normal β-odixation intermediates.

(i) Δ^3-cis-Δ^2-trans-enoyl-CoA isomerase (EC 5.3.3.−)

This isomerase is probably identical with the enzyme vinylacetyl-CoA isomerase (EC 5.3.3.3), which was the first to be discovered [110]. The isomerase converts a Δ^3 double bond to a Δ^2-*trans* double bond [111–114]. The reaction is freely reversible, and it should be noted that both Δ^3-*cis* and Δ^3-*trans* bonds are converted to a

Δ^2-*trans* bond. The enzyme therefore is active in the oxidation of unsaturated fatty acids with both *cis* and *trans* double bonds.

(ii) 2,4-Dienoyl-CoA 4-reductase

The mitochondria contain 2 enoyl-CoA reductases, one 2-enoyl reductase (EC 1.3.1.8), and one 2,4-dienoyl-CoA 4-reductase (EC 1.3.1.–) [115]. The 2,4-dienoyl reductase is also present in *E. coli* growing on unsaturated fatty acids [116]. Both enzymes use NADPH to reduce the double bonds. The function of the 2-enoyl-CoA reductase in the mitochondria is not known, but the 2,4-dienoyl-CoA 4-reductase is probably necessary for the degradation of unsaturated fatty acids [116]. Reduction of the 4-double bond in 2,4-dienoyl-CoA generates a normal β-oxidation intermediate, thus permitting the β-oxidation to proceed. The Δ^4 reductase reduces both *cis* and *trans* double bonds. This reaction is striking in two ways. A reducing step is part of a catabolic mitochondrial pathway, and it is NADPH dependent. In the mitochondria NADPH is formed mainly by the energy-dependent NADH:NADP transhydrogenase (EC 1.6.1.1)

$$NADH + NADP \rightarrow NAD + NADPH$$

In uncoupled mitochondria the level of NADPH will therefore be low, and this explains why oxidation of carnitine esters of unsaturated fatty acids with a 4-double bond is strongly inhibited in uncoupled mitochondria while the oxidation of saturated carnitine esters is unaffected by uncoupling [117]. The enzyme has also been found to be present in peroxisomes [118] (see also Fig. 9).

(iii) 3-Hydroxyacyl-CoA epimerase (EC 5.1.2.–)

3-Hydroxyacyl-CoA epimerase converts reversibly D-(–)-3-hydroxyacyl CoA, formed by crotonase from Δ^2-*cis*-enoyl-CoA, to L-(+)-3-hydroxyacyl-CoA which is subsequently oxidized by 3-hydroxyacyl-CoA dehydrogenase [111,119]. The epimerase has been assumed to have a quantitative important function in the oxidation of unsaturated fatty acids. However, the detection of 2,4-dienoyl-CoA 4-reductase, and the old observation that 2,4-dienoyl-CoA is a poor substrate for crotonase [102,103], indicate that the epimerase represents a minor pathway in the oxidation of unsaturated fatty acids.

(d) Functional characteristics of mitochondrial β-oxidation

When isolated mitochondria oxidise palmitoylcarnitine, almost all the mitochondrial CoA can be accounted for as palmitoyl-CoA and acetyl-CoA [120]. Very little free CoA is found, and very low levels of β-oxidation intermediates are present. This is partly explained by the properties of the β-oxidation enzymes which prevent accumulation of intermediates. The lack of intermediates is still surprising when it is considered that the oxidation of palmitoyl-CoA to acetyl-CoA proceeds through a total of 28 intermediates. Careful studies have shown the presence of some of these intermediates in mitochondria [121], and in the presence of free carnitine,

carnitine esters of these intermediates can even pass out of the mitochondria using the carnitine acyltransferase and the carnitine translocase system [122,123]. However, even these low concentrations of intermediates do not behave as true intermediates. Their turnover is too slow, and isotope chase experiments have shown that they show no precursor product relationship [121]. It has been suggested therefore that the β-oxidation enzymes are organized in a complex, and that the intermediates found represent intermediates which escape temporarily from the complex [121]. This complex must be loosely organized since it falls apart when the mitochondria are broken up. The acetyl-CoA formed seems to leave the complex to mix freely in the mitochondrial matrix with the acetyl-CoA formed by the pyruvate dehydrogenase complex, and it is freely available both for citrate synthesis and for ketogenesis in the mitochondrial matrix [124].

(e) Ketogenesis and ketone body utilization

In the liver, and to some extent in the kidneys, the acetyl-CoA formed by β-oxidation of fatty acids can either be completely oxidized to CO_2 and water in the citric acid cycle, or converted to ketone bodies (i.e. to acetoacetate and β-hydroxybutyrate). It can also be hydrolysed to free acetate which physiologically can be considered as a "ketone body". Since thiolase reversibly converts acetyl-CoA to acetoacetyl CoA it was originally assumed that acetoacetyl-CoA is hydrolysed to free acetoacetate. However, no such hydrolase could be isolated, and it was then established that free acetoacetate is formed from acetoacetyl-CoA and acetyl-CoA in a 2-enzyme process (Fig. 5). The first step is a condensation of acetoacetyl-CoA and acetyl-CoA to 3-hydroxy-3-methylglutaryl-CoA by the enzyme hydroxymethylglutaryl (HMG)-CoA synthase (EC 4.1.3.5). In the second step the HMG-CoA is cleaved to free acetoacetate and acetyl-CoA by HMG-CoA lyase (EC 4.1.3.4) [125].

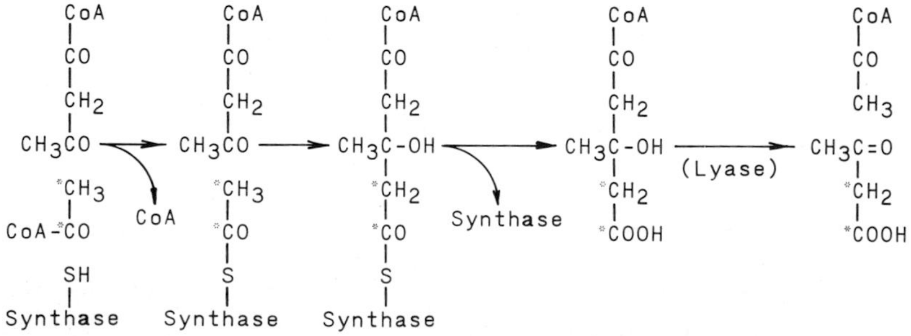

Fig. 5. The formation of acetoacetate from acetoacetyl-CoA and acetyl-CoA. An SH group of hydroxymethylglutaryl-CoA synthase is first acetylated by acetyl-CoA. The acetylated enzyme condenses with acetoacetyl-CoA to a hydroxymethylglutaryl-CoA synthase thioester complex which is hydrolysed to hydroxymethylglutaryl-CoA (HMG-CoA) and free synthase. The free HMG-CoA is finally cleaved to free acetoacetate and acetyl-CoA by the HMG-CoA lyase. Note that carbons of the free acetoacetate formed are not identical with the carbons of the acetoacetyl-CoA used. This explains that free acetoacetate can be asymmetrically labelled from labelled acetyl-CoA (marked with asterisks).

The second ketone body, D-(−)-β-hydroxybutyrate, is formed from acetoacetate and NADH by D-(−)-β-hydroxybutyrate dehydrogenase (EC 1.1.1.30):

$$Acetoacetate + NADH \quad \rightleftharpoons \quad \beta\text{-hydroxybutyrate} + NAD$$

It should be noted that this β-hydroxybutyrate is of a different optical configuration from the L-(+)-hydroxybutyryl-CoA which is formed as a β-oxidation intermediate from butyryl-CoA.

Under conditions with a rapid fatty acid oxidation (diabetes, starvation) significant amounts of free acetate are also formed in the liver by an acetyl-CoA hydrolase [19,126]. The ketone bodies and acetate formed in the liver are transported via the circulation to extrahepatic tissues. Here the acetate is converted back to acetyl-CoA by the acetyl-CoA synthase (EC 6.2.1.1). 3-Hydroxybutyrate is converted back to acetoacetate by the 3-hydroxybutyrate dehydrogenase, and the acetoacetate to acetoacetyl-CoA by the succinyl-CoA:acetoacetate-CoA transferase (EC 2.8.3.5). The action of thiolase generates 2-acetyl-CoA which is oxidized to CO_2 and water in the citric acid cycle.

Thus, an incomplete oxidation of fatty acids in the liver furnishes the extrahepatic tissues with readily oxidizable substrates. The oxidation of the fatty acids is thus completed.

(i) 3-Hydroxy-3-methyl glutaryl-CoA synthase (HMG-CoA synthase) (EC 4.1.3.5)

This synthase is found mainly in the matrix of liver mitochondria [127], but an immunologically different HMG synthase is also found in the cytosol of liver and other tissues [128]. The mitochondrial enzyme is active in ketogenesis, while the cytosolic enzyme has its main function in the biosynthesis of cholesterol.

In the formation of HMG-CoA an SH group on the enzyme is first acetylated by acetyl-CoA. The bound acetyl group then condenses with acetoacetyl-CoA to give a HMG-CoA-enzyme–thioester complex. The acyl-enzyme thioester bond is then hydrolysed to give free HMG-CoA [129,130] (Fig. 5). The K_m for acetoacetyl-CoA in this reaction is exceedingly low. The lowest value reported from direct enzyme kinetic studies is 0.35 μM [131].

However, under the assumption that the thiolase reaction is close to equilibrium in the mitochondria or in mitochondrial extracts, an assumption which is reasonable because of the high activity of the thiolase in the mitochondria [127], the K_m for acetoacetyl-CoA can be calculated to be less than 10^{-8} M (Fig. 6) [132,133]. The K_m for acetyl-CoA has been found to be approximately 0.1 mM. Thus, the rate of HMG-CoA formation and therefore ketogenesis is determined by the acetoacetyl-CoA concentration which again is determined by the acetyl-CoA/CoA ratio in the mitochondria. The acetyl-CoA concentration as such is probably of little importance since the enzyme will be nearly saturated with this substrate even under conditions when the rate of ketogenesis is slow. The correlation of a high rate of ketogenesis with a high acetyl-CoA/CoA ratio has been demonstrated both in whole liver and in isolated mitochondria [134,135].

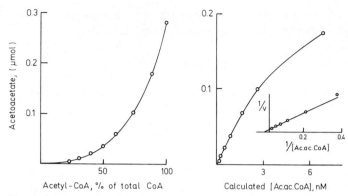

Fig. 6. The effect of acetyl-CoA/CoA ratio on the rate of ketogenesis in disrupted mitochondria. The acetyl-CoA/CoA ratio was varied by adding variable ratios of acetylcarnitine/carnitine and carnitine acetyl transferase. The acetyl-CoA/CoA ratio was calculated from the acetylcarnitine/carnitine ratio and the equilibrium constant of the reaction acetyl-CoA + carnitine $\rightleftharpoons$ acetylcarnitine + CoA ($K_{eqv} \approx 1.5$). The acetoacetyl-CoA concentrations was calculated from the equilibrium constant of the reaction: 2-acetyl-CoA $\rightleftharpoons$ acetoacetyl-CoA + CoA ($K_{eqv} \approx 10^{-5}$). Based on these calculations the inserted Lineweaver–Burk plot gave a K_m value for acetoacetyl-CoA of approximately 10^{-8} M. (Reproduced from ref. 132 with the permission of Academic Press.)

(ii) 3-Hydroxy-3-methylglutaryl-CoA lyase (EC 4.1.3.4)

This lyase is localized exclusively in the matrix of the mitochondria of the liver and the kidneys [136]. This localization is in agreement with the potential for ketogenesis in these organs [137]. Its K_m for HMG-CoA has been determined to be approximately 10 μM in the presence of Mg^{2+} which is required by the enzyme [138].

(iii) Hydroxybutyrate dehydrogenase (EC 1.1.1.30)

Hydroxybutyrate dehydrogenase is found firmly bound to the inner mitochondrial membrane in all tissues. The purified enzyme requires the presence of the phospholipid phosphatidyl choline to be active [139,140]. The reaction is freely reversible, and at pH 7.0 the $K_{eqv} = 5 \times 10^{-2}$. 3-Hydroxybutyrate is therefore easily formed [141]. In the inner mitochondrial membrane the enzyme "faces" inward toward the matrix [142]. Because of this, its has generally been assumed that the 3-hydroxybutyrate/acetoacetate ratio in the liver is in equilibrium with the NADH/NAD ratio in the matrix of the mitochondria [141]. This equilibrium has been utilized in studies of the mitochondrial redox status and the regulation of ketogenesis.

(iv) Acetyl-CoA hydrolase

This enzyme is present both in the mitochondria [126] and in the cytosol of the liver [143]. The mitochondrial enzyme can catalyse a relatively rapid formation of acetate in ketotic conditions. Free acetate is also formed as a major end-product of fatty acid oxidation in brown adipose tissue of the hamster. The brown adipose tissue hydrolase is strongly inhibited by free CoA. Thus, acetate is formed only when the acetyl-CoA/CoA ratio is high [144,145].

(v) Succinyl-CoA:acetoacetate-CoA transferase (EC 2.8.3.5)

Succinyl-CoA:acetoacetate-CoA transferase in the mitochondrial matrix has been isolated from pig heart [146]. Its activity is low in the liver [147]. It catalyses the reaction:

$$\text{succinyl-CoA} + \text{acetoacetate} \;\rightleftharpoons\; \text{acetoacetyl-CoA} + \text{succinate}$$

The enzyme with covalently bound CoA is an intermediate. The reaction is freely reversible, but the V_{max} is about 25 times faster in the direction of succinyl-CoA formation than in the direction of acetoacetyl-CoA formation, and the K_{eqv} of the reaction also favours succinyl-CoA formation. In spite of the unfavourable equilibrium acetoacetate is efficiently converted to acetoacetyl-CoA in extrahepatic tissues, and relatively high acetoacetyl-CoA concentrations have been found in hearts of diabetic rats [131] and in isolated hearts perfused with acetoacetate [148].

In the mitochondria the CoA transferase competes for succinyl-CoA with the reversed reaction of succinyl-CoA synthase (EC 6.2.1.4) [149]. Thus, the efficient uptake of acetoacetate in the heart evidently requires a high succinyl-CoA/succinate ratio in the mitochondria.

The presence of succinyl-CoA:acetoacetate-CoA transferase in the liver, which normally does not utilize ketone bodies is surprising. It has been suggested that it has a function in the regulation of ketogenesis [147].

5. Peroxisomal fatty acid oxidation

The presence of a β-oxidation system outside the mitochondrial compartment was first described in glyoxysomes from germinating castor bean endosperm [150,151], and subsequently in peroxisomes in Tetrahymena [152] and Euglena [153], and finally in rat-liver peroxisomes [68]. Peroxisomal β-oxidation is probably also present in other mammalian tissues [154–157].

Although the reactions involved during peroxisomal β-oxidation are identical to those of mitochondrial β-oxidation, the enzymes are quite distinct from their mitochondrial counterparts. No requirement for $(-)$-carnitine has been observed in peroxisomal β-oxidation, fatty acyl-CoA esters formed by peroxisomal acyl-CoA synthase appear to be immediate substrates for oxidation [158,159]. However, peroxisomes contain a medium-chain carnitine acyltransferase as well as carnitine acetyltransferase [67]. It has been assumed that these enzymes have a role in the transfer of β-oxidation products from the peroxisomes to the mitochondria.

(a) β-Oxidation enzymes of peroxisomes

(i) Acyl-CoA oxidase

This is the initial enzyme of the β-oxidation sequence and catalyses the following reaction [160]:

$$\text{fatty acyl-CoA} + O_2 \rightarrow \textit{trans}\text{-2-enoyl-CoA} + H_2O_2$$

The enzyme is an oxygenase and has FAD as the prosthetic group. This is reduced to $FADH_2$ during the reaction, and reoxidized to FAD by direct interaction with O_2. This cycle leads to the formation of H_2O_2. The enzyme has a very high affinity for O_2 ($K_m = 5$ μM). The FAD may be relatively loosely bound to the enzyme. The K_m for acetyl-CoA esters is about 10 μM for substrates of chain lengths of 14–18 carbon atoms. With shorter acyl-CoA esters the K_m increases markedly (about 60 μM for octanoyl-CoA).

Denaturing conditions revealed 3 different polypeptides, although this may be due to proteolytic cleavage of a single polypeptide chain [161,162].

(ii) 2-Enoyl-CoA hydratase and β-hydroxyacyl-CoA dehydrogenase

The 2-enoyl-CoA hydratase activity and the β-hydroxyacyl-CoA dehydrogenase activity of peroxisomes have been shown to copurify on one single polypeptide [163,164]. This is markedly different from the mitochondrial activities which reside on separate protein molecules. The reactions catalysed are:

$$trans\text{-}2\text{-}enoyl\text{-}CoA \xrightarrow{\;H_2O\;} L\text{-}(+)\text{-}hydroxyacyl\text{-}CoA \xrightarrow{\;NAD^+\;\;NADH\;} \beta\text{-}ketoacyl\text{-}CoA$$

This enzyme has been identified as the polypeptide which increases markedly in rat liver and kidney cortex on treatment with hypolipidaemic drugs like clofibrate and with di(2-ethyl-hexyl)phthalate [165,166]. These substances are known to cause induction of peroxisomal β-oxidation (Section 8.c). In comparison to mitochondrial hydratase the peroxisomal hydratase activity shows relatively higher rates of reaction with 2-enoyl-CoA ester of carbon chain length 12, as compared to a chain length of 4 carbon atoms [167]. The K_m is higher with the shorter chain length substrates [164]. The β-hydroxyacyl-CoA dehydrogenase activity has been shown to be unable to utilize acetoacetyl-pantetheine as a substrate in the reversed reaction, in contrast to the mitochondrial dehydrogenase [168].

(iii) Acetyl-CoA acyltransferase (thiolase)

The peroxisomal β-ketoacyl-CoA thiolase has been isolated and shown to be immunologically different from both the two mitochondrial thiolases and the cytosolic acetoacetyl-CoA thiolase. The apparent K_m values for β-keto-octanoyl-CoA and acetoacetyl-CoA are about 8 μM. The thiolase is about 20 times more active towards β-keto-octanoyl-CoA than to acetoacetyl-CoA. With the general β-keto-acetyl-CoA thiolase from mitochondria this ratio of activities is only about 4-fold [169]. The peroxisomal thiolase is therefore maximally active only with substrates of long chain lengths.

(b) Functional characteristics of peroxisomal β-oxidation

Because peroxisomal β-oxidation does not depend on any direct connection with an electron-transport chain, it is possible to have active β-oxidation in detergent-solubilized peroxisomal preparations. With mitochondrial β-oxidation this is nearly impossible since the flow of electrons from the acyl-CoA dehydrogenase to the electron-transport chain is disrupted on solubilization. Peroxisomal β-oxidation is even stimulated by solubilization [159]. The use of solubilized preparations therefore provides a means of detecting this activity with maximal sensitivity.

In solubilized peroxisomes, addition of both CoA and NAD is required for β-oxidative activity [68]. With intact peroxisomes incubated in an iso-osmotic medium, however, no requirement for exogenous CoA was found [159], but added NAD was still essential. Thus, the peroxisomes, like mitochondria, have a separate CoA pool and they can function without having to compete for CoA with cytosolic CoA-requiring reactions [170,171].

The finding of a peroxisomal pool of CoA implies a peroxisomal membrane with regulated permeability for CoA and acyl-CoA, and a carrier for acyl-CoA in the peroxisomal membrane has been suggested [172]. The activity of this permease may be influenced by the acyl-CoA/CoA ratio in the cytosol since the oxidation of palmitoyl-, myristoyl-, and lauroyl-CoA is inhibited by free CoA. However, it is striking that added CoA has little or no effect on peroxisomal oxidation of longer acyl-CoA esters like erucoyl- and eladioyl-CoA, both of which are poorly oxidized by mitochondria [159,173,174]. Thus, the peroxisomes may show a certain preference for the longest fatty acids in the intact cell.

One outstanding difference between peroxisomal and mitochondrial β-oxidation is that fatty acids are incompletely oxidized by peroxisomes. Both with solubilized and intact peroxisomes, long-chain acyl-CoA has been found to undergo 2–5 cycles

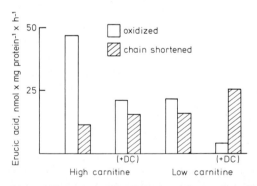

Fig. 7. Effect of carnitine and of (+)-decanoylcarnitine, 2 mM, (+DC), an inhibitor of carnitine-dependent acyl transfer through the mitochondrial membrane on the metabolism of [14-^{14}C]erucic acid (C$_{22:1}$) in isolated hepatocytes. The "high-carnitine" hepatocytes contained approximately 2 nmoles carnitine/mg protein, the "low-carnitine" hepatocytes approximately 0.3 nmole/mg protein. Chain shortening represent the sum of C$_{16}$, C$_{18}$, and C$_{20}$ radioactive fatty acids recovered from the cellular lipids. Oxidation products represent acid-soluble reaction products. The figure shows that the complete oxidation of erucic acid is carnitine dependent, while the extramitochondrial, peroxisomal shortening is not. When mitochondrial oxidation is inhibited, more of the shortened products are incorporated into the cellular lipids. (Reproduced from ref. 249 with the permission of Biochim. Biophys. Acta.)

of β-oxidation [68,158,174,175]. In accordance with these properties of peroxisomes it is established that very-long-chain fatty acids (e.g. erucic acid, $C_{22:1}$) are subjected to extramitochondrial chain shortening both by perfused livers [176], isolated hepatocytes [177] (Fig. 7), and by isolated peroxisomes [178].

Since C_{22} fatty acids are poor substrates for mitochondria, chain shortening of these fatty acids leads to fatty acids which are more easily oxidized by the mitochondria. Peroxisomal β-oxidation of these fatty acids therefore becomes a mechanism by which poorly oxidizable fatty acids are converted to metabolically more palatable products. As this is achieved by chain shortening, rather than complete oxidation, a minimum of metabolic energy is wasted.

Peroxisomal β-oxidation has also been suggested to be involved in the chain shortening of the cholesterol side-chain taking place during biosynthesis of bile acids [179]. It is also possible that β-oxidation in the peroxisomes may be a chain-shortening mechanism for long-chain dicarboxylic acids formed during fatty acid ω-oxidation (see Section 7).

(c) Hepatic capacities for peroxisomal β-oxidation

In terms of capacity to generate acetyl groups, the capacity of the peroxisomes is relatively low, being around 10% of the mitochondrial capacity in rats treated with clofibrate or fed on partially hydrogenated marine oil diet [174,180]. This may not provide the most relevant estimate of peroxisomal β-oxidative capacity. If chain shortening of fatty acids is considered a major function of peroxisomal β-oxidation, then it is the peroxisomal capacity to chain shorten e.g. a $C_{22:1}$ fatty acid which is significant. The peroxisomal capacity to chain shorten a $C_{22:1}$ fatty acid may be as much as 100–300% of the mitochondrial capacity to oxidize this fatty acid. Hence there appears to be a peroxisomal capacity which would be of significant physiological value.

Patients suffering from the inheritable disease adrenoleukodystrophy show accumulation of very long fatty acids (C_{25} and C_{26}) in adrenals as well as in the central nervous system. This may be due to a defect in peroxisomal β-oxidation [181].

6. α-Oxidation of fatty acids

Several systems for α-oxidation of fatty acids have been found in nature. In plant leaves α-oxidation of long-chain fatty acids by oxygenase(s) has been found to be a quantitative important pathway for shortening of fatty acids [182] (see Chapter 7).

A related, but apparently different reaction sequence using hydrogen peroxide as oxidizing substrate has been found in peanut cotyledon [183]. In the animal brain, relatively great amounts of α-hydroxy acids (cerebronic acid, 1-hydroxy-C_{24}) are found in the cerebrocides and other complex lipids. In brain microsomes, lignoceric acid (C_{24}) and lignoceroyl-CoA is converted to cerebronic acid by a mixed-function oxygenase, which requires O_2 and NADPH. In vitro the cerebronic acid is recovered in ceramide. Lignoceroyl-CoA as such does not seem to be a direct substrate in the hydroxylation [184].

The breakdown of the α-hydroxy fatty acids also takes place in brain microsomes. In the presence of NAD and O_2 the hydroxy acid is converted to the $n-1$ carboxylic acid and CO_2. The α-keto acid is assumed to be an intermediate in the reaction [185].

In liver and kidney an α-oxidation system different from that of brain is present. This α-oxidizes branched-chain fatty acids which cannot be β-oxidized because of a methyl group in the 3-position, e.g. phytanic acid, (3,7,11,15-tetramethyl palmitic acid). Phytanic acid is formed in the animal body from phytol, the alcohol side-chain of chlorophyll [186]. Small amounts of phytanic acid are also present in butter [187].

Tracer studies have shown that 3-methyl fatty acids are first chain shortened by 1 carbon by α-oxidation. Then they can undergo β-oxidation, presumably giving propionyl-CoA as a reaction product [188,189].

$$RCH_2 - \underset{\underset{CH_3}{|}}{CH} - CH_2 - COOH \xrightarrow{\alpha - ox} RCH_2 - \underset{\underset{CH_3}{|}}{CH} - COOH \xrightarrow{\beta - ox}$$

$$RCO\underset{\underset{CH_3}{|}}{CH} - COOH \longrightarrow RCOOH + CH_3CH_2COOH$$

It is not known whether it is the CoA ester which is α-oxidized. The α-oxidation of phytanic acid has been shown to take place in isolated liver mitochondria where it is stimulated by O_2, NADP(H) and ferric ions. α-Hydroxyphytanic acid was isolated as a reaction product, as were products of subsequent β-oxidation [190].

An inborn error of metabolism (Refsum's disease) has been described where the ability to oxidize phytanic acid is lacking. In these patients phytanic acid accumulates in blood and tissues [191].

7. ω-Oxidation of fatty acids

Ordinary straight-chain free fatty acids can be ω-oxidized to dicarboxylic acids in the animal body. The long-chain dicarboxylic acids are subsequently shortened by β-oxidation, and excreted as C_6-C_{10} dicarboxylic acids in the urine [192]. The rate of ω-oxidation is stimulated during starvation and in diabetes [193–195]. However, for normal straight-chain fatty acids the ω-oxidation is quantitatively a minor pathway [196,197].

The pathway acquires more significance for branched-chain or substituted fatty acids which are poorly, or not at all oxidized by normal β-oxidation [198,199].

2,2-Dimethylstearic acid can only be ω-oxidized, and nearly 100% of the ingested fatty acid is excreted in the urine as 2,2-dimethyladipic acid, which evidently is formed by ω-oxidation followed by β-oxidation from the ω end [200]. The first reaction step in ω-oxidation is the ω-hydroxylation of the free fatty acid. This is catalysed by a mixed-function oxidase system in the endoplasmic reticulum. The system is related to, or identical with, the drug-hydroxylating enzyme system [201,202] and involves cytochrome P-450 and a cytochrome P-450 reductase (a flavoprotein). It requires NADPH and O_2 for activity:

$$\text{NADPH} \diagdown \quad \diagup \text{P-450} \qquad\qquad \xleftarrow{\quad H_2O \quad} \quad \text{—CH}_2\text{OH}$$
$$\text{NADP} \diagup \quad \diagdown \text{P-450 red.} \qquad \xrightarrow{\quad O_2 \quad} \quad \text{—CH}_3$$

In microorganisms (Pseudomonas) a different system involving rubredoxin, (a non-haem iron protein) and rubredoxin reductase, requiring NADH and oxygen, is active [203]. The main reaction product is an ω-hydroxy fatty acid, but some ($\omega - 1$)-hydroxy fatty acid is also formed [204]. The ω-hydroxy fatty acids are subsequently oxidized to dicarboxylic acids by alcohol and aldehyde dehydrogenases present in the endoplasmic reticulum and the cytosol of the cell [205].

The long-chain dicarboxylic acids formed can be activated to the corresponding mono-CoA esters, presumably by the long-chain acyl-CoA synthase in the endoplasmic reticulum or the mitochondria [206,207]. Monocarboxyl esters of carnitine can also be formed. These have been shown to be oxidized in the mitochondria, although at a slow rate as compared to carnitine esters of monocarboxylic acids [208].

A second possibility for the β-oxidation of the dicarboxylic mono-CoA esters is the chain-shortening β-oxidation system of the peroxisomes. This possibility has not been investigated. However, studies of the source of extramitochondrial acetyl-CoA for the hepatic acetylation of 2-amino-4-phenylbutyric acid may be taken to indicate that the peroxisomes are active in the chain shortening of dicarboxylic acids [209].

Theoretically ω-oxidation of fatty acids can give succinate and therefore net production of glucose. It is unlikely that this mechanism is of any quantitative importance for gluconeogenesis [195].

8. Regulation of fatty acid oxidation

Numerous studies on perfused livers, isolated liver cells, and perfused hearts have shown that the rates of fatty acid oxidation and of ketogenesis depend on the concentration of free fatty acids offered to the tissues [210–214].

The rate of fatty acid oxidation also correlates with high levels of long-chain acyl-CoA and long-chain acylcarnitine esters in the tissues [215,216]. Hence lipolysis in adipose tissue is an important regulatory process as regards rates of fatty acid oxidation in all animal tissues. However, especially in the liver, the rate of fatty acid oxidation and ketogenesis also depends on the nutritional and hormonal state of the tissue. This is illustrated by the findings that isolated, perfused livers from fasted, fat-fed, diabetic, or thyrotoxic animals oxidize more, and esterify less, of incoming fatty acids than do livers from normal animals fed on carbohydrates. In the following, some main characteristics of regulatory mechanisms of fatty acid oxidation and ketogenesis are discussed.

(a) Effect of competing substrates

The slow rate of oxidation of fatty acids in the liver, and other tissues, in the fed state might be due to relative abundance of other substrates, primarily pyruvate and extramitochondrial NADH from glycolysis, and intermediates in the citric acid cycle, which all compete with β-oxidation of fatty acids for NAD and for access to a shared electron-transport chain. However, experiments with isolated mitochondria have shown that it is difficult to suppress oxidation of fatty acids once they have reached the mitochondrial matrix. Pyruvate and most of the citric acid cycle intermediates have only a weak ability to suppress fatty acid oxidation [122,217], while fatty acids have the ability to inhibit pyruvate [218] and citrate oxidation almost completely [219–221]. This domination by the β-oxidation sequence, when activated fatty acids are available in the matrix of the mitochondria, will accelerate acetyl-CoA formation and the electron-transport chain will become more reduced. Consequently the NADH/NAD ratio increases. This increased NADH/NAD ratio inhibits the NAD-dependent oxidation of isocitrate and α-ketoglutarate and displaces the malate/oxaloacetate equilibrium towards malate. The increased rate of acetyl-CoA formation, and the decreased availability of oxaloacetate for citrate formation, will increase the acetyl-CoA/CoA ratio and the rate of ketogenesis. Hence ketogenesis can be seen as an automatic "overflow" phenomenon [222].

Paradoxically, extramitochondrial NADH is a stronger competing substrate against fatty acid oxidation than is the NADH generated intramitochondrially from citric acid cycle intermediates [223]. This is explained by the active transfer of reducing equivalents into the mitochondria via the malate–aspartate and glycerophosphate shuttles. The active transport of aspartate out of the mitochondria combined with transamination will very efficiently remove oxaloacetate from the mitochondria and increase the NADH/NAD ratio by pulling the malate dehydrogenase reaction towards oxaloacetate formation. However, the citric acid cycle is even more inhibited than is β-oxidation. This mechanism explains why alcohol, which generates rapid extramitochondrial NADH formation via alcohol dehydrogenase, inhibits fatty acid oxidation [224]. However, the preferential oxidation of fatty acid carnitine esters in mitochondria suggests that fatty acid oxidation is regulated mainly by their rate of synthesis in the cell.

(b) Effect of metabolites and cofactors

(i) Malonyl-CoA
Malonyl-CoA has been found to be a strong inhibitor of the outer carnitine palmitoyl transferase [225]. When animals are fed carbohydrates, acetyl-CoA carboxylation is stimulated. The level of malonyl-CoA is increased, and fatty

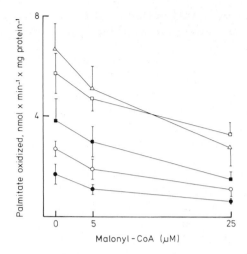

Fig. 8. Effect of fasting, thyroid state and of malonyl-CoA on the carnitine-dependent oxidation of palmitoyl-CoA in isolated liver mitochondria. [1-^{14}C]Palmitoyl-CoA (70 μM), carnitine (1 mM) and malate (5 mM), were incubated in the presence of 1% bovine serum albumin with liver mitochondria from normal rats (■), normal, fasted rats (□), hypothyroid rats treated with thiouracil (●), hypothyroid, fasted rats (○), and hyperthyroid rats treated with triiodothyronine (△). Malonyl-CoA was added as shown. Oxidation was measured as acid-soluble radioactivity. For experimental details, see refs. 230 and 273. The bars represent standard deviation of results obtained with 3–5 different mitochondrial preparations.

oxidation is inhibited. Studies have shown that there is an inverse correlation between the level of malonyl-CoA and the rate of fatty acid oxidation. The outer carnitine palmitoyl transferase is sensitive to malonyl-CoA in all tissues tested, and it is striking that the enzyme is most readily inhibited in muscle and adipose tissue [226].

The malonyl-CoA inhibition is overcome by high concentrations of long-chain acyl-CoA. The effect of malonyl-CoA in the liver appears to be modified by changes in the mitochondria themselves (Fig. 8). In liver mitochondria isolated from fasted rats, oxidation of fatty acids is relatively less inhibited by malonyl-CoA, as compared to mitochondria from fed animals [227–229]. This is explained both by a selective increase in the activity of the outer carnitine palmitoyl transferase and by a decreased sensitivity of the enzyme to the inhibitor. The total carnitine palmitoyl transferase activity is unchanged [230]. The cause of this change in sensitivity is not known. Both different ions [231], thiol group reagents [232], and phospholipase [233] have been shown to change the activity of the outer carnitine palmitoyl transferase.

(ii) Glycerophosphate

It has been speculated that variations in the tissue concentration of glycerophosphate primarily regulate the rate of triglyceride formation, and therefore indirectly the rate of fatty acid oxidation. However, in the liver no general inverse correlation between the concentration of glycerophosphate and the rate of fatty acid oxidation has been found [234]. However, the enzyme glycerophosphate acyltransferase shows changes in activity. This enzyme is found both in endoplasmic reticulum and in the outer mitochondrial membrane [235]. The activity of the mitochondrial glycerophosphate acyltransferase decreases on fasting, while the activity of the outer carnitine acyltransferase increases [236,237]. The glycerophosphate acyltransferase apparently has a K_m for palmitoyl-CoA which is lower than that of carnitine palmitoyl transferase. In accordance with these observations glycerophosphate has a trapping effect on fatty acids in isolated mitochondria [236] and in isolated liver cells [238]. This decreases formation of acylcarnitine, and hence the rate of fatty acid oxidation.

The microsomal glycerophosphate acyltransferase shows no corresponding variations in activity [237]. This hypothesis therefore depends on the assumption that there is no homogenous extramitochondrial pool of long-chain acyl-CoA and that it is primarily the long-chain acyl-CoA synthase of the outer mitochondrial membrane, which activates fatty acids for oxidation. This idea has gained support from the observation that separate acyl-CoA synthases are active in the oxidation and esterification of fatty acids in *Candida lipolytica* [31].

(iii) Carnitine

In the liver the concentration of carnitine increases in fasting and in diabetic animals [73,87,239]. Since carnitine can stimulate fatty acid oxidation in isolated hepatocytes [213] this can contribute to the increased rate of fatty acid oxidation observed in the liver of fasting animals. However, no essential correlation between fatty acid oxidation rate and carnitine level exists [234]. The effect of carnitine, therefore, is evidently modified by e.g. malonyl-CoA. Carnitine is both actively taken up from the plasma and relased by the liver. The uptake of carnitine in the liver is stimulated by glucagon [82,239]. It is therefore likely that the distribution of carnitine in the body is under hormonal control.

(iv) Coenzyme A

In the liver the total concentration of CoA approximately doubles both in the whole tissue and in the mitochondria during fasting [240]. The initial, and rate-limiting, step in the biosynthesis of coenzyme A is pantothenate kinase (EC 2.7.1.33). The enzyme is inhibited by acetyl-CoA [241]. This seems paradoxical as the concentration of acetyl-CoA in the liver goes up in fasting animals [242]. However, it is the mitochondrial acetyl-CoA which goes up in fasting and ketotic states, while the cytosolic acetyl-CoA/CoA ratio is decreased [243]. Thus, the activity of pantothenate kinase will increase and more phosphopantothenate, phosphopantetheine, and CoA will be formed. The mitochondrial CoA is synthesized from extramitochondrial phosphopantetheine which is transferred to the mitochondria, where the synthesis of mitochondrial CoA is completed [244]. Since there is a close correlation between the level of long-chain acyl-CoA in tissues and the rate of fatty acid oxidation [242–245] it seems likely that the availability of CoA is of importance.

(c) Inducible changes in peroxisomal and mitochondrial β-oxidation

High-fat diets, particularly diets containing a high proportion of fatty acids which are poorly oxidized by mitochondria, lead to induction of peroxisomal β-oxidation [180,246]. Starvation and diabetes have the same effect [247,248]. All these conditions cause increased hepatic influx of fatty acids and consequently increased β-oxidation. Hence, peroxisomal β-oxidation is induced under conditions requiring high β-oxidative capacity, and it can be considered as an inducible, auxiliary system under these conditions.

The greater induction obtained with high-fat diets containing large amounts of fatty acids which are poorly oxidized by the mitochondria [180], suggests that the peroxisomal β-oxidation plays a specific role by shortening these fatty acids. In accordance with such a function, animals adapted to diets containing long-chain *trans* fatty acids and C_{22} fatty acids show an increased hepatic capacity to shorten and oxidize such fatty acids [8,176,249].

Peroxisomal β-oxidation is also induced by a number of non-physiological substances, all of which are hypolipidaemic [168,250]. The best known example is probably clofibrate [58], which has been used clinically to treated various hyperlipidaemic disorders. Another such substance is the commonly used plasticizer di(2-ethylhexyl)phthalate [76]. These compounds cause peroxisomal proliferation [251,252] and increase hepatic peroxisomal β-oxidation 5–10-fold [68]. Peroxisomal β-oxidation is therefore a highly inducible activity. A diet which is deficient in vitamin E also leads to induction of hepatic peroxisomal β-oxidation in rats [253].

However, not only the peroxisomal activity is inducible. The mitochondrial β-oxidative activity is also affected, but to a lesser extent. A high-fat diet increases the rates of oxidation of acyl-CoA esters by isolated mitochondria by at least 50% [180]. Treatment of rats with hypolipidaemic agents causes induction of additional carnitine acetyl transferase [254], carnitine palmitoyl transferase [254], acyl-CoA dehydrogenase [255], 2,4-dienoyl-CoA 4-reductase [117] and electron-transfer protein [255] in liver mitochondria. The total mitochondrial mass is also increased [256].

Mitochondrial rates of oxidation of short-chain fatty acids (per mg of mitochondrial protein) are increased in rats given low doses of clofibrate (0.3% in the diet) while the oxidation of long-chain fatty acids is nearly unaffected [257]. However, with higher levels of clofibrate in the diet a doubling of the rate of long-chain fatty acid oxidation can be observed (H. Osmundsen, unpublished results).

Altogether, it is striking that hypolipidaemic drugs and high-fat diets have remarkably similar effects on the metabolism of fatty acids in the liver and trigger similar adaptative mechanisms.

(d) Effect of hormones

(i) Insulin and glucagon
Metabolic states associated with a rapid rate of fatty acid oxidation (starvation,

diabetes) always correlate with low insulin/glucagon ratios.

There is no known unambiguous, direct effect of insulin on fatty acid oxidation. Indirectly, however, it has marked effects. In adipose tissue it inhibits lipolysis, thus decreasing the concentration of free fatty acids in the blood and availability of fatty acids for oxidation. It stimulates acetyl-CoA carboxylation and lipogenesis in the liver, thus inhibiting fatty acid oxidation by the malonyl-CoA mechanism [255,258]. It also increases the activity of the mitochondrial glycerophosphate acyltransferase [259] and may thus divert fatty acids from oxidation to esterification.

Glucagon and cyclic AMP stimulate fatty acid oxidation in perfused livers [260] and in isolated hepatocytes [213]. Also with glucagon the effect appears to be mainly indirect. It stimulates gluconeogenesis which will drain citric acid cycle intermediates (oxaloacetate) from the mitochondria, and accordingly stimulate ketogenesis. It inhibits acetyl-CoA carboxylase. Therefore the tissue level of malonyl-CoA is decreased, and inhibition of fatty acid oxidation is relieved. In isolated hepatocytes it also decreases the concentration of glycerophosphate, probably via a stimulated gluconeogenesis [238,261,262]. This may decrease the rate of fatty acid esterification, and make more acyl-CoA available for oxidation.

Pretreatment of rats with glucagon in vivo has been reported to have a long series of stimulatory effects on metabolism in subsequently isolated liver mitochondria [263]. Among these effects are increased rates of octanoate and octanoylcarnitine oxidation. The latter may be due to an increased activity of the carnitine translocase [264]. The activity of the liver translocase is also increased in fasting and diabetic rats [87].

(ii) Vasopressin

Vasopressin inhibits fatty acid oxidation in isolated hepatocytes, and this inhibition is dependent on the presence of Ca^{2+} ions in the medium [265]. The mechanism of vasopressin action may be complex. It stimulates glycolysis and lactate formation in hepatocytes, and it also stimulates the activity of acetyl-CoA carboxylase, increasing the formation of malonyl-CoA [266]. Lactate is an inhibitor of fatty acid oxidation [210], partly by furnishing extramitochondrial reducing equivalents for oxidation in the mitochondria [223]. Vasopressin is believed to increase the cytosolic concentration of Ca^{2+} [267]. Ca^{2+} in physiological concentrations is also a strong inhibitor of fatty acid oxidation in isolated mitochondria (Borrebaek, unpublished; J. McMillin Wood, personal communication).

Ca^{2+} has no effect on the carnitine palmitoyl transferase. The mechanism of the Ca^{2+} effect on β-oxidation is not known, and the importance of this effect on fatty acid oxidation in relation to other regulatory mechanisms of fatty acid oxidation is still uncertain.

(iii) Thyroid hormones

Thyroid hormones facilitate the release of free fatty acids in adipose tissue [268], and they also influence metabolism of fatty acids in the liver. In thyrotoxic livers the rates of fatty acid oxidation are increased, and the rate of esterification is decreased

[269–272]. These effects correlate with an increased activity of the outer carnitine palmitoyl transferase in liver mitochondria isolated from rats treated with triiodothyronine [273]. When thiouracil-treated hypothyroid rats and triiodothyronine-treated rats are compared, the activity of the outer carnitine palmitoyl transferase in liver mitochondria is 4 times higher in the triiodothyronine-treated animals (Fig. 8). The total carnitine palmitoyl transferase was nearly unchanged. This hormone therefore has an effect on the distribution of this enzyme in the inner membrane of the liver mitochondria, and these results confirm that the activity of the outer carnitine palmitoyl transferase has a dominating effect on the rate of fatty acid oxidation. No corresponding effect of triiodothyronine has been found in heart mitochondria.

(iv) Adrenal cortex hormones

The glucocorticoid hormones have an ambiguous effect on fatty acid oxidation. They facilitate the release of free fatty acids from adipose tissue [274], making fatty acids available for oxidation, but at the same time corticoids make the animal more resistant against ketosis during fasting [275]. Perfused livers from adrenalectomized rats produce more ketone bodies than do livers from normal rats, or from rats treated with cortisol [276]. Corticoids increase the activity of lipogenic enzymes in the liver [275], and it is also observed that adrenalectomy increases the activity of the outer carnitine palmitoyl transferase [229]. It is therefore possible that corticoids decrease the rate of fatty acid oxidation in the liver by increasing the level of malonyl-CoA.

(v) Sex hormones

Isolated perfused livers from female rats esterify relatively more and oxidize relatively fewer fatty acids than do livers from male rats [277]. These differences have been found to correlate with the content of a specific fatty-acid-binding protein in the liver. The formation of this protein is increased by estradiol and inhibited by testosterone [278]. Its formation is also increased by high-fat diets [279]. With isolated hepatocytes it has been found that the presence of flavispidic acid, a competitive inhibitor of fatty acid binding to this protein, leads to inhibition of fatty acid esterification, while oxidation is increased. Flavispidic acid also inhibits the acyl-CoA synthase in endoplasmic reticulum, but appears to activate the mitochondrial enzyme [280]. The fatty-acid-binding protein, therefore, seems to channel fatty acids for esterification in the endoplasmic reticulum. The acyl-CoA formed here may not be available for acylcarnitine formation and subsequent oxidation.

9. Fatty acid β-oxidation in various tissues

Most studies of mitochondrial β-oxidation have been carried out with tissue preparations from liver, and a great deal of what has been described in the preceding sections relates to liver studies. In the following we give a brief outline of some main characteristics of β-oxidation in various other tissues.

(a) Heart and skeletal muscle

Due to the large muscle mass, fatty acid oxidation in muscle tissues is quantitatively very important. It is this tissue which is responsible for oxidation of a major fraction of circulating fatty acids and ketone bodies. Oxidation of fatty acids in skeletal muscle and the heart is mainly controlled by the supply of fatty acids, i.e. the concentration of free fatty acids in the circulation [281,282], but also by work load [214], and by adaptative changes [283].

In the heart about 85% of the tissue content of CoA is found in the mitochondria, while only about 9% of tissue carnitine is associated with mitochondria [37]. This constellation is likely to cause activated fatty acids to be quickly converted to acylcarnitine esters, funnelling fatty acids toward oxidation, rather than to lipid synthesis. This way of reasoning is supported by observations on pathological conditions demonstrating that intracellular accumulation of triacylglycerol (lipidosis) is associated with carnitine-depleted muscle tissue. Diphtheria toxin causes the heart to lose carnitine and to develop lipidosis [284]. The heart lipidosis in diphtheric animals is decreased by administration of carnitine. An inborn error of metabolism characterized by a low carnitine content of skeletal muscle is also associated with lipidosis in this tissue [285,286]. Depletion of muscle carnitine can also occur during intermittent haemodialysis [287]. The oxidation of fatty acids in skeletal and heart mitochondria is more sensitive to inhibition by malonyl CoA than is oxidation in liver mitochondria [226]. The metabolic significance of this finding is, however, not clear since muscle tissue has very little fatty acid synthesis, and its content of malonyl-CoA is unknown.

Foetal bovine heart mitochondria appear to have an impaired ability to β-oxidize long-chain acyl-CoA esters, although oxidation of acylcarnitines is similar to that found in mature tissue [288].

The absence of ketogenesis in muscle tissue couples β-oxidation rigidly to citric acid cycle activity. It has been suggested that β-oxidation in the heart is inhibited by a high intramitochondrial concentration of acetyl-CoA or a high acetyl-CoA/CoA ratio [214]. This in turn will depend on work load, and citric acid cycle activity. Acetyl-CoA is a product inhibitor of the general thiolase [289]. This inhibition may be propagated backwards in the β-oxidation sequence since β-ketoacyl-CoA is an inhibitor of the acyl-CoA dehydrogenases [93,98].

Fatty acid oxidation in muscle is subjected to adaptive changes. Following physical training, β-oxidation activity is increased, as are activities of long-chain acyl-CoA synthase, carnitine palmitoyl transferase and palmitoyl-CoA dehydrogenase [283].

Both ketone bodies and fatty acids, when present in sufficient concentrations in the blood, can suppress glucose oxidation almost completely [290,291]. In the fasted rat, ketone bodies and fatty acids together provide as much energy as does glucose in the fed animal [292].

As far as skeletal muscle is concerned, the preferred utilization of fatty acids and ketone bodies to carbohydrates appears to be restricted to red muscle fibres [293]. White fibres in contrast, are dependent on glycolysis for their energy supply [294].

(b) Kidney

Kidney cortex mitochondria possess a very active β-oxidative system, and they have a low, although detectable, ketogenetic capacity [137]. Kidney cortex can also utilize ketone bodies as an energy source [292]. Renal medulla, however, appears to be an essential glycolytic tissue [296].

(c) Gastrointestinal tissues

Studies with rat tissues suggest that β-oxidation is present in these tissues, but at a low level. The rate of oxidation of oleate has been estimated to be less than $1/400$ of that of glucose. These tissues, and in particular the stomach, appear well able to utilize ketone bodies [295].

(d) White adipose tissue

Although this tissue has a massive capacity for triglyceride synthesis (and lipolysis), its mitochondria have a β-oxidative activity which is comparable to that of liver mitochondria [297]. It has been suggested that long-chain fatty acid oxidation in white adipose tissue may be regulated by the activity of the inner carnitine palmitoyl transferase [297]. However, the outer carnitine palmitoyl transferase is strongly inhibited by malonyl-CoA [226] which therefore may regulate the rate of fatty acid oxidation.

(e) Brown adipose tissue

Brown adipose tissue possesses a highly active mitochondrial β-oxidative system [298]. In this tissue mitochondrial metabolism is unusual in that the mitochondria physiologically can operate in a loosely coupled state [299,300]. This is the mechanism for non-shivering thermogenesis [301]. The extent of uncoupling appears to be regulated by GTP and a specific translocase protein which renders the inner mitochondrial membrane permeable to hydrogen ions [302].

Lipolysis and fatty acid oxidation in brown adipose tissues are stimulated by catecholamines [303]. The availability of free fatty acids therefore regulates the rate of oxidation in the cold-adapted tissue, and probably also the proton conductance protein of the inner mitochondrial membrane [304].

In brown adipose tissue from cold-adapted hamsters, acetate can be the end-product of β-oxidation. This is due to induction of an acetyl-CoA hydrolase activity in the mitochondrial matrix of animals being subjected to cold adaptation [144].

(f) Brain

Brain is usually assumed to depend mainly on glucose for its energy supply. There are, however, several reports in the literature which show that brain mitochondria oxidize labelled fatty acids to CO_2 and water-soluble products with about 25% of the rate of liver mitochondria [305]. The water-soluble radioactivity was recovered mainly in aspartate and glutamate, but also in succinate and citrate [306]. The metabolic significance of these findings remains to be established.

The brain is able to use ketone bodies as a major source of energy during periods of fasting or starvation, when the supply of glucose is limited [296]. After 48 h of fasting ketone bodies account for about 20% of the brain's fuel requirement in the rat [307] (the remainder being filled by glucose). In humans this value increases to 75% during prolonged starvation [296]. The normal brain contains adequate amounts of enzyme activities required for ketone body utilization: β-hydroxybutyrate dehydrogenase, CoA transferase, and acetoacetyl-CoA thiolase [308]. The mechanism which facilitates the switch in brain metabolism from total dependence of glucose for energy, to partial dependence on ketone bodies, is therefore not clear.

10. Inhibitors of fatty acid β-oxidation

Inhibitors of β-oxidation have always attracted appreciable interest, both from a biochemical and a pharmacological point of view. To selectively inhibit β-oxidation has been a tempting target for pharmacologists searching for substances which could control ketosis, e.g. in diabetes. Very few inhibitors of β-oxidation e.g. 2-tetradecylglycerate and some other substituted oxiran-2-carboxylic acids appear to act exclusively on β-oxidation. Most inhibitors of β-oxidation, when administered to fasting experimental animals, also cause hypoglycaemia. This may be caused by a direct effect of the inhibitor (or a metabolite of the inhibitor) on some key gluconeogenic enzyme, or as a secondary effect due to inhibited β-oxidation.

All effects described here refer to studies carried out with mitochondrial β-oxidation. There is at present no information regarding their effects on peroxisomal β-oxidation.

(a) Inhibitors of transport of acyl groups across the inner mitochondrial membrane

2-Bromo-substituted fatty acids are inhibitors of the carnitine acyltransferases. Bromoacetylcarnitine is a very potent inhibitor of carnitine acetyltransferase. The inhibition, which entails alkylation of CoA on the enzyme in the presence of CoA, or alkylation of a histidine residue near the active site in the absence of CoA, is essentially irreversible [309,310].

A similar inhibition of the outer carnitine palmitoyl transferase is achieved with 2-bromopalmitoyl-CoA or 2-bromopalmitoylcarnitine [311,312]. The inner carnitine palmitoyl transferase, however, appears able to use 2-bromopalmitoylcarnitine as a substrate, generating intramitochondrial 2-bromopalmitoyl-CoA which presumably causes rapid inhibition of β-oxidation [56]. Maximal inhibition can be observed with less than 10 μM concentrations of these inhibitors. It is noteworthy that the carnitine–acylcarnitine exchange carrier [82,83] does not appear to be inhibited by these 2-bromo fatty acyl esters.

With isolated hepatocytes, 2-bromopalmitate inhibits fatty acid oxidation without affecting the mitochondrial metabolism directly. Both the long-chain acyl-CoA synthetase and the carnitine acyltransferase activities were unperturbed in hepatocytes exposed to 2-bromopalmitate [313]. It is suggested that 2-bromopalmitate competes reversibly with the transport of fatty acids across the hepatocyte cell membrane. This may involve 2-bromopalmitate competing with fatty acids for binding on the fatty-acid-binding protein in the cytosol, a process which is thought essential for fatty acid transport across the cell membrane [314].

11-Trimethylamino-hexadecanoyl ester of D,L-*carnitine* inhibits the carnitine translocase with a K_i value of about 1 μM [311]. The inhibitory action may be due to the inability of the carnitine–acylcarnitine exchange carrier to transport the cationic acyl group through the inner mitochondrial membrane.

Sulfobetaines (*N*-alkyl-*N*, *N*-dimethyl-3-ammonio-1-propanesulphonates) are also potent inhibitors of the carnitine–acylcarnitine exchange carrier [315]. These compounds are consequently potent inhibitors of mitochondrial fatty acid oxidation.

Acyl esters of (+)-D-carnitine are potent inhibitors of fatty acid oxidation in isolated mitochondria [316], in isolated hepatocytes [177], and in perfused livers [317]. The solubilized carnitine palmitoyl transferase is not inhibited [316]. With isolated mitochondria the inhibition apparently is due to an inhibition of the carnitine translocase [52].

Pyrenebutylcarnitine, which has useful spectroscopic properties, has been reported to be a very potent inhibitor of the inner carnitine palmitoyl transferase, and also of the acylcarnitine–carnitine exchange [318].

2-Tetradecyl glycidate is a potent inhibitor of the outer carnitine palmitoyl transferase, and hence of β-oxidation. At a concentration of 1 μM this substance has been shown to cause 80–90% inactivation of the transferase [319]. The CoA ester of 2-tetradecyl glycidic acid is probably the active inhibitor.

2-Substituted oxiran-2-carbonyl-CoA esters are potent inhibitors of the outer carnitine palmitoyl transferase [320]. Some of these CoA esters are reported to cause 50% inhibition of palmitoyl-CoA oxidation by isolated liver mitochondria at concentrations of 30–300 nM, which shows that these compounds are some of the most potent inhibitors of the outer transferase which have been described. The inner transferase is not inhibited, as judged by absence of inhibition of oxidation of palmitoylcarnitine [320].

Palmitoyl-CoA analogues in which the fatty acyl carbonyl group, or CoA-thioester moiety, has been replaced by a methylene group also are potent inhibitors of the outer carnitine palmitoyl transferase [321].

(b) Inhibitors of acyl-CoA dehydrogenase

The only clearly established inhibitor of an acyl-CoA dehydrogenase is the hypoglycine metabolite methylencyclopropylacetyl-CoA. This CoA ester has been shown to irreversibly inhibit the butyryl-CoA dehydrogenase and isovaleryl-CoA dehydrogenase in rat-liver and skeletal-muscle mitochondria [322]. The palmitoyl-CoA dehydrogenase does, however, not appear to be inhibited. Consequently this inhibitor causes partial inhibition of e.g. palmitate oxidation (usually by about 50%), even though the butyryl-CoA dehydrogenase, and butyrylcarnitine oxidation, are virtually 100% inactivated [323,324]. Both butyrate, and isovalerate from the degradation of leucine, accumulate in the circulation of animals treated with hypoglycine [325].

2-Mercaptoacetate, following injection into rats, has been shown to powerfully inhibit fatty acid oxidation in subsequently isolated liver mitochondria [326]. This effect is thought to be due to inhibition of the palmitoyl-CoA dehydrogenase.

(c) Inhibitors of thiolase

Compounds of different structure inhibit thiolase by a similar mode of action. The thiolases possess an active SH group which is acetylated during the reaction cycle. It is this SH group which usually is thought to be modified through a reaction with one of the thiolase inhibitors.

2-Bromo-octanoate is a very potent inhibitor of β-oxidation both in perfused rat-liver [327] and in isolated rat-liver mitochondria [328]. With perfused livers, 2-bromo-octanoate inhibits gluconeogenesis from lactate and pyruvate, while this is not so as regards gluconeogenesis from dihydroxyacetone-phosphate [327]. In mitochondrial oxidative metabolism the action of this inhibitor appears markedly restricted to β-oxidation. Oxidation of succinate, 2-ketoglutarate, and pyruvate plus malate is nearly unaffected by concentrations of 2-bromo-octanoate which completely inhibits oxidation of palmitate or oleate [328].

The mechanism of inhibition involves partial β-oxidation to 2-bromo-3-keto-octanoyl-CoA. During the thiolytic cleavage of this metabolite, a 2-bromo-acetyl group irreversibly inactivates the general thiolase by covalently modifying the SH group which is acetylated during the normal catalytic cycle. The acetoacetyl-CoA thiolase is not significantly inhibited. The inhibitory metabolite of 2-bromo-octanoate is an α-haloketone. A similar group of irreversible thiolase inhibitors, the chloro-methyl-ketone derivatives, has also been described [329,330].

Pent-4-enoate is a very potent inhibitor of β-oxidation. With the (−)-carnitine ester, close to 100% inhibition in liver mitochondria is observed with concentrations of 100 μM or less [324,331].

Pent-4-enoic acid is often referred to as an analogue of the hypoglycaemic toxin hypoglycine. Although both substances are hypoglycaemic in fasted animals and inhibit mitochondrial β-oxidation, it is now clear that they do so by different mechanisms [325,332].

To become inhibitory, pent-4-enoate requires activation to the CoA ester, and subsequent metabolism [331]. It is in this manner very analogous to 2-bromo-octanoate. Pent-4-enoyl-CoA is an excellent substrate for the acyl-CoA dehydrogenases, which convert it to penta-2,4-dienoyl-CoA. This metabolite inhibits the acetoacetyl-CoA thiolase [102,329].

Penta-2,4-dienoyl-CoA is probably converted to 3-oxo-pent-4-enoyl-CoA which may be a much more potent inhibitor of the thiolases than penta-2,4-dienoyl-CoA [333]. Pent-4-enoic acid is unusual in that it is readily metabolized at low concentrations while at higher concentrations it becomes inhibitory to β-oxidation, and is no longer metabolized itself [117,334,335]. This metabolism of pentenoate depends on a reduction of the pent-2,4-dienoyl-CoA to pent-2-enoyl-CoA with NADPH by the 2,4-dienoyl-CoA reductase followed by a normal β-oxidation [117,336]. NADPH can be supplied here from NADH via the energy-dependent transhydrogenase in mitochondria. This is analogous to the function of this enzyme in the metabolism of unsaturated fatty acids (see Section 4.c.ii). These findings explain why clofibrate treatment, which increases the activity of 2,4-dienoyl-CoA reductase dramatically, protects against toxic effects of pent-4-enoate [337] and that uncoupling increases

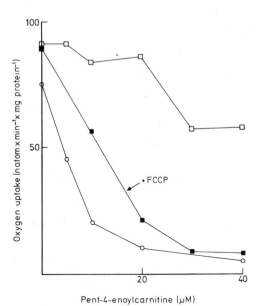

Fig. 9. The effect of pent-4-enoylcarnitine on the oxidation of palmitoylcarnitine by liver mitochondria. Isolated mitochondria from normal rats (○) and rats treated for 2 weeks with 0.25% clofibrate in the diet (□, ■) were preincubated for 1 min with pent-4-enoylcarnitine as shown with and without an uncoupler of oxidative phosphorylation (FCCP, carbonylcyanide p-trifluoromethoxyphenylhydrazone). The curves show the rates of oxygen uptake after addition of (−)-palmitoylcarnitine (40 μM). Clofibrate induces a 5-fold increase in the activity of 2,4-dienoyl-CoA reductase in the mitochondria, the rate-limiting enzyme in the breakdown of pent-4-enoate. (Reproduced from ref. 117 with the permission of Biochem. Biophys. Res. Commun.)

the inhibitory effect of pent-4-enoylcarnitine in isolated mitochondria (Fig. 9) [117].

Arsenite has been shown to inhibit ketogenesis in isolated rat liver mitochondria [338]. This inhibitory action is due to arsenite-induced inactivation of the thiolases and is presumed to be due to a reaction between arsenite and the active SH group of the enzymes. Arsenite is also strongly inhibitory to other mitochondrial enzymes [338,339], notably pyruvate and α-ketoglutarate dehydrogenases. This effect is unrelated to the inhibition of thiolase.

References

1 Geelmuyden, H.C. (1897) Z. Physiol. Chem. 23, 431–475.
2 Knoop, F. (1904) Beitr. Chem. Physiol. Pathol. 6, 150–162.
3 Lynen, F. and Decker, K. (1957) Ergebnisse der Physiologie, Biologische Chemie und Experimentelle Pharmacologie, Vol. 49, Springer, Berlin, pp. 327–424.
4 Stern, J.R., Del Campillo, A. and Raw, I. (1956) J. Biol. Chem. 218, 971–983.
5 De Duve, C., Pressman, B.C., Gianette, R., Wattiaux, R. and Appelmans, F. (1955) Biochem. J. 60, 604–617.
6 Friedman, S. and Frenkel, G. (1955) 59, 491–505.
7 Fritz, I.B. (1955) Acta Physiol. Scand. 34, 367–385.
8 Bremer, J. and Norum, K.R. (1982) J. Lipid Res. 23, 243–256.
9 McGarry, J.D. and Foster, D.W. (1971) J. Biol. Chem. 246, 1149–1159.
10 Aas, M. (1971) Biochim. Biophys. Acta 231, 32–47.
11 Scholte, H.R. and Groot, P.H.E. (1975) Biochim. Biophys. Acta 409, 283–296.
12 Vessey, D.A. (1979) J. Biol. Chem. 254, 2059–2063.
13 Groot, P.H.E. (1975) Biochim. Biophys. Acta 380, 12–20.
14 Lee, K.Y. and Schulz, H. (1979) J. Biol. Chem. 254, 4516–4523.
15 Berge, R.K. and Farstad, M. (1979) Eur. J. Biochem. 95, 89–97.
16 Webster Jr., L.T. (1965) J. Biol. Chem. 240, 4158–4163.
17 Webster Jr., L.T. (1965) J. Biol. Chem. 240, 4164–4169.
18 Bergman, E.N., Reid, R.S., Murray, M.G., Brockway, J.M. and Whitelaw, F.G. (1965) Biochem. J. 97, 53–58.
19 Seufert, C.D., Graf, M., Janson, G., Kuhn, A. and Söhing (1974) Biochem. Biophys. Res. Commun. 57, 901–909.
20 Groot, P.H.E. (1976) Biochim. Biophys. Acta 441, 260–267.
21 Smith, R.M. and Russel, G.R. (1967) Biochem. J. 102, 39c–41c.
22 Webster Jr., L.T., Gerowin, L.D. and Rakita, L. (1965) J. Biol. Chem. 240, 29–33.
23 Mahler, H.R., Wakil, S.J. and Bock, R.M. (1953) J. Biol. Chem. 204, 453–467.
24 Bremer, J. (1955) Acta Chem. Scand. 9, 268–271.
25 Forman, W.B., Davidson, E.D. and Webster Jr., L.T. (1971) Mol. Pharmacol. 7, 247–259.
26 Kornberg, A. and Pricer, W.E. (1953) J. Biol. Chem. 204, 453–468.
27 Norum, K.R., Farstad, M. and Bremer, J. (1966) Biochem. Biophys. Res. Commun. 24, 797–804.
28 Garland, P.B., Yates, D.W. and Haddock, B.A. (1970) Biochem. J. 119, 553–564.
29 Krisans, S.K., Mortensen, R.M. and Lazarow, P.B. (1980) J. Biol. Chem. 255, 9599–9607.
30 Shindo, Y. and Hashimoto, T. (1978) J. Biochem. 84, 1177–1181.
31 Numa, S. (1981) TIBS 6, 113–115.
32 Groot, P.H.E., Van Loon, C.M.I. and Hülsmann, W.C. (1974) Biochim. Biophys. Acta 337, 13–21.
33 Maes, E. and Bar-Tana, J. (1977) Biochim. Biophys. Acta 480, 527–530.
34 Philip, D.B. and Parson, P. (1979) J. Biol. Chem. 254, 10776–10784.
35 Tanaka, T., Hosaka, K., Hoshimaru, M. and Numa, S. (1979) Eur. J. Biochem. 98, 165–172.
36 Normann, P.T., Thomassen, M.S., Christiansen, E.N. and Flatmark, T. (1981) Biochim. Biophys. Acta 664, 416–427.

148

37 Oram, J.F., Wenger, J.I. and Neely, J.R. (1975) J. Biol. Chem. 250, 73–78.
38 Berg, P. (1956) J. Biol. Chem. 222, 991–1013.
39 Berg, P. (1956) J. Biol. Chem. 222, 1015–1023.
40 Webster Jr., L.T. (1963) J. Biol. Chem. 238, 4010–4014.
41 Graham, A.B. and Park, M.V. (1969) Biochem. J. 111, 257–262.
42 Rose, G., Bar-Tana, J. and Shapiro, B. (1979) Biochim. Biophys. Acta 573, 126–135.
43 Rossi, C.R. and Gibson, D.M. (1964) J. Biol. Chem. 239, 1694–1699.
44 Rossi, C.R., Aexande, A., Galzigna, L., Sartorelli, L. and Gibson, D.M. (1970) J. Biol. Chem. 245, 3110–3114.
45 Pande, S.V. and Mead, J.F. (1968) Biochim. Biophys. Acta 152, 636–638.
46 Lippel, K. and Beattie, D.S. (1970) Biochim. Biophys. Acta 218, 565–573.
47 Batenburg, J.J. and van den Bergh, S.G. (1973) Biochim. Biophys. Acta 316, 136–142.
48 Fritz, I.B. and Yue, K.T.N. (1963) J. Lipid Res. 4, 279–284.
49 Bremer, J. (1962) J. Biol. Chem. 237, 3628–3632.
50 Yates, D.W. and Garland, P.B. (1970) Biochem. J. 119, 547–552.
51 Norum, K.R. and Bremer, J. (1967) J. Biol. Chem. 242, 407–411.
52 Pande, S.V. (1975) Proc. Natl. Acad. Sci. (U.S.A.) 72, 883–887.
53 Ramsay, R.R. and Tubbs, P.K. (1975) FEBS Lett. 54, 21–25.
54 Bremer, J. (1962) J. Biol. Chem. 237, 2228–2231.
55 Childress, C.C., Sacktor, B. and Traynor, D.R. (1966) J. Biol. Chem. 242, 754–760.
56 Chase, J.F.A. and Tubbs, P.K. (1972) Biochem. J. 129, 55–65.
57 Hoppel, C.L. and Tomec, R.J. (1972) J. Biol. Chem. 247, 832–841.
58 Edwards, Y.H., Chase, J.F.A., Edwards, M.R. and Tubbs, P.K. (1974) Eur. J. Biochem. 46, 209–215.
59 Bergstrom, J.D. and Reitz, R.C. (1980) Arch. Biochem. 204, 71–79.
60 Solberg, H.E. (1971) FEBS Lett. 12, 134–136.
61 Kopec, B. and Fritz, I.B. (1971) Can. J. Biochem. 49, 941–948.
62 Choi, Y.R., Fogle, P.J., Clarke, P.R.H. and Bieber, L.L. (1977) J. Biol. Chem. 252, 7930–7931.
63 Clarke, P.R.H. and Bieber, L.L. (1981) J. Biol. Chem. 256, 9869–9873.
64 Kahonen, M.T. (1976) Biochim. Biophys. Acta 428, 690–701.
65 Kawamoto, S., Ueda, N., Nozaki, C., Yamamura, N., Tanaka, A. and Fukui, S. (1978) FEBS Lett. 96, 37–40.
66 Reddy, J.K. and Kumar, N.S. (1979) J. Biochem. 85, 847–856.
67 Bieber, L.L., Krahling, J.B., Clarke, P.R.H., Valkner, K.J. and Tolbert, N.E. (1981) Arch. Biochem. 211, 599–604.
68 Lazarow, P.B. and De Duve, C. (1976) Proc. Natl. Acad. Sci. (U.S.A.) 73, 2043–2046.
69 Chase, J.F.A., Pearson, D.J. and Tubbs, P.K. (1965) Biochim. Biophys. Acta 96, 162–165.
70 Chase, J.F.A. and Tubbs, P.K. (1966) Biochem. J. 99, 32–40.
71 Chase, J.F.K. (1967) Biochem. J. 104, 510–518.
72 Marquis, N.R. and Fritz, I.B. (1965) J. Biol. Chem. 240, 2193–2196.
73 Snoswell, A.M. and Henderson, G.D. (1970) Biochem. J. 119, 59–65.
74 Davis, E.J. and Bremer, J. (1973) Eur. J. Biochem. 38, 86–97.
75 Bieber, L.L. and Choi, Y.R. (1977) Proc. Natl. Acad. Sci. (U.S.A.) 74, 2795–2798.
76 Clarke, P.R.H. and Bieber, L.L. (1981) J. Biol. Chem. 256, 9861–9868.
77 Bremer, J. and Norum, K.R. (1967) J. Biol. Chem. 242, 1744–1748.
78 Bremer, J. and Norum, K.R. (1967) Eur. J. Biochem. 1, 427–433.
79 Bremer, J. and Norum, K.R. (1967) J. Biol. Chem. 242, 1749–1755.
80 McGarry, J.D. and Foster, D.W. (1979) J. Biol. Chem. 254, 8163–8168.
81 Normann, P.T., Ingebretsen, O.C. and Flatmark, T. (1978) Biochim. Biophys. Acta 501, 286–295.
82 Ramsay, R.R. and Tubbs, P.K. (1976) Eur. J. Biochem. 69, 299–303.
83 Pande, S.V. and Parvin, R. (1976) J. Biol. Chem. 251, 6683–6691.
84 Pande, S.V. and Parvin, R. (1978) J. Biol. Chem. 253, 1944–1946.
85 Pande, S.V. and Parvin, R. (1980) J. Biol. Chem. 255, 2994–3001.
86 Idell-Wenger, J.A. (1981) J. Biol. Chem. 256, 5597–5603.

149

87 Parvin, R. and Pande, S.V. (1979) J. Biol. Chem. 254, 5423–5429.
88 Christiansen, R.Z. and Bremer, J. (1976) Biochim. Biophys. Acta 448, 562–577.
89 Haddock, B.A., Yates, D.W. and Garland, P.B. (1970) Biochem. J. 119, 565–573.
90 Crane, F.L., Mii, S., Hauge, J.G., Green, D.E. and Beinert, H. (1956) J. Biol. Chem. 218, 701–716.
91 Hauge, J.G., Crane, F.L. and Beinert, H. (1956) J. Biol. Chem. 219, 727–733.
92 Furuta, S., Miyasawa, S. and Hashimoto, T. (1981) J. Biochem. 90, 1739–1750.
93 Davidson, B. and Schulz, H. (1982) Arch. Biochem. 213, 155–162.
94 Crane, F.L. and Beinert, H. (1956) J. Biol. Chem. 218, 717–731.
95 Garland, P.B., Chance, B., Ernster, L., Lee, C. and Wong, W. (1967) Proc. Natl. Acad. Sci. (U.S.A.) 58, 1696–1702.
96 Bremer, J. and Davis, E.J. (1972) Biochim. Biophys. Acta 275, 298–301.
97 Hauge, J.G. (1956) J. Am. Chem. Soc. 73, 5266–5272.
98 Schmidt, J., Reinsch, J. and McFarland, J.T. (1981) J. Biol. Chem. 256, 11667–11670.
99 Stern, J.R. and Del Campillo, A. (1956) J. Biol. Chem. 218, 985–1002.
100 Schulz, H. (1974) J. Biol. Chem. 249, 2704–2709.
101 Wakil, S.J. (1956) Biochim. Biophys. Acta 19, 497–504.
102 Holland, P.C., Senior, A.E. and Sherratt, H.S.A. (1973) Biochem. J. 136, 173–184.
103 Hiltunen, J.K. and Davis, E.J. (1981) Biochem. J. 194, 427–432.
104 El-Fakhri, M. and Middleton, B. (1979) Biochem. Soc. Trans. 7, 392–393.
105 Nayes, B. and Bradshaw, P.A. (1973) J. Biol. Chem. 248, 3052–3059.
106 Middleton, B. (1973) Biochem. J. 132, 717–730.
107 Staack, H., Binstock, J.F. and Schulz, H. (1978) J. Biol. Chem. 253, 1827–1831.
108 Huth, W., Jonas, R., Wunderlich, I. and Seufert, W. (1975) Eur. J. Biochem. 475–489.
109 Middleton, B. (1974) Biochem. J. 139, 109–121.
110 Rilling, H.C. and Coon, M.J. (1960) J. Biol. Chem. 235, 3087–3092.
111 Stoffel, W., Ditzer, R. and Caesar, H. (1964) Z. Physiol. Chem. 339, 167–182.
112 Struijk, C.B. and Beerthuis, R.K. (1966) Biochim. Biophys. Acta 116, 12–22.
113 Davidoff, F.D. and Korn, E.I. (1965) J. Biol. Chem. 240, 1549–1558.
114 Stoffel, W. and Schiefer, H.-G. (1965) Z. Physiol. Chem. 341, 84–90.
115 Kunau, W.-H. and Dommes, P. (1978) Eur. J. Biochem. 91, 533–544.
116 Mizugaki, M., Nishimaki, T., Yamamoto, H., Nishimura, S., Sagi, M. and Yamanaka, H. (1982) J. Biochem. 91, 1453.
117 Borrebaek, B., osmundsen, H. and Bremer, J. (1980) Biochem. Biophys. Res. Commun. 93, 1173–1180.
118 Dommes, V., Baumgart, C. and Kunau, W.-H. (1981) J. Biol. Chem. 256, 8259–8262.
119 Stern, J.R., Del Campillo, A. and Lehninger, A.L. (1955) J. Am. Chem. Soc. 77, 1073–1074.
120 Garland, P.B., Shepherd, D. and Yates, D.W. (1965) Biochem. J. 97, 587–594.
121 Stanley, K.K. and Tubbs, P.K. (1975) Biochem. J. 150, 77–88.
122 Bremer, J. and Wojtczak, A.B. (1972) Biochim. Biophys. Acta 280, 515–530.
123 Lopes-Cardozo, M., Klazinga, W. and van den Bergh, S.G. (1978) Eur. J. Biochem. 83, 629–634.
124 Lopes-Cardozo, M., Klazinga, W. and van den Berg, S.G. (1978) Eur. J. Biochem. 83, 635–640.
125 Lynen, F., Henning, U., Bublitz, C., Sörbo, B. and Kröplin-Rueff, L. (1958) Biochem. Z. 330, 269–295.
126 Seufert, C.D., Grigat, K.P., Koppe, K. and Söling, H.D. (1978) in: H.D. Söling and C.D. Seufert (Eds.), Biochemical and Clinical Aspects of Ketone Body Metabolism, Georg Thieme, Stuttgart, pp. 23–40.
127 Williamson, D.H., Bates, M.W. and Krebs, H.A. (1968) Biochem. J. 108, 353–361.
128 Klinkenbeard, K.D., Reed, W.D., Mooney, R.A. and Lane, M.D. (1975) J. Biol. Chem. 250, 3108–3116.
129 Stewart, P.R. and Rudney, H. (1966) J. Biol. Chem. 241, 1222–1225.
130 Miziorko, H.M. and Lane, M.D. (1977) J. Biol. Chem. 252, 1414–1420.
131 Menahan, L.A., Hron, W.T., Hinkelman, D.G. and Miziorko, H.M. (1981) Eur. J. Biochem. 119, 287–294.
132 Bremer, J. and Aas, M. (1969) FEBS Symp. 17, 127–135.

150

133 Lee, L.P.K. and Fritz, I.B. (1972) Can. J. Biochem. 50, 120–127.
134 Wieland, O. and Weiss, L. (1963) Biochem. Biophys. Res. Commun. 10, 333–339.
135 Shepherd, D., Yates, D.W. and Garland, P.B. (1965) Biochem. J. 97, 38c–40c.
136 Clinckenbeard, K.D., Reed, W.D., Mooney, R.A. and Lane, M.D. (1975) J. Biol. Chem. 250, 3108–3116.
137 McGarry, J.D. and Foster, D.W. (1969) J. Biol. Chem. 244, 4251–4256.
138 Stegink, L.D. and Coon, M.J. (1968) J. Biol. Chem. 243, 5272–5279.
139 Grover, A.K., Slotboom, A.J., de Haas, G.H. and Hammes, G.G. (1975) J. Biol. Chem. 259, 31–38.
140 Jurshuk, P., Sekuzu, I. and Green, D.E. (1963) J. Biol. Chem. 238, 3595–3605.
141 Williamson, D.H., Lund, P. and Krebs, H.A. (1967) Biochem. J. 103, 512–527.
142 Bendall, D.S. and de Duve, C. (1960) Biochem. J. 74, 445–450.
143 Prass, R.L., Isohashi, F. and Utter, M.F. (1980) J. Biol. Chem. 255, 5215–5223.
144 Bernson, V.S.M. and Nichols, D.G. (1974) Eur. J. Biochem. 47, 517–525.
145 Bernson, V.S.M. (1976) Eur. J. Biochem. 67, 403–410.
146 Stern, J.R., Coon, M.J., Del Campillo, A. and Schneider, M.C. (1956) J. Biol. Chem. 221, 15–31.
147 Zammit, V.A., Beis, A. and Newsholm, E.A. (1979) FEBS Lett. 103, 212–215.
148 Menahan, L.A. and Hron, W.T. (1981) Eur. J. Biochem. 119, 295–299.
149 Cha, S. and Parks Jr., R.E. (1961) J. Biol. Chem. 239, 1968–1977.
150 Cooper, T.G. and Beevers, H. (1969) J. Biol. Chem. 244, 3507–3513.
151 Cooper, T.G. and Beevers, H. (1969) J. Biol. Chem. 244, 3514–3520.
152 Blum, J.J. (1973) J. Protozool. 20, 688–692.
153 Graves, L.B. and Becker, W.M. (1974) J. Protozool. 21, 771–774.
154 Murphy, P.A., Krahling, J.B., Gee, R., Kirk, J.R. and Tolbert, N.E. (1979) Arch. Biochem. Biophys. 193, 179–180.
155 Brontman, M., Inestrosa, N.C. and Leighton, F. (1979) Biochem. Biophys. Res. Commun., 91, 108–113.
156 Kramar, R., Hüttinger, M., Gweiner, B. and Goldenberg, H. (1978) Biochim. Biophys. Acta 531, 353–355.
157 Nedergaard, J., Alexson, S. and Cannon, B. (1980) Am. J. Physiol. 239, C208–C216.
158 Lazarow, P.B. (1978) J. Biol. Chem. 253, 1522–1528.
159 Osmundsen, H. and Neat, C.E. (1979) FEBS Lett. 107, 81–85.
160 Kawaguchi, A., Tsubotani, S., Seyama, Y., Yamakawa, T., Osumi, T., Hashimoto, T., Kikuchi, T., Ando, M. and Okuda, S. (1980) J. Biochem. (Tokyo) 88, 1481–1486.
161 Osumi, T., Hashimoto, T. and Vi, N. (1980) J. Biochem. 87, 35–1746.
162 Inestrosa, N.C., Bronfman, M. and Leighton, F. (1980) Biochem. Biophys. Res. Commun. 95, 7–12.
163 Osumi, T. and Hashimoto, T. (1979) Biochem. Biophys. Res. Commun. 89, 580–584.
164 Furuta, S., Miyazawa, S., Osumi, T., Hashimoto, T. and Ui, N. (1980) J. Biochem. 88, 1059–1070.
165 Kumudavalli, M., Qupeshi, S.A., Hollenberg, P.F. and Reddy, J.K. (1981) J. Cell. Biol. 89, 406–417.
166 Lalwani, N.D., Reddy, M.K., Mangkornkanok-Mark, M. and Reddy, J.K. (1981) Biochem. J. 198, 177–186.
167 Lazarow, P.B. (1981) Arch. Biochem. Biophys. 206, 342–345.
168 Osumi, T. and Hashimoto, T. (1979) Biochim. Biophys. Acta 574, 258–267.
169 Miyazawa, S., Osumi, T. and Hashimoto, T. (1980) Eur. J. Biochem. 103, 589–596.
170 Van Broekhoven, A., Peeters, M.C., Debeer, L.J. and Mannaerts, G.P. (1981) Biochem. Biophys. Res. Commun. 100, 305–312.
171 Mannaerts, G.P., van Veldhoven, P., van Broekhoven, A., Vandebroek, G. and DeBeer, L.J. (1982) Biochem. J. 204, 17–23.
172 Appelkvist, E.L. and Dallner, G. (1980) Biochim. Biophys. Acta 617, 156–170.
173 Osmundsen, H. (1982) Int. J. Biochem., 14, 905–914.
174 Osmundsen, H. (1982) Ann. N.Y. Acad. Sci., 386, 13–29.
175 Osmundsen, H., Neat, C.E. and Borrebaek, B. (1980) Int. J. Biochem. 12, 625–630.
176 Christiansen, E.N., Thomassen, M.S., Christiansen, R.Z., Osmundsen, H. and Norum, K.R. (1979) Lipids 14, 829–835.

151

177 Christiansen, R.Z. (1978) Biochim. Biophys. Acta 530, 314–320.
178 Osmundsen, H., Christiansen, R.Z. and Bremer, J. (1980) in: R.A. Frenkel and J.D. McGarry (Eds.), Carnitine Biosynthesis, Metabolism and Functions, Academic Press, New York, pp. 127–139.
179 Pedersen, J.C. and Gustavsson, S. (1980) FEBS Lett. 121, 345–348.
180 Neat, C.E., Thomassen, M.S. and Osmundsen, H. (1981) Biochem. J. 196, 149–159.
181 Singh, I., Moser, H.W., Moser, A.B. and Kishimoto, Y. (1981) Biochem. Biophys. Res. Commun. 102, 1223–1229.
182 Hitchcock, C., Morris, L.J. and James, A.T. (1966) Biochim. Biophys. Acta 116, 413–424.
183 Martin, R.O. and Stumpf, P.K. (1959) J. Biol. Chem. 234, 2448–2554.
184 Akanuma, H. and Kishimoto, Y. (1979) J. Biol. Chem. 254, 1050–1056.
185 Levis, G.M. and Mead, J.F. (1964) J. Biol. Chem. 239, 77–80.
186 Steiberg, D., Avigan, J., Mize, C., Eldjarn, L., Try, K. and Refsum, S. (1965) Biochim. Biophys. Res. Commun. 19, 783–789.
187 Sonneveld, W., Begemann, P.H, van Beers, G.J., Keyning, R. and Schogt, J.C.M. (1962) J. Lipid Res. 3, 351–355.
188 Stokke, O. (1969) Biochim. Biophys. Acta 176, 54–59.
189 Mize, C.E., Steinberg, D., Avigan, J. and Falls, H.M. (1966) Biochem. Biophys. Res. Commun. 25, 359–365.
190 Tsai, S.-C., Avigan, J. and Steinberg, D. (1969) J. Biol. Chem. 2682–2692.
191 Klenk, E. and Kahlke, W. (1963) Z. Physiol. Chem. 333, 133–139.
192 Verkade, P.E. and Van der Lee, J. (1934) Z. Physiol. Chem. 227, 213–222.
193 Pettersen, J., Jellum, E. and Eldjarn, L. (1972) Clin. Chim. Acta 38, 17–24.
194 Bjørkhem, I. (1972) Eur. J. Biochem. 40, 415–422.
195 Mortensen, P.B. and Gregersen, N. (1981) Biochim. Biophys. Acta 666, 394–404.
196 Björkhem, I. (1978) J. Lipid Res. 19, 585–590.
197 Kam, W., Kumaran, K. and Landau, B.R. (1978) J. Lipid Res. 19, 591–600.
198 Weitzel, G.Z. (1951) Z. Physiol. Chem. 287, 254–296.
199 Yamakawa, T. (1950) J. Biochem. 37, 343–353.
200 Bergström, S., Borgström, B., Tryding, N. and Westö, G. (1954) Biochem. J. 58, 604–608.
201 Lu, A.Y.H., Junk, K.W. and Coon, M.J. (1969) J. Biol. Chem. 244, 3714–3721.
202 van der Hoeven, T.A. and Coon, M.J. (1974) J. Biol. Chem. 249, 6302–6310.
203 Petterson, J.A., Basu, D. and Coon, M.J. (1966) J. Biol. Chem. 241, 5159–5164.
204 Hamberg, M. and Björkhem, I. (1971) J. Biol. Chem. 246, 7411–7416.
205 Björkhem, I. and Danielson, H. (1970) Eur. J. Biochem. 17, 450–459.
206 Adach, H., Mitsuhashi, O. and Imai, Y. (1974) J. Biol. Chem. 76, 1281–1286.
207 Pettersen, J.E. and Aas, M. (1974) J. Lipid Res. 15, 551–556.
208 Pettersen, J.E. (1973) Biochim. Biophys. Acta 306, 1–14.
209 Hemmelgarn, E., Kumaran, K. and Landau, B.R. (1977) J. Biol. Chem. 252, 4379–4383.
210 McGarry, J.D. and Foster, D.W. (1971) J. Biol. Chem. 246, 6247–6253.
211 McGarry, J.D. and Foster, D.W. (1973) J. Biol. Chem. 248, 270–278.
212 Ontko, J.A. (1972) J. Biol. Chem. 247, 1788–1800.
213 Christiansen, R.Z. (1977) Biochim. Biophys. Acta 488, 249–262.
214 Oram, J.F., Bennetch, S.L. and Neely, J.R. (1973) J. Biol. Chem. 248, 5299–5309.
215 Böhmer, T., Norum, K.R. and Bremer, J. (1966) Biochim. Biophys. Acta 125, 244–251.
216 Pearson, D.J. and Tubbs, P.K. (1967) Biochem. J. 105, 953–963.
217 Bremer, J. (1965) Biochim. Biophys. Acta 104, 581–590.
218 Hansford, R.G. and Cohen, L. (1978) Arch. Biochem. 191, 65–81.
219 Nichols, P.G. and Garland, P.B. (1969) Biochem. J. 114, 215–225.
220 Lenartowicz, E., Winter, C., Kunz, W. and Wojtczak, A.B. (1976) Eur. J. Biochem. 67, 137–144.
221 Lopes-Cardozo, M. and van den Berg, S.G. (1972) Biochim. Biophys. Acta 283, 1–15.
222 Lopes-Cardozo, M. and van den Bergh, S.G. (1974) Biochim. Biophys. Acta 357, 53–62.
223 Lumeng, L., Bremer, J. and Davis, E.J. (1976) J. Biol. Chem. 251, 277–284.
224 Ontko, J.A. (1973) J. Lipid Res. 14, 78–86.

225 McGarry, J.D. and Foster, D.W. (1980) Annu. Rev. Biochem. 49, 395–420.
226 Saggerson, E.D. and Carpenter, C.A. (1981) FEBS Lett. 129, 229–232.
227 Cook, G.A., Otto, D.A. and Cornell, N.W. (1980) Biochem. J. 192, 955–958.
228 Ontko, J.A. and Johns, M.L. (1980) Biochem. J. 192, 959–962.
229 Saggerson, E.D. and Carpenter, C.A. (1981) FEBS Lett. 129, 225–228.
230 Bremer, J. (1981) Biochim. Biophys. Acta 665, 628–631.
231 Saggerson, E.D. (1982) Biochem. J. 202, 397–405.
232 Saggerson, E.D. and Carpenter, C.A. (1982) FEBS Lett. 137, 124–128.
233 McMillin Wood, J. (1975) J. Biol. Chem. 250, 3062–3066.
234 Zammit, V.A. (1981) Biochem. J. 198, 75–83.
235 Daae, L.N.W. and Bremer, J. (1970) Biochim. Biophys. Acta 210, 92–104.
236 Borrebaek, B. (1975) Acta Physiol. Scand. 95, 448–456.
237 Bates, E.J. and Saggerson, E.D. (1979) Biochem. J. 182, 751–762.
238 Lund, H., Borrebaek, B. and Bremer, J. (1980) Biochim. Biophys. Acta 620, 364–371.
239 McGarry, J.D., Robles-Valdes, O. and Foster, D.W. (1975) Proc. Natl. Acad. Sci. (U.S.A.) 72, 4385–4388.
240 Smith, C.M., Cano, M.L. and Potyraj, J. (1978) J. Nutr. 108, 854–862.
241 Halvorsen, O. and Skrede, S. (1982) Eur. J. Biochem. 124, 211–215.
242 Tubbs, P.K. and Garland, P.B. (1964) Biochem. J. 93, 550–556.
243 Siess, E.A., Brocks, D.G. and Wieland, O.H. (1978) Z. Physiol. Chem. 359, 785–798.
244 Skrede, S. and Halvorsen, O. (1979) Biochem. Biophys. Res. Commun. 91, 1536–1542.
245 Bortz, W.M. and Lynen, F. (1963) Biochem. Z. 339, 77–82.
246 Neat, C.E., Thomassen, M.S. and Osmundsen, H. (1980) Biochem. J. 186, 369–371.
247 Ishii, H., Horie, S. and Suga, T. (1980) J. Biochem. (Tokyo) 87, 1855–1858.
248 Horie, S., Ishii, H. and Suga, T. (1981) J. Biochem. 90, 1691–1696.
249 Christiansen, R.Z., Christiansen, E.N. and Bremer, J. (1979) Biochim. Biophys. Acta 573, 417–429.
250 Lazarow, P.D. (1977) Science 197, 580–581.
251 Svoboda, J., Grady, H. and Azarnoff, D.L. (1967) J. Cell. Biol. 35, 127–152.
252 Reddy, J.K., Azarnoff, D.L., Svoboda, J. and Prasad, D. (1974) J. Cell. Biol. 61, 344–358.
253 Reddy, J.K., Lalwani, N.D., Dabholkar, A.S., Reddy, M.K. and Qunshi, S.A. (1981) Biochemistry, I Int. 3, 41–49.
254 Solberg, H.E., Aas, M. and Daae, L.N.W. (1972) Biochim. Biophys. Acta 280, 434–439.
255 Furuta, S., Miyazawa, S. and Hashimoto, T. (1982) J. Biochem. 90, 1751–1756.
256 Kurup, C.K.R., Aithal, H.N. and Ramasarma, T. (1970) Biochem. J. 116, 773–779.
257 Christiansen, R.Z., Osmundsen, H., Borrebaek, B. and Bremer, J. (1978) Lipids 13, 487–491.
258 Beynen, A.C., Vaartjes, W.J. and Geelen, M.J.H. (1979) Diabetes 28, 828–835.
259 Bates, E.J., Topping, D.L., Sooranna, S.P., Saggerson, D. and Mayes, P.A. (1977) FEBS Lett. 84, 225–228.
260 Heimberg, M., Weinstein, J. and Kohnt, M. (1969) J. Biol. Chem. 244, 5131–5139.
261 Christiansen, R.Z. (1979) FEBS Lett. 103, 89–92.
262 Pilkis, S.J., Riou, J.P. and Claus, T.H. (1976) J. Biol. Chem. 251, 7853–7862.
263 Siess, E.A., Fahimi, F.M. and Wieland, O.H. (1981) Z. Physiol. Chem. 362, 1643–1651.
264 Zammit, V.A. (1980) Biochem. J. 190, 293–300.
265 Edwards, M.W., Cawthorne, M.A. and Williamson, D.H. (1981) Biochem. J. 198, 239–242.
266 Assimacopoulos-Jeannet, F., Denton, R.M. and Jeanrenaud, B. (1981) Biochem. J. 198, 458–490.
267 Denton, R.M. and McCormack, J.G. (1981) Clin. Sci. 61, 135–140.
268 Pfeifle, B., Pfeifle, R., Faulhaber, J.-D. and Ditschureit, H. (1980) Hormone Metab. Res. 12, 711–713.
269 Bartels, P.D. and Sestoft, L. (1980) Biochim. Biophys. Acta 633, 56–67.
270 Keyes, W.G., Wilcox, H.G. and Heimberg, M. (1981) Metabolism 30, 135–146.
271 Laker, M.E. and Mayes, P.A. (1981) Biochem. J. 196, 247–255.
272 Müller, M.J., Köster, H. and Seitz, H.J. (1981) Biochim. Biophys. Acta 666, 475–481.
273 Stakkestad, J.A. and Bremer, J. (1982) Biochim. Biophys. Acta 711, 90–100.

274 Leung, K. and Munck, A. (1975) Annu. Rev. Physiol. 37, 245–272.

275 Shafrir, E. (1978) in: H.-D. Söling and C.-D. Seufert (Eds.), Biochemical and Clinical Aspects of Ketone Body Metabolism, Georg Thieme, Stuttgart, pp. 127–136.

276 Klausner, H. and Heimberg, M. (1967) Am. J. Physiol. 212, 1236–1246.

277 Soler-Argilaga, C. and Heimberg, M. (1976) J. Lipid Res. 17, 605–615.

278 Ockner, R.K., Lysenko, N., Manning, J.A., Monroe, S.E. and Burnett, D. (1980) J. Clin. Invest. 65, 1013–1023.

279 Ockner, R.K. and Manning, J.A. (1974) J. Clin. Invest. 54, 326–338.

280 Wu-Rideout, M.Y.C., Elson, C. and Shrago, E. (1976) Biochem. Biophys. Res. Commun. 71, 809–816.

281 Carlson, L.A. and Pernow, B. (1959) J. Lab. Clin. Med. 53, 833–841.

282 Friedberg, S.J., Sher, P.B., Bogdonoff, M.D. and Esters, E.H. (1963) J. Lipid Res. 4, 34–38.

283 Molé, P.A., Oscai, L.B. and Holleszy, J.O. (1971) J. Clin. Invest. 50, 2323–2330.

284 Bressler, R. and Wittels, B. (1965) Biochim. Biophys. Acta 104, 39–45.

285 Engel, A.E. and Angelini, C. (1973) Science 179, 899–901.

286 Markesbery, M.D., McQuillin, M.P., Procopis, P.C., Harrison, A.K. and Engel, A.G. (1974) Arch. Neurol. 31, 320–324.

287 Böhmer, T., Bergrem, H. and Eiklid, K. (1978) Lancet 1, 126–128.

288 Tomec, R.J. and Hoppel, C.L. (1975) Arch. Biochem. Biophys. 170, 716–723.

289 Olowe, Y. and Schulz, H. (1980) Eur. J. Biochem. 109, 425–429.

290 Hall, L.M. (1961) Biochem. Biophys. Res. Commun. 6, 177–179.

291 Randle, P.J., Garland, P.B., Hales, C.N., Newsholme, E.A., Denton, R.M. and Pogson, C.I. (1966) Recent Progr. Hormone Res. 22, 1–44.

292 Krebs, H.A. (1967) Adv. Enzyme Regul. 4, 339–353.

293 Rennie, M.J., Winder, W.W. and Holloszy, J.O. (1976) Biochem. J. 156, 647–655.

294 Baldwin, K.M., Klinkerfuss, G.H., Terjung, R.L., Mole, R.A. and Holloszy, J.O. (1972) Am. J. Physiol. 222, 373–378.

295 Hanson, P.J. and Carrington, J.M. (1981) Biochem. J. 200, 349–355.

296 Cahill, G.F. and Owen, O.E. (1968) in: F. Dickens, P.J. Randle and W.J. Whelan (Eds.), Carbohydrate Metabolism and its Disorders, Vol. I. pp. 497–528.

297 Harper, R.D. and Saggerson, E.D. (1975) Biochem. J. 152, 485–494.

298 Hittelman, K., Lindberg, O. and Cannon, B. (1969) Eur. J. Biochem. 11, 183–192.

299 Christiansen, E.N., Pedersen, J.I. and Grav, H.J. (1969) Nature (London) 222, 857–860.

300 Nicholls, D.G. (1979) Biochim. Biophys. Acta 549, 1–29.

301 Smith, R.E. and Horwitz, B.A. (1969) Physiol. Rev. 49, 330–425.

302 Nicholls, D.G. (1976) Eur. J. Biochem. 62, 223–228.

303 Prusiner, S.B., Cannon, B. and Lindberg, O. (1968) Eur. J. Biochem. 6, 15–22.

304 Locke, R.M. and Nicholls, D.G. (1981) FEBS Lett. 135, 249–252.

305 Vignais, P.M., Gallagher, C.H. and Zabin, I. (1958) J. Neurochem. 2, 283–287.

306 Kawamura, N. and Kishimoto, Y. (1981) J. Neurochem. 36, 1786–1791.

307 Hawkins, F.A., Williamson, D.H. and Krebs, H.A. (1971) Biochem. J. 122, 13–18.

308 Williamson, D.H., Bates, M.W., Page, M.A. and Krebs, H.A. (1971) Biochem. J. 121, 41–47.

309 Chase, J.F.A. and Tubbs, P.K. (1969) Biochem. J. 111, 225–235.

310 Chase, J.F.A. and Tubbs, P.K. (1970) Biochem. J. 116, 731–720.

311 Tubbs, P.K., Ramsay, R.R. and Edwards, M.R. (1980) in: R.A. Frenkel and J.D. McGarry (Eds.), Carnitine Biosynthesis, Metabolism and Function, Academic Press, New York, pp. 207–217.

312 West, D.W., Chase, J.F.A. and Tubbs, P.K. (1971) Biochem. Biophys. Res. Commun. 42, 912–917.

313 Mahadevan, S. and Sauer, F. (1971) J. Biol. Chem. 246, 5862–5867.

314 Goresky, C.A., Daly, D.S., Mishkin, S. and Arias, I.M. (1978) Am. J. Physiol. 234, E542–E553.

315 Parvin, R., Goswami, T. and Pande, S.V. (1980) Can. J. Biochem. 58, 822–829.

316 Fritz, I.B. and Marquis, N.R. (1965) Proc. Natl. Acad. Sci. (U.S.A.) 54, 1226–1233.

317 McGarry, J.D. and Foster, D.W. (1974) Diabetes 23, 485–493.

318 Wolkowicz, P.E., Pownall, H.J. and McMillin-Wood, J.B. (1982) Biochemistry 21, 2990–2996.

154

319 Tutwiler, G.F., Ho, W. and Mohrbacher, R.J. (1981) Methods Enzymol. 72, 533–551.
320 Bartlett, K., Bone, A.J., Koundakjian, P.P., Meredith, E., Turnbull, D.M. and Sherratt, H.S.A. (1981) Biochem. Soc. Trans. 9, 574–575.
321 Ciardelli, Th., Stewart, Ch.J. and Wieland, Th. (1981) Liebigs Ann Chem. 828–841.
322 Sherratt, H.S.A. and Osmundsen, H. (1976) Biochem. Pharmacol. 25, 743–753.
323 Osmundsen, H. and Sherratt, H.S.A. (1976) FEBS Lett. 55, 38–42.
324 Osmundsen, H. (1978) FEBS Lett. 88, 219–222.
325 Billington, D., Osmundsen, H. and Sherratt, H.S.A. (1978) Biochem. Pharmacol. 27, 2879–2890.
326 Bauche, F., Sabourault, D., Guidicelli, Y., Nordmann, J. and Nordmann, R. (1981) Biochem. J. 196, 803–809.
327 Brunengraber, H., Boutry, M. and Lowenstein, J.M. (1973) J. Biol. Chem. 248, 2656–2664.
328 Raaka, B.M. and Lowenstein, J.M. (1979) J. Biol. Chem. 254, 6755–6762.
329 Bloxham, D.P. and Chalkly, R.A. (1976) Biochem. J. 159, 201–211.
330 Bloxham, D.P., Chalkly, R.A., Coghlin, S.J. and Salam, W. (1978) Biochem. J. 175, 999–1011.
331 Holland, P.C. and Sherratt, H.S.A. (1973) Biochem. J. 136, 157–171.
332 Foug, J.C. and Schulz, H. (1978) J. Biol. Chem. 253, 6916–6922.
333 Schulz, H. and Foug, J.C. (1981) Methods Enzymol. 72, 604–610.
334 Williamson, J.R., Rognstad, S.G. and Peterson, M.J. (1970) J. Biol. Chem. 245, 3242–3249.
335 Hiltunen, J.K., Kaupinen, R.A., Nuutinen, E.M., Peuhkurinen, K.J. and Hassinen, I. (1980) Biochem. J. 188, 725–729.
336 Hiltunen, J.K. and Davis, E.J. (1981) Biochem. J. 194, 427–432.
337 Van Hoof, F., Hue, L. and Sherratt, H.S.A. (1979) Biochem. Soc. Trans. 7, 163–165.
338 Rein, K.A., Borrebaek, B. and Bremer, J. (1979) Biochim. Biophys. Acta 574, 497–504.
339 Lynen, F. (1953) Fed. Proc. 12, 683–691.

S. Numa (Ed.) Fatty Acid Metabolism and Its Regulation
© 1984 Elsevier Science Publishers B.V.

CHAPTER 6

Fatty acid biosynthesis in higher plants

P.K. STUMPF

Department of Biochemistry and Biophysics, University of California, Davis, CA 95616, U.S.A.

1. Introduction

In this chapter, the present status of the biosynthesis of fatty acids in higher plants will be examined.

For a number of years, the general outline of fatty acid biosynthesis in extracts or isolated organelles derived from a variety of plant tissues has become quite well defined. However, precise knowledge concerning the localization of the fatty acid synthetase (FAS) systems was not available until the techniques of protoplast isolation and disruption were developed. More recently with the advent of sensitive assay systems and the development of methods for the chemical and enzymic synthesis of acyl acyl carrier protein (ACP), research into the individual enzymes of the FAS could be conducted. By using these and other techniques, investigators have recently shown that higher-plant FAS systems are prokaryotic in molecular structure, i.e. are non-associated enzyme proteins — both in the leaf cell and in the seed cell.

This chapter will, therefore, describe these results as they apply to a variety of plant tissues.

2. Initial steps

(a) Origin of acetyl-CoA

(i) Leaf cell

Although CO_2 is the ultimate carbon precursor of acetyl-CoA in the leaf cell, the immediate precursor is probably pyruvic acid.

Pyruvic acid is derived from the conversion of either dihydroxyacetone phosphate (DHAP) or 3-phosphoglyceraldehyde to pyruvic acid by the glycolytic enzyme triose phosphate dehydrogenase, phosphoglycerokinase, phosphoglyceromutase, enolase and pyruvic kinase all of which are present in the cytosolic compartment of the leaf cell. The triose phosphates, namely dihydroxyacetone phosphate and 3-phosphoglyceraldehyde, are generated in the stroma phase of the chloroplast by the Calvin cycle and are then transported into the cytosol via the phosphate translocator of the outer envelope of the chloroplast [1].

There is, at present, still some uncertainty as to whether the necessary glycolytic enzymes are present in the chloroplast for the conversion of DHAP to pyruvic acid. In addition, the presence of the pyruvic dehydrogenase complex (PDC) in the chloroplast is also in dispute [1]. Whereas some investigators have presented evidence in support of a complete glycolytic enzyme system in chloroplasts, others have shown consistently that enolase is absent in the chloroplast but present in the cytosol.

It could be quite possible that enolase and PDC are present in the developing chloroplast and then lost in the mature chloroplast, or that chloroplasts derived from other plant species might have variable concentrations of these enzymes. It should be pointed out, however, that it would be to the leaf cell's advantage not to have a complete glycolytic system in its chloroplasts. If the complete system were present, phosphoglyceric acid would be converted to pyruvic acid and thence to acetyl-CoA in the chloroplast. Thus, one of the principal functions of the chloroplast, namely the export of DHAP into the cytosol for the synthesis of sucrose would be negated. The flow of carbon from DHAP to pyruvate in the chloroplast must be prevented either by the absence of a key enzyme(s) or by a careful regulation of the enzyme(s) during CO_2 fixation. This appears to be the case.

Pyruvate, formed in the cytosol from DHAP, now enters the mitochondrion, there to be oxidatively decarboxylated by PDC to form acetyl-CoA + CO_2 [2,3]. At this point, acetyl-CoA may enter the TCA cycle to be oxidized to CO_2 + water and to generate ATP by oxidative phosphorylation or it may be hydrolyzed by an acetyl-CoA hydrolase, found only in the mitochondrion, to be relased as free acetate [2,3]. Free acetate can then move out of the mitochondrion through the cytosol and into the chloroplast, there to be converted to acetyl-CoA [4]. Free acetate is non-toxic, readily permeable and totally unreactive. The regulatory system that must come into play in the mitochondrion in order for acetyl-CoA to convert either to citrate or to free acetate is at present not well understood. Although it is known that free CoA non-competitively inhibits the hydrolase, its role in the physiological regulation of acetate flow is not clear [2,3]. There are instances where acetyl-CoA must be generated in the cytosolic compartment and this may occur in some tissues either by the cleavage of citrate by citrate : ATP-CoA lyase to acetyl-CoA and oxaloacetate or by a direct conversion of acetate to acetyl CoA by acetyl-CoA synthetase [5].

In the spinach leaf cell, acetyl-CoA synthetase is located exclusively in the stroma phase of the chloroplast [6]. The localization of this enzyme in the chloroplast makes possible a vectorial flow of free acetate from the mitochondrion to the chloroplast and its conversion to acetyl-CoA which is then utilized in several biosynthetic pathways.

The formation of acetyl-CoA, therefore, requires the interaction of the mitochondria with the chloroplast in the spinach leaf cell [2,3]. This conclusion is based on (i) the presence of PDC only in the mitochondrion, (ii) the presence of acetyl-CoA synthetase only in the stroma phase of the chloroplast, and (iii) a reconstituted system in which pyruvate was readily incorporated into fatty acids only when both mitochondria and chloroplast were present in the reaction mixture [3]. It should be emphasized that these conclusions were derived from experiments with spinach mitochondria and chloroplasts. Certainly in leaf or seed cells from other plants where acetyl-CoA must be generated in the cytosol for other metabolic functions, modifications of this system must occur.

(ii) Seed cell

In the developing seed tissue, be it cotyledonous or endosperm tissue, there is now considerable evidence that special organelles identified as proplastids contain all the necessary enzymes to generate ATP, NADPH, NADH, as well as the enzymes to convert pyruvate to acetyl-CoA and the FAS enzymes to utilize acetyl-CoA for oleic acid synthesis [1].

Sucrose, synthesized in the cytosolic compartment of the leaf cell, is transported by the phloem vascular system to the developing seed. There, invertase hydrolyzes sucrose to glucose and fructose. These sugars are then phosphorylated by the proplastid hexokinase to glucose-6-PO_4 and fructose-6-PO_4 which are then converted by glycolytic enzymes to pyruvic acid, generating ATP and NADH. NADPH is generated by the proplastid pentose PO_4 pathway. PDC, present in the proplastids of developing seeds, readily converts pyruvate to acetyl-CoA. Since acetate is also effectively used as a substrate for fatty acid synthesis, acetyl-CoA synthetase is also present.

In summary, in the leaf cell, CO_2 converts to DHAP via the Calvin cycle; DHAP is transported into the cytosol there to be converted to pyruvate. This substrate then enters the leaf mitochondrion to be oxidized to acetyl-CoA, and then in part, hydrolyzed to acetate which is vectorially transported back into the chloroplast, there to be converted to acetyl-CoA. In the seed cell, sucrose serves as the source of pyruvate. All the necessary enzymes to convert sucrose to pyruvate and then to acetyl-CoA are found either in the cytosol or in the matrix of the proplastid. As we shall see, both in the chloroplast and in the proplastid, the major product of fatty acid synthesis is oleic acid.

(b) Formation of malonyl-CoA

Acetyl-CoA carboxylase is the enzyme responsible for the synthesis of malonyl-CoA in all plant tissues. In procaryotic organisms (see Chapter 1 of this volume), the enzyme consists of 3 separable proteins, namely biotin carboxylase, biotin carboxylcarrier protein, and transcarboxylase and these proteins are involved in the following sequence:

$$ATP + HCO_3^- + BCCP \xrightarrow{\text{biotin carboxylase}} CO_2^- BCCP + ADP + P_i$$

$$CO_2^- BCCP + \text{acetyl-CoA} \xrightarrow{\text{transcarboxylase}} \text{malonyl-CoA} + BCCP$$

In animal systems (see Chapter 1 of this volume), the enzyme exists as a polyfunctional inactive protein with a molecular weight of about 240 000 which consists of 3 domains — biotin carboxylase, BCCP and transcarboxylase. These are linked by an exposed polypeptide chain peculiarly susceptible to attack by endogenous proteases. In the presence of citrate this protomer rapidly aggregates to polymers of 7–10 million dalton, and these polymers are active forms of the enzyme. These polymers rapidly depolymerize in the presence of low concentrations of palmitoyl-CoA to the inactive protomer. In addition, there is increasing evidence that a phosphorylation–dephosphorylation cycle is involved in further modulating the activity of this important enzyme [7].

Acetyl-CoA carboxylase was first identified in plant tissues in 1961 when wheat-germ acetyl-CoA carboxylase was purified some 120-fold and some of its properties were described [8]. Acetyl-CoA was the most active substrate whereas propionoyl-CoA and butyryl-CoA were progressively less reactive. Unlike the animal system that was markedly activated by citrate anion, the wheat-germ carboxylase was not affected by a number of mono-, di- and tri-carboxylic acids. In 1969, Heinstein et al. purified the enzyme some 1000-fold and demonstrated that the enzyme had a high molecular weight of approximately 630 000 [9]. In 1979, Nielsen further purified the enzyme and demonstrated a complex relationship between the concentrations of K^+, Mg^{2+}, Mg-ATP and carboxylase activity [10]. More recently, Egin-Bühler et al. [11] have purified both the acetyl-CoA carboxylase from suspension culture cells of parsley and from wheat germ. Their results indicated that the parsley carboxylase had a molecular weight of 840 000 consisting of a large subunit of 210 000 and 105 000 dalton, whereas the wheat germ carboxylase had a molecular weight of 700 000 with a large subunit of 240 000 and a smaller subunit of 98 000 dalton. In both cases, biotin was associated with the larger subunits. The smaller subunits may be proteolytic breakdown products during purification of the enzyme.

The maize carboxylase has recently been examined by Nikolau [12]. While the activity is quite unstable, the kinetic parameters of the carboxylase were nevertheless determined. The avocado mesocarp carboxylase has also been purified to homogeneity [13]. Evidence would suggest that all these carboxylases are oligomeric with a molecular weight ranging from 6.1 to 6.5×10^5. These enzymes when kept in solution rapidly lose their activity and cannot be readily restored. The activity may be stabilized somewhat in the presence of glycerol, citrate, HCO_3^- and bovine serum albumin. The function of all these compounds is not clear.

Recently Eastwell in this laboratory has examined the regulation of wheat-germ and spinach-chloroplast acetyl-CoA carboxylases [14]. He noticed that if crude extracts of wheat germ or spinach were preincubated with ATP, and then assayed by the usual procedures, the activity was much lower than when ATP was omitted from the preincubation mixture. In contrast, partial purification of the carboxylase now yielded preparations which, on preincubation with ATP, did not show any inhibitory effects by ATP. Further examination indicated that all crude plant extracts contained high levels of adenylate kinase and ATPase. Indeed, the inhibitory component turned out to be ADP which has a K_i of 40 μM with the spinach carboxylase. A

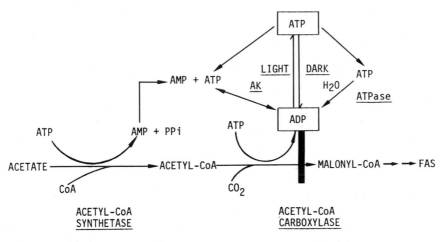

Fig. 1. The regulation of chloroplast acetyl-CoA carboxylase as a function of the control of the levels of ATP, ADP, and AMP in the chloroplast.

regeneration of ATP by such systems as creatine-PO_4 and creatine kinase prevented the preincubation effects. Fig. 1 summarizes a possible regulatory scheme in the chloroplast which would in part explain the long known observation that light is required for fatty acid synthesis from acetate in isolated chloroplasts. In the absence of light, ADP concentrations rise whereas in the presence of light, photophosphorylation will reduce ADP levels [15]. Finlayson and Dennis [16] have recently examined these effects with acetyl-CoA carboxylase from developing castor-bean seeds and have evidence to suggest that 3 dead-end complexes, namely $E \cdot HCO_3 \cdot ADP$, $E \cdot HCO_3 \cdot P_i$ and $E \cdot P_i P_i$ may participate in the inhibition of the enzyme. Thus, the adenylate charge in the chloroplast and in the proplastid may participate in the regulation of acetyl-CoA carboxylase and hence fatty acid biosynthesis in these organelles. There is no evidence to support either a phosphorylation–dephosphorylation cycle, or an inactive monomer transition to an active oligomer form of the enzyme, both of which mechanisms are of considerable importance in the animal systems.

(c) Plant acyl carrier proteins

The demonstration of the presence and requirement of an acyl carrier protein (ACP) in higher plant systems was first reported by Overath and Stumpf [17] working with extracts of avocado mesocarp tissue. Shortly thereafter, Simoni et al. [18] isolated, purified and characterized spinach and avocado ACP; Matsumura and Stumpf [19] elucidated the core amino acid sequence adjacent to the serine residue to which the 4′-phosphopantetheine residue was associated. Although there were marked differences in the composition of the amino acids peripheral to the core amino acid sequence in spinach ACP when compared to the *E. coli* ACP, the core amino acid

TABLE 1

A comparison of plant and bacterial acyl carrier proteins

Source [a]	MW	Amino acid residues	Relative specific activities [a]
Escherichia coli	8 700	77	1.0
Arthrobacter sp.	9 500	81	1.0
Spinach leaf	9 500	88	0.3
Avocado mesocarp	11 500	117	0.3

[a] With spinach chloroplast stroma as the source of the fatty acid synthetase assay system.

sequence of -gly-ala-asp-ser*-asp- was the same.

A number of investigators have now also confirmed the requirement of ACP for de novo fatty acid synthesis in higher plants [5]. Because E. coli ACP is readily available, it is usually employed in experiments dealing with plant fatty acid synthesis. When either E. coli ACP or spinach ACP are employed as the component in FAS extracts, the final products are essentially identical. Of course, there always exists the possibility of fine differences in substrate specificity provided by either E. coli or the endogenous ACP. Table 1 compares some of the characteristics of plant and bacterial ACPs.

The precise role of ACP was defined by the observations of Ohlrogge et al. [20]. They showed that when antibodies raised against spinach ACP were added to extracts of spinach leaves, [^{14}C]malonyl-CoA incorporation into fatty acids was completely blocked. In addition, all the ACP in a spinach protoplast preparation was localized in the chloroplast. Assuming that ACP is a specific marker for the synthesis of C_{16} and C_{18} fatty acids, it can therefore be concluded that only the chloroplast is the site for the synthesis of these fatty acids in the leaf cell.

It has been estimated that ACP is present at approximately 8 μM concentration in the stroma phase of spinach chloroplasts [20]. If ACP only occurs in the stroma phase, the interesting question arises as to the site of the synthesis of this key protein in the leaf cell. Since up to 80% of all chloroplast proteins are encoded for by nuclear DNA, one could assume that the ACP mRNA is present in the cytosol and translated to the protein for transport directly into the chloroplast [21]. This important question should be readily answered in the near future.

The functions of ACP can now be enumerated as follows:

(i) It is the specific thioester component for all the enzymes involved in the conversion of C_2 to C_{18} fatty acids. While both the β-ketoacyl-ACP reductase and the enoyl-ACP reductase have low reactivity with CoA thioester derivatives, β-OH acyl-ACP dehydrase is completely unreactive with corresponding CoA thioester derivatives.

(ii) Oleoyl-ACP hydrolase is a specific enzyme that hydrolyzes the thioester to oleic acid and ACP, thereby regenerating ACP and allowing oleic acid to transfer to another compartment.

(iii) The stroma phase of the chloroplast contains a soluble glycerol 3-PO$_4$ acyl transferase that specifically transfers the acyl compartment of an acyl-ACP to the 1-position to form 1-acyl glycerol-PO$_4$. The acyl component is also very specific in that the oleoyl group is much preferred. The envelope-bound monoacyl glycerol 3-P acyltransferase specifically utilizes palmitoyl-ACP for transfer to the 2-OH function to form a 1-oleoyl, 2-palmitoyl phosphatidic acid [22].

(iv) Stearoyl-ACP desaturase is a highly reactive desaturase [9] located only in the chloroplast of leaf cells and in the proplastid of seed cells to form oleoyl-ACP. Stearoyl-CoA, having a much higher K_m, as a substrate, is far less effective (cf. detailed discussion in Section 4.b) [23].

In summary, ACP participates as the thioester moiety in the synthesis of the C$_{16}$ and C$_{18}$ fatty acids, in their transfer to suitable acceptors, and in the introduction of the first double bond in the hydrocarbon chain, namely at the Δ^9 position. Further elongations, modifications and desaturations occur with CoA derivatives and/or complex lipids at appropriate sites in the cell.

3. The plant fatty acid synthetase (FAS) system

In 1952, the effective incorporation of [^{14}C]acetate into long-chain fatty acid was observed by plant tissues [24] and 5 years later, a particulate preparation obtained from avocado mesocarp was the most effective fraction to incorporate [^{14}C]acetate into [^{14}C]palmitic and [^{14}C]oleic acids [25]. In 1958, it was shown that a soluble enzyme extract prepared from an acetone powder of avocado mesocarp particles required HCO$_3^-$ in addition to Mn^{2+}, ATP, CoA and NADPH for the incorporation of [^{14}C]acetate into free [^{14}C]oleic acid [26]. In 1964, Overath and Stumpf [17] showed for the first time that a heat-stable protein was required for the synthesis of fatty acids from [^{14}C]malonyl-CoA. This protein was identified by Overath as a plant ACP. In the meantime, 3 groups independently demonstrated in 1960–1963 that isolated leaf chloroplasts, in the presence of light, very effectively incorporated [^{14}C]acetate into [^{14}C]palmitic acid and [^{14}C]oleic acid [27–29].

Thus by 1964, the broad outline of de novo plant fatty acid biosynthesis had been laid down. Rather than describe the countless numbers of investigations extending these observations, we shall only describe the current status of the biosynthesis of fatty acids in higher plants.

(a) Sites of synthesis

In prokaryotic cells, fatty acid synthesis appears to occur in the cytosolic compartment. However, it has been observed that ACP in E. coli appears to be somewhat loosely associated with the inner face of the plasma membrane of the cell [30]. Nevertheless, all the activities associated with the synthesis of palmitic acid from acetyl-CoA were readily separated and assigned to individual proteins. These proteins have been purified and their molecular and kinetic characteristics examined in considerable detail [31]. In yeast and animal cells, the fatty acid synthetase responsible for the formation of palmitic acid is always associated with the cytosolic compartment as a hetero- or homodimer, respectively (see Chapter 2 of this volume).

Some years ago Stumpf and Barber [25] described a $10\,000 \times g$ particulate preparation obtained from avocado mesocarp tissue, which synthesized palmitic and oleic acids from [^{14}C]acetate. Later a number of workers [27–29] demonstrated that chloroplasts from a number of leaf tissues could readily synthesize fatty acids from [^{14}C]acetate, the principal products being palmitate and oleate under aerobic conditions and palmitate and stearate under anaerobic conditions. In 1964, Yamada and Stumpf [32] demonstrated that a $10\,000 \times g$ pellet obtained from a homogenate of developing castor bean seeds readily incorporated acetyl-CoA into oleic acid.

Although in the early sixties it was already recognized that a particulate fraction from avocado mesocarp and isolated chloroplasts were active sites of fatty acid synthesis, a precise decision on the actual site of synthesis could not be made. In the isolation of organelles, despite all attempts to preserve the integrity of the structures, disruption to varying extents always occurs. Thus, it was difficult to interpret the observation that supernatant extracts also possessed biosynthetic activity. The question of whether the activity was derived from disrupted organelles or from the cytosolic compartment could therefore not be precisely answered.

Zilkey and Canvin [33,34] clarified the earlier Yamada and Stumpf observations by isolating large particles by sucrose density gradient centrifugation of homogenates of developing castor-bean endosperm which converted [^{14}C]acetyl-CoA to [^{14}C]oleate and gave these particles the name "oleosomes". In 1975, Weaire and Kekwick [35] reported that plastid preparations obtained by density gradient centrifugation of homogenates of avocado mesocarp or cauliflower bud tissue, incorporated [1-^{14}C]acetate into fatty acids, principally palmitate and oleate, whereas the cytosolic protein fraction was essentially inactive. They concluded that the proplastids were the principal site of fatty acid biosynthesis. In the meantime, Yamada and his group in Japan [36] extended his 1964 observations in a series of papers which carefully documented the capacity of a $10\,000 \times g$ particle obtained from developing castor bean endosperm tissue to convert [^{14}C]sucrose to palmitate, stearate and oleate. These studies indicated that proplastids possessed all the enzymes necessary for the conversion of sucrose via a UDPG:fructose transglycosylase to glucose 1-phosphate and thence via glucose-6-P into the pentose phosphate pathway and finally to pyruvate and acetyl-CoA. Simcox et al. [37] extended the Zilkey and Canvin observations [33,34] on proplastids or oleosomes obtained from developing castor bean endosperm tissue. In essence, they determined that hexose phosphate synthesis from sucrose occurred in the cytosol along with the first oxidative step in the pentose phosphate pathway, namely, the glucose-6-P dehydrogenase reaction. The proplastid contained 6-phosphogluconate dehydrogenase, transketolase, transaldolase and the glycolytic enzymes necessary to convert fructose 6-phosphate to pyruvic acid, pyruvic dehydrogenase and the full complement of fatty acid synthetase enzymes responsible for the formation of oleic acid. Oleic acid then is transported out of the proplastid to the cytosol where the oleoyl hydroxylase [38,39] responsible for the conversion of oleoyl to ricinoleoyl moiety and the enzymes for triacylglycerol synthesis were all localized on the endoplasmic reticulum membrane [39,39].

Further support for the compartmentation concept is obtained from the recent work of Ohlrogge et al. [40] with in vivo incorporation of [^{14}C]acetate and [^{14}C]glucose into fatty acids and alcohols by slices of developing jojoba seed. Specifically, whereas [^{14}C]acetate was used exclusively for the elongation of endogenous oleic acid, the ^{14}C from [^{14}C]glucose was uniformly distributed throughout the acyl chain of fatty acids. A reasonable explanation of these entirely different labeling patterns would involve the existence of metabolically separate pools of acetate for de novo synthesis and elongation of acyl chains. These pools could possibly relate to proplastids and to endoplasmic reticulum membranes as two discretely different sites, the first for the de novo synthesis, of stearoyl-ACP, its desaturation to oleoyl-ACP and hydrolysis to free oleic acid, and the second for further elongation, reduction, and condensation of acyl-CoA derivatives for wax ester biosynthesis.

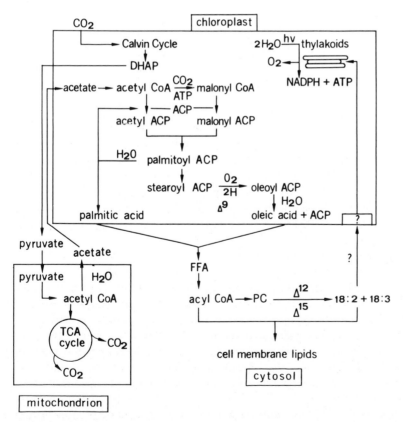

Fig. 2. The interrelationship of various compartments in the biosynthesis of oleic acid in the leaf cell.

164

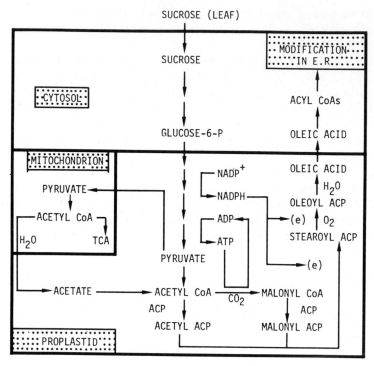

Fig. 3. The interrelationship of various compartments in the biosynthesis of oleic acid in the seed cell.

In addition, Vick and Beever [41] isolated proplastids from endosperm of germinating castor beans and demonstrated that these organelles were sites of fatty acid synthesis. Kleinig and Liedvogel [42] have obtained chromoplasts from daffodil petals and have demonstrated extensive incorporation of [^{14}C]acetate into palmitic acid. Nothelfer et al. [43] have also isolated proplastids from soybean tissue culture suspension cells capable of synthesizing fatty acids from [^{14}C]malonyl-CoA via the ACP track.

If the chloroplast can be considered a variant of a proplastid but with a photosynthetic capability, then this organelle should and does have the same complement of fatty-acid-synthesizing enzymes as the proplastid from non-photosynthetic tissue [5]. Indeed, recent work clearly demonstrated that ACP in a spinach leaf protoplast was exclusively localized in the chloroplast [20]. Since antibodies to spinach ACP completely blocked fatty acid synthesis in a spinach leaf homogenate, it followed that ACP was a specific marker for fatty acid synthesis and thus that the chloroplast was the specific site for the formation of palmitic and oleic acid in the leaf cell. It is conceivable that these acids are transported from the chloroplast to the cytosolic compartment for further modification, etc., and that some of the products of cytosolic modifications (i.e., linoleic and/or α-linolenic acids) are transported back to the chloroplast for final insertion into lamellar membrane lipids [87]. Figs. 2

and 3 outline the interactions of the various compartments in the leaf cell and in the seed cell for the biosynthesis of fatty acids.

(b) Molecular structure of the FAS system

For a number of years, data suggested that the FAS system was not a high molecular weight polyfunctional protein so characteristic of animal eukaryotic systems [5]. These conclusions were based on the fragmentary evidence that prolonged centrifugation at $100\,000 \times g$ did not sediment FAS activity and that ACP had to be added to the reaction mixture for optimal fatty acid synthesis [17]. Work by Jaworski et al. [44] had suggested that the conversion of acetyl-CoA (C_2) to stearic acid (C_{18}) was a 2-step sequence: a de novo system from $C_2 \rightarrow C_{16}$ and an elongation system from $C_{16} \rightarrow C_{18}$. These conclusions were based on the differential effects of the inhibitor, cerulenin, heat stability, and ammonium sulfate fractionation. The traditional assay of the FAS system was the incorporation of [^{14}C]malonyl-CoA into [^{14}C]C_{16} and -C_{18} acids.

The use of acyl-ACP substrates as intermediates in FAS synthesis was hindered by the technical problem of preparing suitable substrates. Acyl carrier protein substrates could be prepared by chemical procedures but there was considerable evidence to suggest that such acyl-ACP substrates were partially inactive. However, in recent years, the preparation of specific ACP substrates by mild procedures was developed by Cronan and his group [45]. These procedures yielded highly reactive substrates.

As a result within the past year (1982) 6 separate laboratories have initiated investigations to elucidate the molecular structure of the FAS system from avocado [46,47], barley [48], safflower [49], spinach [50] tissues, and parsley suspension culture cells [51]. The results from these laboratories complement each other very

TABLE 2

Molecular weights of several plant FAS systems

Enzyme	Molecular weight $\times 10^3$ [a]				
	Safflower [49]	Spinach [50,52–54]	Barley [48]	Avocado [47]	E. coli [3]
Acetyl-CoA : ACP transacylase	–	–	82	–	–
Malonyl-CoA : ACP transacylase	22	22	41	40.5	37
β-Ketoacyl-ACP synthetase I	–	56	92	–	66
β-Ketoacyl-ACP synthetase II	–	57	–	–	–
β-Ketoacyl-ACP reductase (NADPH)	83	97	125	40	–
β-Hydroxyacyl-ACP dehydrase	64	85	–	–	170
Enoyl-ACP reductase (NADH)	83	115	–	62.4	90

[a] Kilodalton.

well. By appropriate protein fractionation procedures, these workers already showed that all these systems are of the non-associated type similar to the FAS system of *E. coli*. Table 2 lists the molecular weights of a number of these systems and compares them to the available molecular weight determinations made with the *E. coli* enzymes. While there is some scattering of molecular weights, the order of magnitude appears to be quite similar.

Rather than examine the FAS systems from the various plant tissues, we shall select the spinach FAS system since this has been examined in considerable detail [50,52–54].

Crude extracts of spinach leaves were fractionated with polyethylene glycol [50]. Three fractions were obtained, i.e. 0–5%, 5–15%, and 15% supernatant. The following major activities were distributed in these fractions: 0–5%, β-ketoacyl-ACP synthetases I and II; 5–15%, β-ketoacyl-ACP reductase; and 15%, acetyl-CoA:ACP-transacylase, and malonyl-CoA:ACP-transacylase. The 5–15% PEG fraction was then chromatographed on a Sephadex G-200 column and there the minor activities of acetyl-CoA:ACP transacylase and malonyl transacylase were well separated but the two reductases and the dehydrase activities were in one rather broad peak. This fraction was then placed on a hydroxyapatite column. The enoyl-ACP reductase eluted early but the β-ketoacyl-ACP reductase and the dehydrase were essentially still in one peak. Finally, this peak was placed on a blue-agarose column and a stepwise elution with increasing salt concentration resulted in a clean-cut separation of the β-ketoacyl-ACP reductase and the dehydrase.

Further work resulted in the purification of the acetyl-CoA:ACP transacylase, the identification and purification of β-ketoacyl-ACP synthetases I and II, the β-ketoacyl-ACP reductase (NADPH), the β-hydroxyacyl-ACP dehydrase and the enoyl-ACP reductase (NADH).

(i) Acetyl-CoA:ACP transacylase and malonyl-CoA:ACP transacylase

Both acetyl-CoA:ACP transacylase and malonyl-CoA:ACP transacylase have been purified but their properties have as yet not been determined in the spinach system [47]. The avocado [47] and the barley chloroplast [48] systems have been described.

(ii) β-Ketoacyl-ACP synthetase I

$$\text{Acyl-ACP}_{(C_2-C_{14})} + \text{malonyl-ACP} \quad \rightarrow \quad \beta\text{-ketoacyl-ACP}_{(C_4-C_{16})} + CO_2 + \text{ACP}$$

This enzyme has been purified some 180-fold from spinach-leaf extracts [53]. Its molecular weight is 56 000 by gel filtration; the K_m for malonyl-ACP was 4 μM. The purified synthetase I was highly active with acyl-ACPs having chain lengths from C_2 to C_{14} with hexanoyl-ACP being the most effective substrate. Palmitoyl-ACP was far less effective and stearoyl-ACP was inactive. Cerulenin at 3 μM concentration caused 50% inhibition of the above reaction. Thus, synthetase I is an integral component of the FAS required for the formation of palmitoyl-ACP.

(iii) β-Ketoacyl-ACP synthetase II

$$\text{Palmitoyl-ACP} + \text{malonyl-ACP} \quad \rightarrow \quad \beta\text{-ketostearoyl-ACP} + CO_2 + \text{ACP}$$

This enzyme was discovered in spinach leaf extracts when it was observed that in crude extracts palmitoyl-ACP was elongated as well as decanoyl-ACP [54]. When the purified synthetase I (with decanoyl-ACP as the assay substrate in the purification procedure) was tested with palmitoyl-ACP, no activity was observed. With palmitoyl-ACP as the assay substrate, a protein was isolated that specifically elongated both myristoyl- and palmitoyl-ACP to β-ketostearoyl-ACP but had no activity for decanoyl-ACP. Synthetase II was purified some 295-fold and has a molecular weight of 57000. In sharp contrast to synthetase I, synthetase II was 50% inhibited only at 40 μM levels of cerulenin. Arsenite at 1 mM level did not inhibit synthetase I but inhibited synthetase II by 42%.

(iv) β-Ketoacyl-ACP reductase

$$\beta\text{-Ketoacyl-ACP} + \text{NADPH} + H^+ \quad \rightarrow \quad \text{D-}\beta\text{-hydroxyacyl-ACP} + \text{NADP}^+$$

This enzyme was purified some 422-fold by employing the PEG fractionation procedure, blue-agarose, Sephadex G-200 and hydroxylapatite chromatographies [52]. The molecular weight was determined by Sephacryl S-300 filtration to be 97000 whereas by SDS-PAGE, a molecular weight of 24200 was observed. These results would indicate that the native enzyme exists as a tetramer. Amino acid analysis showed that 57% of the amino acids were polar and 43% non-polar. Two cysteines were present per monomer. With acetoacetyl-ACP as substrate, NADPH was the reductant with a K_m of 25 μM. The product was the D-isomer. NADH was about 10% as effective as a reductant. While both acetoacetyl-ACP and acetoacetyl-CoA served as substrates, the ACP derivative was the most effective. The K_m values for the ACP derivative and the CoA derivative were 3.7 and 250 μM respectively and the maximal velocities 16.1 and 5.4 μmoles/min/mg protein respectively. Only acetoacetyl-ACP was tested but since the purified reductase functioned in the reconstituted system for the formation of stearoyl-ACP, it is assumed that the reductase has broad β-ketoacyl specificities.

(v) D-β-Hydroxyacyl-ACP dehydrase

$$\text{D-}\beta\text{-Hydroxyacyl-ACP} \quad \rightleftharpoons \quad \textit{trans}\text{-2-enoyl-ACP} + H_2O$$

This enzyme has been purified some 4900-fold to homogeneity [52]. Its molecular weight by gel filtration was determined to be 85000 and on an SDS-PAGE system, 19000. Thus, the native enzyme would appear to be a tetramer. The amino acid composition indicated 62% polar and 38% non-polar amino acid residues. One cysteine was present per monomer. The D-isomer was active whereas the L-isomer was completely inactive. A range of 2-enoyl-ACPs was tested for activity and the single enzyme reacted with substrate ranging from C_4 to C_{16} enoyl-ACPs. No activity was observed with crotonyl-CoA.

(vi) Enoyl-ACP reductase

$$2\text{-Enoyl-ACP} + \text{NADH} + \text{H}^+ \quad \rightleftharpoons \quad \text{acyl-ACP} + \text{NAD}^+$$

This enzyme was purified some 2200-fold to homogeneity [52]. Its molecular weight as determined by gel filtration was 115 000 and 32 500 by the SDS-PAGE procedure. Thus, the enzyme in its native state is probably a tetramer. Its amino acid composition has been determined and 64% of its amino acids are polar and 36% non-polar. It contains 2 cysteine per monomer. The optimum pH was 6.4. NADH was the specific reductant since NADPH was ineffective. The K_m for NADH was 11 μM. Broad substrate specificity was observed with 2-hexenoyl-ACP and 2-octenoyl-ACP as the most effective substrates. Crotonyl-CoA was also active.

(vii) General aspects

The first reduction step in the spinach FAS system catalyzed by β-ketoacyl-ACP reductase was specific for NADPH; similar observations have been made with safflower seeds [49], castor bean [54,55], *E. coli* [56], yeast [57], and animal [58]. However, we have observed that the PEG (5–15%) fraction from developing castor bean seeds contained β-ketoacyl-ACP reductase activity which could employ NADH as a replacement for NADPH but with only 15% of the activity of NADPH at saturating concentrations (T. Shimakata, personal communication). The second reduction step in the spinach system was catalyzed by NADH-dependent enoyl-ACP reductase; in contrast, safflower seed extracts contained both an enoyl-ACP reductase II requiring both NADH and NADPH and a reductase I similar to the spinach reductase [49]. The source of NADH in spinach chloroplasts is probably from electrons flowing through NADP : ferredoxin reductase which can also reduce NAD$^+$. In *E. coli*, 2 distinct enoyl-ACP reductases have been observed, one of which is NADH-specific with broad chain-length specificity and the other is NADPH-specific with limited chain-length specificity (shorter chain specific) [59]. Recently, Saito et al. [55] reported that castor-bean enoyl-ACP reductase was specific for NADPH and that *Chlorella vulgaris* reductase was specific for NADH. The enoyl-thioester reductase in multienzyme complexes of yeast [57] and vertebrates [58] requires NADPH. The spinach β-ketoacyl-ACP reductase and β-hydroxyacyl-ACP dehydrase showed strict stereospecificity (D form) identical to their counterparts in *E. coli* [60]. Although chain-length specificity of the spinach β-ketoacyl-ACP reductase was not tested, it could be suggested that since only a single peak of the activity was observed, albeit only with acetoacetyl-ACP as substrate, presumably the enzyme has a wide specificity. Such is the case with its counterpart in *E. coli* [61]. The β-hydroxyacyl-ACP dehydrase and enoyl-ACP reductase purified from spinach leaves were active to 2-enoyl-ACPs having chain lengths from C_4 to C_{16} [52]. Unlike *E. coli* dehydrase which has its highest activity toward crotonyl-ACP and its lowest activity toward the C_{10} substrate, the spinach dehydrase had the highest activity toward 2-octenoyl-ACP. The spinach enoyl-ACP reductase showed higher activity toward 2-hexenoyl-ACP and 2-octenoyl-ACP as was shown for the NADH-reductase in *E. coli* [59]. 3-Decenoyl-ACP was inactive to both the spinach β-hydroxyacyl-ACP dehydrase and enoyl-ACP reductase.

CoA esters were active to the spinach β-ketoacyl-ACP reductase and enoyl-ACP reductase, but inert to β-hydroxyacyl-ACP dehydrase. The NADPH-reductase of *E. coli* was absolutely specific for the ACP derivatives, whereas the NADH-reductase was active with both ACP and CoA derivatives [59]. The 3 enzymes purified from spinach leaves were sensitive to *p*-CMB but insensitive to NEM and arsenite. This would suggest that the more hydrophobic reagent, *p*-CMB, may penetrate a hydrophobic region of these enzymes where a sulfhydryl group is essential for activity but which cannot be reached by the more hydrophilic reagent, NEM.

Studies on the plant FAS systems have clearly revealed their non-associated nature. These data are now of considerable interest when the endosymbiotic origin of the chloroplast is considered. That the FAS system in the chloroplast appears to be very similar to the *E. coli* system immediately suggests the following questions: (i) what, if any, homology exists between the plant FAS proteins and the prokaryotic FAS proteins; (ii) does the nuclear genome or the chloroplast genome encode for the FAS proteins; and (iii) if the FAS proteins are the gene products of the nuclear genome, by what process of the newly translated proteins do they proceed specifically to the stroma phase of the chloroplast? The availability of these enzymes, purified to homogeneity, will now provide suitable test probes to resolve, in part, these questions.

(c) Termination mechanisms

All chloroplastic fatty acids are of the C_{16} and C_{18} variety, i.e. the principal saturated fatty acid is palmitic and the principal unsaturated fatty acids are linoleic and linolenic. Seed fatty acids, on the other hand, have a more flexible composition of fatty acids ranging in the Cuphea genus from C_8 to C_{18} fatty acids, in the rapeseed from C_{16} to C_{22}, and in other seed lipids, exotic ring and acetylenic fatty acids [63].

The question to be raised here is what determines the chain length of a fatty acid, i.e. why the consistent ratio of $15:85$ for the C_{16} and C_{18} fatty acids in so many leaf lipids? In the safflower species, one variety, US-10 has 6% of its fatty acids as palmitic, 13% as oleic, and 79% as linoleic whereas another variety, UC-1, has 6% palmitic, 75% oleic and 12% linoleic. In both varieties the leaf fatty acids are consistently 19% palmitic, 3% oleic, 27% linoleic and 51% linolenic acid. The ultimate purpose of plant lipid biochemistry is to define precisely the mechanisms that determine fatty acid composition, including the chain length of the acyl moiety and the extent of unsaturation in that acyl moiety.

Now that plant FAS systems have been defined, precise questions can be asked. As described above, β-ketoacyl-ACP synthetases I and II purified from a crude

TABLE 3

Role of synthetases I and II in spinach FAS enzyme system

Expt. No.	Enzymes	[14C]Malonyl-CoA incorporated (cpm)	Distribution of 14C-labeled fatty acids (%)					
			10:0	12:0	14:0	16:0	18:0	20:0
1	FAS enzymes alone	505	–	–	–	–	–	–
2	FAS enzymes + synthetase II	2 846	–	–	–	–	–	–
3	FAS enzymes + synthetase I	18 321	3.1	13.2	17.3	63.9	2.5	0
4	FAS enzymes + synthetases I and II	21 337	1.7	2.3	3.5	7.6	81.9	3.0
5	Crude leaf extract	18 943	0	0	0	17.0	79.8	3.2

For Expts. 1–4, FAS enzymes include purified spinach malonyl-CoA : ACP transacylase, β-ketoacyl-ACP reductase, β-hydroxyacyl-ACP hydratase, and enoyl-ACP reductase. Enzymes were mixed with ACP and dithiothreitol, and the mixture was preincubated. Then the FAS reaction was started by addition of either synthetase I or synthetase II with hexanoyl-ACP as substrate.

extract of spinach leaves had different substrate specificities. In order to examine the role of both synthetases in fatty acid synthesis, the spinach FAS system was reconstituted, employing only the component enzymes purified from spinach extracts. Acetyl-CoA : ACP transacylase was omitted because hexanoyl-ACP served as the primer substrate [54].

As shown in Table 3, when both synthetases were omitted from the reconstituted system, ^{14}C-labeled malonyl-CoA was not converted to [^{14}C]fatty acids. Omission of synthetase I also resulted in low incorporation of [^{14}C]malonyl-CoA into fatty acids (Table 3, Expt. 2). However, when synthetase I was added to the test system, the main product was [^{14}C]palmitate with smaller amounts of shorter-chain [^{14}C]fatty acids also accumulating. The addition of synthetase II alone to the system resulted in no fatty acid synthesis. The addition of synthetases I and II to the test system resulted in [^{14}C]stearate as the main product (Table 3, Expt. 4).

These data clearly demonstrated that (i) synthetase II plays a key role in the synthesis of C_{18} fatty acids, (ii) all the other enzymes, that is, β-ketoacyl-ACP reductase, β-hydroxyacyl-ACP dehydrase, and enoyl-ACP reductase function effectively over the entire C_2–C_{18} range, (iii) earlier suggestions that a special elongation system is responsible for the $C_{16} \rightarrow C_{18}$ conversion can now be reinterpreted in terms of the role of the specific synthetase II activity.

Finally, the products of the completely reconstituted FAS system compare very closely to those synthesized by the crude spinach leaf extract or by isolated chloroplasts in terms of C_{16} and C_{18} fatty acids formed. The regulation of synthetase II may play an important role in determining the relative amounts of C_{16} and C_{18} fatty acids in plant cells.

Not only does the specificity of β-ketoacyl-ACP synthetase II play a role in terminating at the C_{18} level but also the specificity of stearoyl-ACP desaturase is an additional factor limiting fatty acid synthesis at the C_{18} level. As soon as stearoyl-ACP is formed, it is desaturated to oleoyl-ACP. Oleoyl-ACP is now rapidly hydrolyzed by oleoyl-ACP hydrolase to free oleic acid [64] which can then translocate to another site in the cell for further modifications, i.e. hydroxylation, further desaturation or elongation. By the presence of these additional enzymes, the level of stearic acid is kept very low, a common feature of plant fatty acids, and the supply of oleic acid is always provided for further modifications.

The conversion of oleic acid to $C_{20:1}$ and thence to $C_{22:1}$ fatty acids has been examined in a number of tissues including rapeseed, nasturtium [65] and jojoba [66] where these acids occur. The evidence is quite clear that the single double bond in these monounsaturated fatty acids is introduced at the stearoyl-ACP → oleoyl-ACP level, that oleic acid is transferred from its synthesizing compartment to a modifying compartment, presumably the endoplasmic reticulum located in the cytosol, there to be elongated to C_{20} and C_{22} fatty acids. In these elongation reactions, the substrates are all CoA thioesters involving malonyl-CoA. ACP is not required. This system is referred to as a CoA track system in contrast to the $C_2 \rightarrow C_{18}$ system which is called the ACP track system.

Equally intriguing is the problem of the synthesis of the shorter-chain fatty acid, namely C_8, C_{10}, C_{12} and C_{14} acids by seed tissues of the genus Cuphea [67]. It is now known that these acids are synthesized from acetyl-ACP and malonyl-ACP by an ACP track system (M. Pollard, personal communication). But why Cuphea species accumulate very significant levels of medium-chain fatty acids is not known. Possible mechanisms to be considered would include:

(i) A specific acyl-ACP thioesterase for each particular species. Thus, as normal synthesis occurs, a specific acyl-ACP would have a major portion of the carbon flow diverted from C_{16} and C_{18} synthesis by hydrolysis of the appropriate medium-chain-length acyl-ACP by a highly specific thioesterase. The free acid would be converted to a CoA derivative and then transferred to an appropriate acceptor.

(ii) A specific acyl-ACP: acyltransferase will intercept the newly synthesized acyl-ACP and transfer to a specific acceptor which then converts to a triglyceride.

(iii) A fatty acid synthetase independent of the C_{16}–C_{18} conventional FAS system.

(iv) Control of levels of malonyl-CoA and ACP available for the synthesis

TABLE 4

Effect of concentrations of malonyl-CoA and ACP on the products of fatty acid synthesis by extract of *Solanum tuberosa* [68]

Component	Concentration	Fatty acids formed (%)				
		C_8	C_{10}	C_{12}	C_{14}	C_{16}
Malonyl-CoA	5 nmoles	19	22	23	24	12
Malonyl-CoA	65 nmoles	2	5	8	30	55
ACP	7 μg	0	2	2	12	84
ACP	275 μg	15	16	16	30	23

reactions. There is some precedent for this suggestion. Employing a partially purified potato tuber FAS system, Huang and Stumpf [68] showed that with low concentrations of malonyl-CoA, large amounts of C_8, C_{10}, C_{12} and C_{14} fatty acids were formed whereas at high concentrations, palmitic acid was the principal fatty acid synthesized. Changing the levels of acetyl-CoA and of NADPH did not markedly alter the composition of labeled fatty acid. However, with low levels of ACP, 90% of the fatty acids formed was palmitic, whereas with high levels, significant amounts of C_8, C_{10}, C_{12} and C_{14} fatty acids were synthesized. Thus, the conditions maximizing the synthesis of palmitic acid were high levels of malonyl-CoA and low levels of ACP and the converse was true for the synthesis of medium-chain fatty acids. These results are summarized in Table 4.

(v) Specific β-ketoacyl-ACP synthetases for each of the species that produce specific medium-chain fatty acids. Since β-ketoacyl synthetases I and II have been described, there is no reason why synthetases IV, V, etc. may not exist. Thus, there would be 2 normal synthetases I and II involved in C_{16} and C_{18} fatty acid synthesis and then a specific synthetase for a given fatty acid.

(vi) Safflower and spinach FAS systems normally produce C_{16} and C_{18} fatty acids. One of the two limiting enzymes is the acetyl-CoA : ACP transacylase [49,50]. The possibility could exist that in plants with shorter-chain fatty acid compositions, this enzyme is present in high concentrations thereby flooding the FAS system with primer substrates and kinetically making possible the formation of the shorter-chain fatty acids.

These and other possibilities are being at present explored in different laboratories.

4. Biosynthesis of unsaturated fatty acids

(a) Introduction

Plants are the principal sources of the polyunsaturated fatty acids, linoleic and α-linolenic acids. When we consider that all leaf tissues contain high levels of these acids, it is clear that they are the most abundant unsaturated fatty acids in the world. However, just as the synthesis of cellulose, the most abundant polysaccharide in the world, is poorly understood at present, so the synthesis of these two polyunsaturated fatty acids is not well defined. Oleic acid biosynthesis, in sharp contrast, is quite well documented.

Gurr [69] has thoroughly reviewed the literature on the biosynthesis of unsaturated fatty acids by both prokaryotic and eukaryotic organisms. Roughan and Slack [70] have also recently discussed the synthesis of these acids.

(b) Biosynthesis of oleic acid

There are two principal mechanisms for the introduction of a *cis* double bond into a hydrocarbon chain, the anaerobic and the aerobic mechanisms. As the name implies, the anaerobic mechanism requires no oxygen because the *cis* double bond is introduced by a highly specific β-hydroxydecanoyl-ACP dehydrase in prokaryotic organisms to form a *cis*-β-γ-decenoyl-ACP [71]. This substrate is then elongated by a series of malonyl-ACP additions until the final product, *cis*-vaccenoyl-ACP, is formed. In contrast, the aerobic mechanism requires a reductant, usually NADPH or NADH, an electron carrier, usually ferredoxin in plants and cytochrome b_5 in animals and yeasts, and a desaturase which presumably couples the reductant to molecular oxygen to form a species of oxygen which in turn extracts the H_D atoms at C_9–C_{10} to form *cis* double-bond system [72]. At present, there is no evidence supporting the anaerobic mechanism in plants, whereas all evidence points to the aerobic mechanism as the principal, if not the only, mechanism for the synthesis of unsaturated fatty acids [73].

Nagai and Bloch [74] were the first to demonstrate in Chlorella and in spinach chloroplasts a stearoyl-ACP desaturase; more recently these observations have been extended to include a wide variety of plant tissues. In essence, the stearoyl-ACP desaturase in all plants examined is a soluble protein found either in the proplastid of the cell or in the stroma phase of chloroplasts, unlike its counterpart in yeasts and animal tissues in which the substrate is stearoyl-CoA and the desaturase is membrane bound [69]. An input of two electrons either from NADPH or water via photosystems I and II is required, and the intermediate electron-carrier protein between the electron pair and molecular oxygen in plants is ferredoxin. In fact, spinach ferredoxin has been employed in most studies because of its stability, availability and reactivity. Whether the actual endogenous electron carrier is indeed ferredoxin, or any of a number of non-heme iron proteins, remains to be determined. A number of possible heme and non-heme proteins were tested with the safflower system [76] and spinach ferredoxin seems to be the most effective electron carrier.

Very recently, McKeon and Stumpf [77] have purified the safflower stearoyl-ACP desaturase approximately 200-fold by DEAE and affinity chromatography. The protein exists in the native state as a dimer with a molecular weight of 68 000.

Stearoyl-ACP desaturase is essentially specific for stearoyl-ACP. The desaturase is only 5% as active with stearoyl-CoA and 1% as active with palmitoyl-ACP. The K_ms for the two acyl-ACPs are similar (i.e. palmitoyl-ACP, 0.51 μM; stearoyl-ACP, 0.38 μM), yet the V_{max} for stearoyl-ACP is 100 times greater than that for palmitoyl-ACP. This is in sharp contrast to the acyl-CoA desaturase in mammalian systems where the K_ms and V_{max}s for stearoyl-CoA and palmitoyl-CoA are quite similar [78]. Thus, the plant desaturase virtually requires an 18-carbon chain length for activity. This specificity seems to involve more than mere recognition of chain length, since the K_ms of the acyl-ACPs are similar despite the difference in chain length. Apparently, the longer chain length of stearoyl-ACP allows the formation of a more reactive Michaelis complex.

The specificity of the desaturase toward stearoyl-ACP relative to stearoyl-CoA is of further interest. The specificity is derived from the binding of the thioester to the enzyme since the K_ms differ by 20-fold (stearoyl-ACP, 0.38 μM; stearoyl-CoA, 8.3 μM). Since the V_{max} for stearoyl-CoA is the same (within experimental error) as that for stearoyl-ACP, the substrate concentration plays a critical role. Indeed, the difference in K_m indicates the importance of ACP for substrate recognition.

The spectrum of stearoyl-ACP desaturase reveals no obvious absorption peaks from 325 to 800 nm. However, because the desaturase could not be concentrated without a great loss in activity, the spectra obtained for active enzyme would require a molar absorptivity of greater than 3000 to detect a peak. While this is below the ϵ_{max} for most protein pigments, the possibility of a low absorbance cofactor or a quenched redox pigment cannot be eliminated. The nature of the activation of oxygen by the desaturase therefore remains unresolved. Although cyanide, at a final concentration of 1 mM, was observed by Jaworski and Stumpf [76] to inhibit desaturation, the effect may be on the transport of electrons from NADPH to molecular oxygen via NADPH ferredoxin reductase and ferredoxin, rather than directly on the desaturase.

Since lipids of some plants (though not safflower) are more highly unsaturated when the plants are grown at low temperature [79], this phenomenon has been explained as being related to the decreasing solubility of oxygen with increasing temperature and the requirement of oxygen for desaturation [80]. Thus, oxygen has been considered the rate-limiting factor in fatty acid desaturation in non-photosynthetic tissue [80].

The desaturase shows an oxygen dependency; the oxygen concentration necessary for half-maximal activity was 56 μM, approximately one-fifth the concentration of oxygen in air-saturated water [77]. On the other hand, the reaction requires 400 μM oxygen for saturation. Since only a 2-fold increase in activity would result from a 7-fold increase in oxygen (going from half-maximal to maximal) and assuming similarity to stearoyl-ACP desaturases from other oil seeds, it would seem unlikely that oxygen could be a major controlling factor in the biosynthesis of oleic acid.

All proplastids or chloroplasts synthesize oleic acid as their main unsaturated fatty acid from [14C]acetate. Since Ohlrogge et al. [20] have shown that all the ACP of a leaf cell is localized in the chloroplast, it follows that the only site of stearoyl-ACP desaturase must be the chloroplast. The product of the stearoyl-ACP desaturase in crude extracts is always free oleic acid whereas in highly purified desaturase, oleoyl-ACP accumulates. It was shown by Shine et al. [64] and Ohlrogge et al. [81] that a highly specific acyl-ACP thioesterase occurs in both chloroplasts and proplastids which has a marked preference for oleoyl-ACP, converting this product to free oleic acid and ACP. This reaction is significant because it releases ACP for recycling into the FAS system and it forms free oleic acid that can readily move to other compartments for further modifications.

The thioesterase has a strong preference for oleoyl-ACP and is essentially inactive with oleoyl-CoA. With acyl-ACPs as substrates, specificity is a function of reaction rate and not binding selectivity. The K_ms for the acyl-ACPs are quite similar, ranging from 0.25 to 0.50 μM. This similarity points to ACP as the principal determinant of binding. The V_{max}s for palmitoyl-ACP, stearoyl-ACP, oleoyl-ACP, stearoyl-CoA and oleoyl-CoA are 140, 296, 1650, 0 and 0 nmoles/min/mg protein, respectively. The difference in V_{max}, therefore, implies a specific recognition of the acyl chain-bound to the enzyme. It also seems that the double bond of oleate is a more important recognition site than chain length, since the thioesterase has a 5-fold preference for the unsaturated and only a 2-fold preference for the longer of the saturated fatty acyl moieties.

In summary, 3 different enzymes interrelate to guarantee the formation of oleic acid, namely the β-ketoacyl-ACP synthetase II, stearoyl-ACP desaturase, and the acyl-ACP thioesterase. Because of the high specificity of these enzymes, the only product is free oleic acid.

(c) Biosynthesis of linoleic and α-linolenic acids

The introduction of the first double-bond system into a hydrocarbon chain is now quite well understood. The substrate is defined, and the characteristics of the enzyme system reasonably well described [74,76,77].

However, a remarkable change occurs in the systems involved in the introduction of the second and third double bonds into the hydrocarbon chain. The substrates are not clearly defined, and the enzyme systems appear to be membrane-bound. In addition, while the major site of linoleic and α-linolenic acids in leaf cells is the chloroplast lamellar membrane lipids, numerous workers have demonstrated that intact chloroplasts only synthesize oleic acid, although small amounts of linoleic and α-linolenic synthesis have been noted. One is forced to conclude that (i) chloroplasts and proplastids can only synthesize oleic acid or (ii) in the isolation of these organelles, a soluble effector is lost which under in vivo conditions modulates rigidly the oleic → linoleic → linolenic reactions or activities of an enzyme (acyl-ACP hydrolase?) which channels the appropriate substrate away from further desaturation or (iii) linoleic acid is synthesized in a cytosolic compartment and then transported back to the chloroplast for desaturation to α-linolenic acid. Superimposed on this problem is the very good possibility that the expression of activity of the two enzymes, namely, oleoyl desaturase and linoleoyl desaturase, is related to the type of tissue examined and the previous history of the tissue, i.e., the age of the tissue, the temperature at which the tissue was grown, and the light regime the tissue was exposed to. For example, some etiolated tissues such as maize leaves possess a high capacity for the conversion of oleate to linoleic acid and linolenate [82], whereas etiolated germinating cucumber cotyledons are essentially totally devoid of such activities until exposed to a light regime [83]. Non-photosynthetic tissues such as developing safflower seeds possess a high capacity for conversion of oleate to linoleic acid [84] and potato tubers on aging in the dark show a remarkable induction of capacity to convert oleate to linoleate [85,86]. Thus, there appears to be a wide variation among different plant tissues to form linoleic and α-linolenic acids. Unfortunately, there does not appear to be a consistent pattern. Moreover, all attempts to obtain systems which can be purified and thereby fully characterized have met with failure.

The problem of elucidating the biosynthesis of these two important polyunsaturated fatty acids is therefore complex. What is known about the problem is based mostly on intact tissue investigations or experiments with membrane fragments (i.e., microsomal preparations).

Two types of substrates are now considered the most likely candidates for the conversion of oleoyl to a linoleoyl product. The first may be an oleoyl thioester (either as a CoA or ACP moiety). The second substrate is usually considered to a β-oleoyl phosphatidylcholine. Evidence for acyl-CoA as a substrate derives from the investigations of Vijay and Stumpf [84], Abdelkader [86], and Dubacq et al. [87]. These workers employed microsomes from developing safflower seeds, "aged" potato slices, and leaf microsomes, respectively, and they observed that oleoyl-CoA was rapidly desaturated to linoleoyl-CoA in the presence of NADH and molecular oxygen. Both the substrate and the product were very rapidly transferred to the β position of endogenous phosphatidylcholine of the microsomal lipids. The system was very specific in that any substrate other than the oleoyl group, namely, elaidoyl, stearoyl, palmitoleoyl, palmitoyl and cis-vaccenoyl, was completely unreactive. Recently Styme and Appelqvist [88] have provided evidence that with the safflower system the primary substrate for desaturation is not oleoyl-CoA but β-oleoyl phosphatidylcholine. These workers suggest that oleoyl-CoA is the precursor of the formation of the actual substrate β-oleoyl phosphatidylcholine. The cofactor requirements, as would be expected, were the same as reported by earlier investigators. These results are very similar to those reported previously by Gurr [69] and Slack et al. [89] in plants, and by Talamo et al. [90] and Pugh and Kates [91] in yeast microsomal preparations, although these two groups observed very considerable desaturation of oleoyl-CoA to linoleoyl-CoA when compared to a slower desaturation rate with β-oleoyl phosphatidylcholine. One puzzle in all this work is the observation that only 30–50% of oleoyl phosphatidylcholine is converted to linoleoyl phosphatidylcholine; if indeed oleoyl phosphatidylcholine is the true substrate for desaturation, then all the β-oleoyl component should be desaturated to the β-linoleoyl component. This is never observed. Another interpretation suggests that only the boundary β-oleoyl phosphatidylcholine adjacent to the desaturase is the functional substrate, whereas β-oleoyl phosphatidylcholine remote from the desaturase cannot serve as a substrate.

The problem becomes even more confusing when one considers the evidence for the final desaturation in plants, namely, the conversion of linoleic acid to α-linolenic acid. Based mostly on in vivo rates of appearance of [14C]linolenate in complex lipids when the substrate is [14C]acetate, [14C]oleate, or [14C]linoleate, a number of workers concluded that the substrate was β-linoleoyl phosphatidylcholine and the product β-linolenoyl phosphatidylcholine (see review by Roughan and Slack [70]). Other workers have shown that, while β-linoleoyl phosphatidylcholine accumulates under in vivo conditions, β-linolenoyl phosphatidylcholine cannot be detected; in contrast, β-linolenoyl monogalactosyldiglyceride appears to be the primary product [70].

In order to clarify this puzzle, Murphy and Stumpf [83] employed greening cucumber (Cucumis sativus L.) cotyledons as the experimental tissue. Greening cucumber cotyledons exhibited dramatic increases in the ability to desaturase exogenously added [1-^{14}C]oleic acid and [1-^{14}C]linoleic acid after 2–3 h of illumination. These increases were effectively inhibited by 10 μg/mg cycloheximide. Oleate desaturation remained at a high level in constant light for 5–6 days after induction and then declined by ca. 50%; when returned to the dark, the tissue showed a sharp decrease in the conversion of [^{14}C]oleate to [^{14}C]linoleate ($t_{1/2} = 96$ h). Linoleate desaturation reached a maximum ca. 15 h after light induction and declined immediately therefore, while the tissue still was in the light; after induction had peaked, return of the tissue to the dark showed a dramatic fall in linoleate desaturation ($t_{1/2} = 3.6$ h). The changes in desaturation were correlated with the conversion of endogenous linoleate to α-linolenate in the etiolated cotyledons, and with the assembly of the chlorophyll-containing photosynthetic membranes. The incorporation of [1-^{14}C]acetate into lipids showed no significant light stimulation.

In sharp contrast to these experiments, Hawke and Stumpf [82] have clearly shown that both etiolated and greened maize leaf tissue rapidly convert oleic acid to linoleic acid and thence linolenate. Thus, the kinetics of the appearance and disappearance of oleate desaturase and linoleate desaturase differ markedly in different tissues, namely, cucumber cotyledonous tissue and maize leaf tissue. It becomes of obvious importance therefore that, in future research, the type of tissue, the history of the tissue, and the regime of conditions impinging on these tissues be taken into consideration before broad generalities can be stated.

In addition to the sequential desaturation pathway in which stearic acid → oleic acid → linoleic acid → linolenate conversions were observed, Jacobson et al. [92] provided direct evidence that soluble stromal elongation system in spinach chloroplasts elongated a pre-existing endogenous $\Delta^{7,10,13}$-hexadecatrienoic acid with acetyl-CoA to form α-linoleic acid. In addition, $\Delta^{5,8,11}$-tetradecatrienoic acid, which also occurred in low amounts in chloroplast lipid, was elongated. While this system can be demonstrated in vitro, recent in vivo studies do not support the earlier proposal of a specific formation of 12 : 3 and its elongation to 18 : 3 [93].

In summary, the site of oleate desaturation is most likely the endoplasmic reticulum. This organelle contains, in addition, all the enzymes involved in phospholipid biosynthesis. Whether or not a specific polar lipid or an acyl-CoA or an acyl-ACP is directly or indirectly involved for linoleic synthesis remains for further investigations to clarify. There is indirect evidence suggesting that the monogalactosyldiglyceride in the outer envelope of the chloroplast may be involved in the conversion of linoleic acid to linolenic acid. Once linoleic acid and linolenate are formed, these acyl moieties must be transported to their specific sites. In the leaf cell, the principal site of these acids is the chloroplast lamellar membrane. At present, there is no direct evidence for the occurrence of polyunsaturation in these specific membranes or even in chloroplasts themselves. Thus, these acyl moieties must be presumably transferred directly or indirectly to their final site from their synthesizing site.

Obviously, much more research with in vitro systems must be carried out before a final definition of these desaturation systems can be made.

References

1 Dennis, D.T. and Miernyk, J.A. (1982) Annu. Rev. Plant Physiol. 33, 27–50.
2 Murphy, D.J. and Stumpf, P.K. (1981) Arch. Biochem. Biophys. 212, 730–739.
3 Liedvogel, B. and Stumpf, P.K. (1982) Plant Physiol. 69, 897–903.
4 Jacobson, B.S. and Stumpf, P.K. (1970) Arch. Biochem. Biophys. 153, 656–663.
5 Stumpf, P.K. (1980) in: P.K. Stumpf and E.E. Conn (Eds.), The Biochemistry of Plants, Vol. 4, Academic Press, New York, pp. 177–204.
6 Kuhn, D.N., Knauf, M. and Stumpf, P.K. (1981) Arch. Biochem. Biophys. 209, 441–450.
7 Hardie, D.T. and Cohen, P. (1978) FEBS Lett. 91, 1–7.
8 Hatch, M.D. and Stumpf, P.K. (1961) J. Biol. Chem. 236, 2879–2885.
9 Heinstein, P.K. and Stumpf, P.K. (1969) J. Biol. Chem. 244, 5374–5381.
10 Nielsen, N.C., Adee, A. and Stumpf, P.K. (1979) Arch. Biochem. Biophys. 192, 446–456.
11 Egin-Bühler, B., Loyal, R. and Ebel, J. (1980) Arch. Biochem. Biophys. 203, 90–100.
12 Nikolau, B.J. (1981) Ph.D. Thesis, Massey University, Palmerston North, New Zealand.
13 Mohan, S.B. and Kekwick, R.G.O. (1980) Biochem. J. 187, 667–676.
14 Eastwell, K.C. and Stumpf, P.K. (1982) Plant Physiol. 72, 50–55.
15 Stitt, M., Lilley, R.McC. and Heldt, H.W. (1982) Plant Physiol. 70, 971–977.
16 Finlayson, S. and Dennis, D.T., in preparation.
17 Overath, P. and Stumpf, P.K. (1964) J. Biol. Chem. 239, 4103–4110.
18 Simoni, R.D., Criddle, R.S. and Stumpf, P.K. (1967) J. Biol. Chem. 242, 573–581.
19 Matsumura, S. and Stumpf, P.K. (1968) Arch. Biochem. Biophys. 125, 932–941.
20 Ohlrogge, J.B., Kuhn, D.N. and Stumpf, P.K. (1979) Proc. Natl. Acad. Sci. (U.S.A.) 76, 1194–1198.
21 Grossman, A.R., Bartlett, S.G., Schmidt, G.W., Mullet, J.E. and Chua, N.-H. (1982) J. Biol. Chem. 257, 1558–1563.
22 Frentzen, M., Heinz, E., McKeon, T.A. and Stumpf, P.K. (1983) Eur. J. Biochem. 129, 629–636.
23 McKeon, T.A. and Stumpf, P.K. (1982) J. Biol. Chem., 257, 12141–12147.
24 Newcomb, E.H. and Stumpf, P.K. (1953) J. Biol. Chem. 200, 233–239.
25 Stumpf, P.K. and Barber, G.A. (1957) J. Biol. Chem. 227, 407–417.
26 Squires, C.L., Stumpf, P.K. and Schmid, C. (1958) Plant Physiol. 33, 364–366.
27 Smirnov, B.P. (1960) Biokhimia 25, 419–422.
28 Mudd, J.B. and McManus, T.T. (1962) J. Biol. Chem. 237, 2057–2063.
29 Stumpf, P.K. and James, A.T. (1963) Biochim. Biophys. Acta 70, 20–32.
30 van den Bosch, H., Williamson, J.R. and Vagelos, P.R. (1970) Nature (London) 228, 338–341.
31 Vagelos, P.R. (1974) in: T.W. Goodwin (Ed.), MTP International Review of Science, Biochem. of Lipids, Vol. 4, Butterworths, London, pp. 100–140.
32 Yamada, M. and Stumpf, P.K. (1964) Biochem. Biophys. Res. Commun. 14, 165–171.
33 Zilkey, B.F. and Canvin, D.T. (1969) Biochem. Biophys. Res. Commun. 34, 646–653.
34 Zilkey, B.F. and Canvin, D.T. (1971) Can. J. Bot. 50, 323–336.
35 Weaire, P.J. and Kekwick, R.G.O. (1975) Biochem. J. 146, 425–437 and 439–445.
36 Yamada, M. and Nakamura, Y. (1975) Plant Cell Physiol. 16, 151–162; Yamada, M., Usami, Q. and Kazuyo, N. (1974) Plant Cell Physiol. 15, 49–58; Yamada, M. and Usami, Q. (1975) Plant Cell Physiol. 16, 879–889.
37 Simcox, P.D., Reid, E.E., Canvin, D.T. and Dennis, D.T. (1977) Plant Physiol. 59, 1128–1132.
38 Galliard, T. and Stumpf, P.K. (1966) J. Biol. Chem. 241, 5806–5812.
39 Moreau, R.A. and Stumpf, P.K. (1981) Plant Physiol. 67, 672–676.
40 Ohlrogge, J.B., Pollard, M.R. and Stumpf, P.K. (1978) Lipids 13, 203–210.
41 Vick, B. and Beever, H. (1978) Plant Physiol. 62, 173–178.
42 Kleinig, H. and Liedvogel, B. (1978) Eur. J. Biochem. 83, 499–506.
43 Nothelfer, H.G., Barckhaus, R.H. and Spener, F. (1977) Biochim. Biophys. Acta 489, 370–380.
44 Jaworski, J.G., Goldschmidt, E.E. and Stumpf, P.K. (1974) Arch. Biochem. Biophys. 163, 769–776.
45 Cronan Jr., J.E. and Klages, A.L. (1981) Proc. Natl. Acad. Sci. (U.S.A.) 78, 5440–5444.

46 Stapleton, S.R. and Jaworski, J.G. (1982) Fed. Proc. 41 (Abstr.), 1193.
47 Caughey, I. and Kekwick, R.G.O. (1982) Eur. J. Biochem. 12, 553–561.
48 Høj, P.B. and Mikkelsen, J.D. (1982) Carlsberg Res. Commun. 47, 119–141.
49 Shimakata, T. and Stumpf, P.K. (1982) Arch. Biochem. Biophys. 217, 144–154.
50 Shimakata, T. and Stumpf, P.K. (1982) Plant Physiol. 69, 1257–1262.
51 Schüz, R., Ebel, J. and Hahlbrock, K. (1982) FEBS Lett. 140, 207–209.
52 Shimakata, T. and Stumpf, P.K. (1982) Arch. Biochem. Biophys. 218, 77–91.
53 Shimakata, T. and Stumpf, P.K. (1982) Arch. Biochem. Biophys., 220, 39–45.
54 Shimakata, T. and Stumpf, P.K. (1982) Proc. Natl. Acad. Sci. (U.S.A.) 79, 5808–5812.
55 Saito, K., Kawaguchi, A., Okuda, S., Siyama, Y., Yamakawa, T., Nakamura, Y. and Yamada, M. (1980) Plant Cell Physiol. 21, 9–19.
56 Alberts, A.W., Majerus, P.W., Talamo, B. and Vagelos, P.R. (1964) Biochemistry 3, 1563–1571.
57 Lynen, F. (1980) Eur. J. Biochem. 112, 431–442.
58 Stoops, J.K. and Wakil, S.J. (1981) J. Biol. Chem. 256, 5128–5133.
59 Weeks, G. and Wakil, S.J. (1968) J. Biol. Chem. 243, 1180–1189.
60 Majerus, P.W., Alberts, A.W. and Vagelos, P.R. (1965) J. Biol. Chem. 240, 618–621.
61 Birge, C.H. and Vagelos, P.R. (1972) J. Biol. Chem. 247, 4921–4929.
62 Birge, C.H. and Vagelos, P.R. (1972) J. Biol. Chem. 247, 4930–4938.
63 Harwood, J.L. (1980) in: P.K. Stumpf and E.E. Conn (Eds.), Biochemistry of Plants, Vol. 4, Academic Press, New York, pp. 1–55.
64 Shine, W.E., Mancha, M. and Stumpf, P.K. (1976) Arch. Biochem. Biophys. 172, 110–116.
65 Pollard, M.R. and Stumpf, P.K. (1980) Plant Physiol. 66, 641–648.
66 Pollard, N.M., McKeon, T.A., Gupta, L. and Stumpf, P.K. (1979) Lipids 14, 651–662.
67 Graham, S.A., Hirsinger, F. and Röebelen, G. (1981) Am. J. Bot. 68, 243–250.
68 Huang, K.P. and Stumpf, P.K. (1971) Arch. Biochem. Biophys. 143, 412–427.
69 Gurr, M.I. (1974) in: T.W. Goodwin (Ed.), MTP International Review of Science, Biochemistry of Lipids, Vol. 4, Butterworths, London, pp. 181–235.
70 Roughan, P.G. and Slack, C.R. (1982) Annu. Rev. Plant Physiol. 33, 97–132.
71 Bloch, K. (1971) in: P.D. Boyer (Ed.), The Enzymes, 3rd edn., Vol. 5, Academic Press, New York, pp. 441–464.
72 Morris, L.J., Harris, R.V., Kelly, W. and James, A.T. (1968) Biochem. J. 109, 673–678.
73 Hawke, J.C. and Stumpf, P.K. (1965) J. Biol. Chem. 240, 4746–4752.
74 Nagai, J. and Bloch, K. (1968) J. Biol. Chem. 243, 4626–4633.
75 Jacobson, B.S., Jaworski, J.G. and Stumpf, P.K. (1974) Plant physiol. 54, 484–486.
76 Jaworski, J.G. and Stumpf, P.K. (1974) Arch. Biochem. Biophys. 162, 158–165.
77 McKeon, T.A. and Stumpf, P.K. (1982) J. Biol. Chem., 257, 12141–12147.
78 Enoch, H.G., Catala, A. and Strittmatter, P. (1976) J. Biol. Chem. 251, 5095–5103.
79 Canvin, D.T. (1965) Can. J. Bot. 43, 63–69.
80 Harris, P. and James, A.T. (1968) Biochem. J. 112, 325–330.
81 Ohlrogge, J.B., Shine, W.E. and Stumpf, P.K. (1978) Arch. Biochem. Biophys. 189, 382–391.
82 Hawke, J.C. and Stumpf, P.K. (1980) Arch. Biochem. Biophys. 203, 296–306.
83 Murphy, D.J. and Stumpf, P.K. (1980) Plant Physiol. 66, 660–665.
84 Vijay, I.K. and Stumpf, P.K. (1972) J. Biol. Chem. 247, 360–366.
85 Willemot, C. and Stumpf, P.K. (1967) Can. J. Bot. 45, 579–584.
86 Abdelkader, A.B., Cherif, A., Demandre, C. and Mazliak, P. (1973) Eur. J. Biochem. 32, 155–165.
87 Dubacq, J.P., Mazliak, P. and Tremoliere, A. (1976) FEBS Lett. 66, 183–186.
88 Styme, S. and Appelqvist, L.A. (1978) Eur. J. Biochem. 90, 223–229.
89 Slack, C.R., Roughan, P.G. and Terpetra, J. (1976) Biochem. J. 155, 71–80.
90 Talamo, B., Chang, N. and Bloch, K. (1973) J. Biol. Chem. 248, 2738–2742.
91 Pugh, E.L. and Kates, M. (1973) Biochim. Biophys. Acta 316, 305–316.
92 Jacobson, B.S., Kannangara, C.G. and Stumpf, P.K. (1973) Biochem. Biophys. Res. Commun. 51, 487–493.
93 Murphy, D.J. and Stumpf, P.K. (1972) Plant Physiol. 64, 428–430.

S. Numa (Ed.) Fatty Acid Metabolism and Its Regulation
© *1984 Elsevier Science Publishers B.V.*

CHAPTER 7

Lipid degradation in higher plants *

H. KINDL

Institut für Biochemie, Fachbereich Chemie, Philipps-Universität, D-3550 Marburg,
F.R.G.

1. Introduction

Acyl lipids can constitute a major portion of storage compounds in plants. Phospholipids and glycolipids contain fatty acyl groups which are subjects of turnover. Beyond that, a broad spectrum of compounds with diverse hydrophobic structures exists which can be seen as plant lipids and may also be degradable. But in this contribution, they are not dealt with for either their turnover is not known or they do not contribute significantly to the intermediary metabolism.

2. Metabolic situations of lipid degradation

Most of our knowledge about lipid degradation in plants has been gathered from cells intensively involved in the mobilization of fat reserves. This sort of catabolism occurs almost exclusively during germination of seeds. A quantitatively less important, but nevertheless essential, kind of lipid degradation is the constant turnover of membrane material and the response to wounding.

(a) Coupling of triglyceride hydrolysis, fatty acid β-oxidation, glyoxylate cycle and gluconeogenesis

A feasible, imaginable and very effective manner in which an organism could construct an apparatus for a long reaction sequence would be to concentrate the respective enzymes in one compartment or in compartments cooperating closely. It would be advantageous, for one type of cell to do the whole job. Many seeds are characterized by large deposits of lipids. These are stored during seed development and are needed as nutriment during seed germination. These lipid reserves consist almost exclusively of triglycerides, with oleic acid, linoleic and palmitic acid being the major acid components [1,2]. By the concerted action of lipases, fatty acid

---

* Dedicated to Professor Peter Karlson on the occasion of his 65th birthday.

β-oxidation and glyoxylate cycle the building blocks for carbohydrate synthesis are provided. Transport forms of carbohydrates are exported by the cell and eventually reach meristematic tissues where new cells are being actively synthesized.

Seeds of sunflower, cucumber, or rapeseed contain their storage tissue within the cotyledons. In castor beans or coconuts, the fat reserves are housed in the endosperm. Pericarp is the lipid-rich tissue in avocados. Aleurone layers (bran) are the tissues distinguished by the occurrence of lipids, lipases and glyoxysomes in cereal seeds. In these instances, triglycerides mobilized in lipid bodies furnish fatty acids and glycerol. In a few special cases, long-chain alcohols are the products besides the fatty acids, e.g., in Simmondsia species. Jojoba plants (*Simmondsia chinensis*) tolerate extreme desert temperatures and are drought resistant. The seeds contain high amounts of lipid in the form of wax. The storage wax is located within wax bodies and accounts for more than 50% of the dry weight. It consists of C_{20} and C_{22} acids, e.g. eicosanoic acid, and alcohols, and thus resembles the sperm whale oil. Jojoba oil offers an alternative to the sperm whale oil being used as lubricant for machinery under high pressure.

The close arrangement of fatty acid β-oxidation and glyoxylate cycle is a good example of the principle of effective channeling. It is also an example of enzymes being used for mobilization of storage material and for anabolism leading to building blocks for new structures being housed in one type of cell. Therefore, in all cases where massive lipid degradation is used to form building blocks for other carbon skeletons, the β-oxidation enzymes and the enzymatic machinery for the glyoxylate cycle are concentrated in one organelle, the glyoxysomes.

Fig. 1 emphasizes the close arrangement and interrelationship between fatty acid β-oxidation and glyoxylate cycle. As cosubstrates usually are present in limiting concentrations, it is an advantage for the cell, in terms of kinetics, that products of one sequence are not shuttled to the next pathway taking place at another site or organelle. In this way, coenzymes are rather released and thus immediately available in the same compartment. By the tight arrangement of β-oxidation and glyoxylate cycle, the oxidation of fatty acids is highly effective in yielding succinate and NADH. For the latter obviously exists no effective mechanism of reoxidation in situ. Redox equivalents produced in glyoxysomes have to be shuttled to mitochondria.

Substrates for the reaction sequence summarized in Fig. 1 are provided in close vicinity to glyoxysomes. Lipid bodies pressed to the glyoxysomes and cooperating with them furnish fatty acids.

Lipid bodies (also named spherosomes, oleosomes, oil bodies, lipid-containing vesicles) are particles found in low-fat tissues and dominate in high-fat tissues. Their size ranges from 0.4 μm to over 2 μm in diameter [3,4]. Lipid bodies are bound by a single fine-line membrane [5–7], and it is undecided whether or not the membrane originates, during seed maturation, from the ER membrane [8–10]. Biochemical analysis of membrane proteins does not support a direct ontogeny of lipid body membrane from an already differentiated ER membrane [8]. During fat mobilization, lipid body membranes participate in the degradation process by providing lipases.

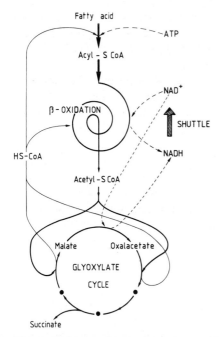

Fig. 1. Tight coupling between fatty acid β-oxidation and glyoxylate cycle. The flow of carbon compounds is stressed by thick lines, the reflux of coenzymes marks the tight association of the two pathways.

Fatty acids were thus generated already on the way between the lipid droplet of the lipid body matrix and the matrix of glyoxysomes. Following β-oxidation and glyoxylate cycle in glyoxysomes, succinate, the final product of the reaction sequence in the glyoxysomes, has to be oxidized in mitochondria. Succinate dehydrogenase and fumarase are enzymes present only in mitochondria. Malate is used in the cytoplasm, for gluconeogenesis.

As the cofactors for lipid degradation (CoA, NAD$^+$) are not available in the cell in unlimited amounts, and as pronounced piling up of intermediates may be dangerous and does therefore not occur, we have to consider lipolysis, β-oxidation, glyoxylate cycle and part of gluconeogenesis as rather tightly coupled processes.

(b) Lipid turnover in green leaves

It is likely that also green leaves possess temporary energy stores in the form of lipid bodies (oleosomes). If this is a more general phenomenon, work of Parker and Murphy [11] may be exemplary in demonstrating the intracellular location and morphology of the organelles. They found that in wheat leaves the lipid bodies are primarily composed of triacylglycerols (palmitoyl groups dominating), sterols and wax esters. As similar results were also obtained with other leaves [12] and cell cultures [7], we may hypothesize that tissues other than storage tissues in seeds produce triacylglycerides and use them as short-time reserves. Whether lipid synthesis or its subsequent degradation is in response to fungal attack [11,19] is an unsolved problem.

In leaves, lipid acyl hydrolases [14], enzymes of galactolipid metabolism [15], phospholipases as well as enzymes of β-oxidation have been found. Very limited data are available that these enzymes, e.g. enoyl-CoA hydratase activity, also occur in etiolated leaves, hypocotyls and roots.

Leaf peroxisomes are known to possess the capacity to degrade fatty acids by β-oxidation [16]. Work of Thomas and McNeil [17], however, using pea cotyledons and demonstrating enhancement of β-oxidation by carnitine suggests that mitochondria are the intracellular sites where β-oxidation proceeds. As green leaves lack a fully active glyoxylate cycle, it is postulated that acetyl-CoA produced in peroxisomes has to be transferred into mitochondria or other organelles (plastids) for further conversions.

(c) Lipid catabolism in respiratory active tissue

Mechanical damage of roots and storage organs (e.g. potato tubers) induces, in a rapid response, marked degradation of membrane lipids. Laties [18] reported 40% loss of membrane lipids within minutes of slicing potato tubers. Following the attack by acylhydrolases, α-oxidation is assumed to be the dominant degradation process. This is the origin of fatty-acid-based respiration.

3. Mechanisms of lipid degradation

In general, hydrolytic enzymes cleaving the ester bonds between fatty acids and glycerol as well as enzymes of fatty acid β-oxidation are required for lipid degradation. But other oxidative pathways are also known, and even peroxidative steps followed by breakage of the C skeleton.

(a) Hydrolytic enzymes

(i) Lipase

Lipases (triacylglycerol acylhydrolases, EC 3.1.1.3) attack triacylglycerides (Fig.

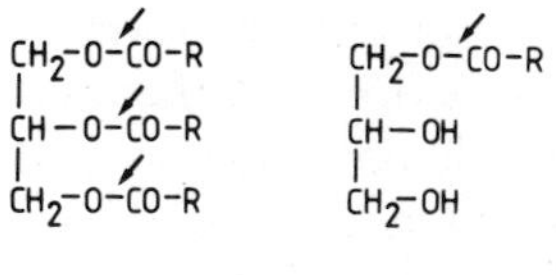

$$CH_2-O-CO-R \qquad CH_2-O-CO-R$$
$$CH-O-CO-R \qquad CH-OH$$
$$CH_2-O-CO-R \qquad CH_2-OH$$

Fig. 2. Position at which triacylglyceride lipases function (left side) in contrast to several alkaline lipases which preferably deacylate monoacyl glycerides.

2) and function as membrane-bound enzymes at the interphase between the hydrophobic region and the surrounding water compartment.

(ii) Lipases of lipid bodies

Since fats are stored in lipid bodies, it is reasonable to expect that the enzyme responsible for their degradation are linked to lipid body membranes. Well characterized is the castor bean lipase exhibiting an optimal activity in the pH range of 4–5. This "acid" lipase was described to catalyze the sequence of reactions:

$$\text{Triacylglycerol} \rightarrow 1,2\text{-diacylglycerol} \rightarrow 1\text{-monoacylglycerol} \rightarrow \text{glycerol}$$

It was found that the primary ester group was attacked preferentially but the total reaction has not a pronounced specificity for the position of the acyl group on the glycerol molecule. In the case of castor bean endosperm, 90% of the reserve seed lipids are triricinoleoylglycerol which is totally mobilized during germination before the endosperm fades. Ory [4] demonstrated the involvement of a low-molecular-weight cofactor formed from 4 molecules of ricinoleic acid. Membranes of lipid bodies have been prepared [19] and analyzed for their protein components. But it remains unclear at present which M_r has to be attributed to the lipase.

Lipid in the form of wax can be the storage material as exemplified by the seeds of Simmondsia species. In this case, the esters of long-chain fatty acids and C_{20}–C_{22} alcohols are housed in wax bodies which possess, in their delimiting membrane, an alkaline lipase [20]. The membrane-bound enzyme was found to hydrolyze monoglycerides, e.g. monolaurin, more effectively than myristyl myristate. The enzyme exerts low activities on diglycerides or triglycerides. The enzyme exhibits optimum activity at pH 9.0 and its activity peaks at the stage of seed germination that is characterized by maximal gluconeogenesis from lipid. No lipase was found in the glyoxysomes of germinating Simmondsia seeds.

(iii) Lipases of glyoxysomes

Alkaline lipases which preferentially hydrolyze di-acyl- and mono-acyl-glycerols have been found in the membranes of glyoxysomes. The alkaline lipase from *Arachis hypogaea* has been purified and reported [28] to exhibit an M_r of 50000. The findings of Huang and Moreau [22] and Muto and Beevers [23] seem to indicate that alkaline lipases tightly integrated in the membrane are a general feature of glyoxysomes. Glyoxysomal membranes prepared by osmotic shock of purified glyoxysomes and analyzed by isopycnic density gradient centrifugation contained almost all alkaline lipase and malate synthase of endosperm cells. The situation of two lipases occurring in the membranes of lipid bodies and glyoxysomes appears to be unique to the castor bean endosperm. In other fat-containing tissues, e.g. peanut cotyledons, the acid lipase is absent and only the alkaline lipase dominates during the peak of fat degradation [23].

(iv) Other lipases

Theimer and Rosnitschek [24] working with rapeseed cotyledons, found a tri-glycerol lipase which was neither associated with lipid bodies nor with glyoxysomes or the ER but was rather contained in a light microsomal fraction. The enzyme has an alkaline pH optimum.

Cereal seeds contain their embryo (germ) and in the outer layers of the grain (aleurone, bran) lipases with slightly alkaline pH optimum. Although their properties were partially elucidated [25], the intracellular location has not been investigated.

(v) Lipolytic acyl hydrolases

The term lipolytic acylhydrolase is used for enzymes deacylating glycerolipids, mono- and di-acylglycerol as well as lysophosphatidyl glycerol or glycosyl di-acylglycerol. But their substrate specificities have not really been established and unfortunately different names have been proposed. It is not unequivocally proved but very likely, that these lipolytic activities are housed in the lytic compartment (vacuoles, lysosomes). The enzyme from leaves [14] did not hydrolyze esters of high alcohols or acylated steryl glucosides and it had only low activities towards phosphatidyl choline and digalactosyl diacylglycerol. It worked, however, efficiently in deacylating monoacylglycerol and lysophosphatidyl choline. Optimal activity was in the pH range of 5–6, while the presence of detergents shifted the pH optimum to pH 7. Another acylhydrolase was purified from potato tubers [26]. The striking feature of this enzyme (M_r 70 000) was its high activity in hydrolyzing acylstearylglucosides.

Lipid acylhydrolases of the lytic compartment are very active and destroy membranes, even at 0°C when they are freed during cell fractionation. Their activity can cause drawbacks in many cell-free systems. Free fatty acids released by the enzyme can disrupt membrane structures and facilitate the excess of the enzyme to other substrates.

(vi) Galactolipase in chloroplasts

Lipases which cause extensive breakdown of galactolipids have been localized in chloroplasts. The galactolipase prepared from bean chloroplasts [27] hydrolyzed monogalactosyl diglyceride at a rate 10 times higher than that of dipalmitoyl-phosphatidyl choline hydrolysis. Envelopes of chloroplasts appear to be the site of enzymes of galactolipid metabolism in leaves [15].

(vii) Other lipolytic activities

A calcium-stimulated acylhydrolase has been detected in membranes of potato mitochondria. Bligny and Douce [28] failed to demonstrate monoacyl intermediates as products. This indicates that the enzyme does not preferably hydrolyze one of the two acyl groups of the endogenous diacyl lipids.

Lipid polymers as cutin and suberin are extracellularly located and are, therefore, not assumed to be subject to turnover during the life time of a plant. As an exception can be regarded an extracellular enzyme from pollen which is an SH hydrolase and capable of degrading cutin.

Cutinases have an important physiological role for fungi, plant pathogens attacking the plant at its surface. Then, the fungal cutinase released into extracellular space is the enzyme of the first attack on the hydrophobic part of the plant cell wall.

(viii) Phospholipase D

Phospholipase D (EC 3.1.4.4) is one of the most intensively studied plant enzymes [29]. It hydrolyzes the choline–phosphate bond in phosphatidyl choline, but has been shown to catalyze also the hydrolysis of most of the common phospholipids. The enzyme is dependent of Ca^{2+}, has an isoelectric point of 4.7 and an M_r of 200 000. Its activity of transphosphatidylation is well documented. Several primary alcohols, even methanol, are suitable as acceptors of the phosphatidyl group. Phosphatidyl transfer can be demonstrated by the following reactions:

phosphatidylcholine + glycerol = phosphatidylglycerol + choline

phosphatidylglycerol + phosphatidylglycerol = diphosphatidylglycerol + glycerol

The physiological role of the enzyme is unclear, the enzyme's subcellular location is not established. Generally, phospholipase D activity is highest in storage tissues (tubers, seeds), but, surprisingly, is almost absent in potato tubers.

(b) Fatty acid β-oxidation

The pathway of fatty acid β-oxidation in microbodies was at first discovered, and then intensively studied, in glyoxysomes. These findings had strong impact on studies with other microbodies. There is direct experimental evidence that the set of enzymes responsible for β-oxidation in glyoxysomes and the respective enzymes in leaf peroxisomes, or in liver peroxisomes, is very similar or almost identical [30,31].

A divergent path took nature by evolving the mitochondrial β-oxidation apparatus. It differs from the way how β-oxidation in glyoxysomes is organized in many important details. In mitochondria, each step of β-oxidation is catalyzed by an independent enzyme usually constructed from several identical subunits. In this respect, the β-oxidation enzymes of mitochondria have many similarities with the corresponding catalysts in the gram-positive bacterium Clostridium. Gram-negative bacteria, however, exemplified by *Escherichia coli* [32], possess an enzyme complex for the task of β-oxidation, and this complex contains one protein which carriers out at least 2 functions. This monomeric multifunctional protein is also a typical component of glyoxysomal and peroxisomal β-oxidation. It is remarkable that these principles, and by and large the subunit M_r of the proteins too, have been preserved during evolution from *E. coli* to microbodies and from gram-positive bacteria to mitochondria.

Plant microbodies may not only differ from each other in principle, in their capability of fatty acid degradation and in the kind of final products afforded by the organelle. Comparing glyoxysomes, leaf peroxisomes and other peroxisomes, quantitative differences may also be found, as were detected in the case of liver peroxisomes: in mice, the proportion of fatty acid β-oxidation in peroxisomes versus degradation in mitochondria is much greater than in rats.

β-Oxidation in germinating seeds seems to be exclusively located in glyoxysomes [33]. In many cases it was actually demonstrated that mitochondria are not involved in the chain-shortening process. Neither in degradation of fatty acids originating from wax esters nor in mobilization of fatty acids from triglycerides, as investigated in fat-containing endosperms or cotyledons, were mitochondria found to be capable of β-oxidation. They lack all enzymes necessary for this pathway.

(i) Entry into β-oxidation

β-Oxidation in glyoxysomes starts by conversion of free fatty acids into their CoA esters. In accord with the results given by Tolbert [34] no further steps are implicated for importing the fatty acyl group into the glyoxysomes. It seems to be widely accepted that the glyoxysomal process, and liver peroxisomal β-oxidation too, are carnitine-independent. Unlike mitochondria from pea leaves, little carnitine palmitoyl transferase has been found in glyoxysomes. Although it was stated [34] that plants lack any carnitine transferase enzymes for transport of acyl groups, carnitine is detectable in plants and palmitoyl carnitine can be synthesized enzymatically, at least in etioplasts [35].

As fatty acid degradation is initiated mainly by a lipase in the glyoxysomal membrane, and as the CoA-ligase too, is membrane bound, a carnitine-dependent transfer through the microbody membrane could be difficult to detect.

The molecular properties of long-chain fatty acyl-CoA synthetase are not known. Cooper [36] and Mishina et al. [37,38] carrying out some research on this enzyme reported the requirement of ATP, Mg^{2+} and CoA. They found a pronounced stimulatory effect of phosphatidylcholine.

In several respects, fatty acid β-oxidation in lipid-degrading yeasts is comparable with the process taking place in glyoxysomes in higher plants. Hence, it would be worthwhile to know whether or not mitochondria participate in fatty acid oxidation in fungi; probably not [39].

(ii) Conversion of fatty acyl-CoA into acetyl-CoA

In glyoxysomes, an acyl-CoA oxidase with FAD as coenzyme transfers 2 electrons to O_2. H_2O_2 produced in this way could be involved, along with catalase also present, in peroxidative processes. Probably, most H_2O_2 is just decomposed to H_2O and O_2. Acyl-CoA oxidases of glyoxysomes and leaf peroxisomes are assumed to consist, in analogy to the liver peroxisomal enzyme [40], of 2–3 different subunits.

For catalyzing the next 2 steps in β-oxidation, glyoxysomes and leaf peroxisomes are equipped with a bifunctional or multifunctional protein possessing enoyl-CoA hydratase and L-3-hydroxyacyl-CoA dehydrogenase activities [30,41]. Exemplified by the molecular properties of this protein, the close relationship between several forms of plant microbodies and liver peroxisomes can be demonstrated. Enoyl-CoA hydratases (also called crotonase) of mitochondrial origin have a molecular weight of 160 000 and are composed of 6 polypeptide chains of identical size [42]. The glyoxysomal enoyl-CoA hydratase activity is confined to an M_r 75 000 protein which is a monomer and is distinguished by a remarkably alkaline isoelectric point. Exactly the same properties were described for the protein known to be a component of peroxisomal β-oxidation in liver.

β-Ketoacyl-CoA (C_{n+2}) is cleaved, under the catalysis of a thiolase, with CoA as nucleophile and yielding acetyl-CoA and acyl-CoA (C_n) as products. Thiolase is a dimer composed of 2 identical subunits of M_r 45 000 [43]. It possesses an extremely sensitive SH group which can be the reason why thiolase activity is usually not detectable in crude extracts.

As in the case of the enzyme just discussed, the molecular properties of thiolase and the striking similarities between the liver peroxisomal enzyme and the plant glyoxysomal protein are to be emphasized. Emphasis is put on the clear distinction between the microbody proteins and the respective mitochondrial enzymes [44,45]: tetramers (M_r 154 000) in mitochondria and dimers (M_r 90 000) in all forms of microbodies.

Our present knowledge concerning fatty acid β-oxidation in microbodies is summarized in Fig. 3.

(iii) Utilization of acetyl-CoA and NADH

Glyoxysomes are characterized by a tight intraorganellar coupling of β-oxidation and glyoxylate cycle. By virtue of the close spatial arrangement of the 2 pathways, CoA is split off in the first steps of the glyoxylate cycle and becomes thus again available for β-oxidation (Fig. 1).

Peroxisomal β-oxidation, at least in liver peroxisomes, leads to hexanoyl-CoA and acetyl-CoA which are exported as carnitine esters. In this way, the peroxisomal β-oxidation is carnitine dependent. This process permits CoA to be regenerated at the site of re-use immediately after fatty acid degradation.

Whereas the organization of β-oxidation and utilization of its products in microbodies guarantees a quick regeneration of the limiting amount of coenzyme A,

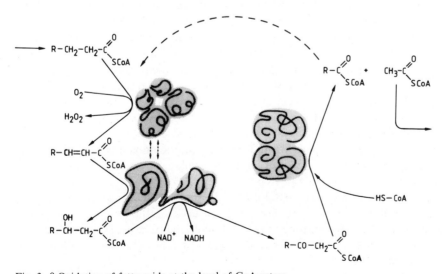

Fig. 3. β-Oxidation of fatty acids at the level of CoA esters.

we have only a rather limited knowledge about the re-oxidation of NADH, the other free-moving coenzyme in β-oxidation.

Although it seems feasible that NADH is oxidized either at the glyoxysomal membrane by a NADH-cytochrome oxidoreductase [46] or exterior to the glyoxysomes by a similar enzyme in the cytoplasm, it is more likely that a shuttle transfers reduction equivalents from microbodies via cytosol into mitochondria [47,48].

Lord and Beevers [49] working with purified organelles have demonstrated that glyoxysomes generated NADH when incubated with palmitoyl-CoA. In the presence of mitochondria, however, no accumulation of NADH was observed. On addition of cyanide, not effecting palmitoyl-CoA-dependent NAD$^+$ reduction in glyoxysomes but inhibiting mitochondrial electron transport, the system responded by immediate accumulation of NADH.

Supply of external aspartate and α-ketoglutarate also effects that NADH does not accumulate during palmitoyl-CoA degradation with isolated glyoxysomes. In the model proposed by Beevers [48], oxaloacetate generated in glyoxysomes by the aminotransferase is the acceptor of reducing equivalents produced by fatty acid β-oxidation. Malate is then eventually re-oxidized to oxaloacetate, but only after transfer to mitochondria, conversion to aspartate via oxaloacetate, and renewed aminotransferase reaction with the aspartate transferred from mitochondria to glyoxysomes [48].

At the state characterized by active glyoxysomes, the fate of acetyl-CoA is clear and β-oxidation of fatty acids is known to take place in glyoxysomes only. But what happens when glyoxysomal activities decrease and leaf peroxisomes take over the task of β-oxidation? Does the mitochondrial β-oxidation then become prevalent, and what happens to the acetyl-CoA formed during β-oxidation in the peroxisomes? Such a situation has to be taken into consideration when cotyledons only partially depleted of fat reserves reach the surface of soil and become photoautotrophic. After a period of transition, glyoxysomal activities of the microbodies disappear while fat is still available for degradation. The catabolism of fatty acid may then proceed similar to β-oxidation in liver peroxisomes, where mitochondria and peroxisomes participate or cooperate in degrading fatty acids. Tetrahymena may be a good model system for studying these problems. While in liver cells it is difficult to assess what percentage of fatty acids is degraded in mitochondria and how much peroxisomes contribute to β-oxidation, in Tetrahymena the measurement of label incorporated into glycogen from fatty acid permits us to assess the peroxisomal contribution to β-oxidation in one type of intact cells. 40–60% of the octanoate β-oxidation takes place in the peroxisomal compartment, and this value was not too significantly changed when cells were exposed to hypoxia. In the presence of glucose, however, peroxisomal β-oxidation was virtually eliminated whereas little effect on the amount of fatty acids oxidized in the mitochondria was observed [50].

It is likely that metabolic situations exist characterized by mitochondria being the only site of fatty acid β-oxidation in plants. Only a few examples are known to support this assumption.

Thomas and McNeil [17] studying mitochondria from cotyledons of dark-grown pea seedlings measured enhanced O_2 uptake and higher values of respiratory control ratio when carnitine was added together with various fatty acids used as substrates. It was suggested that acyl carnitines (e.g. palmitoyl carnitine) formed from acyl-CoA derivatives should more readily penetrate the mitochondrial membranes than free palmitate or palmitoyl-CoA. It is likely that at least for short-chain acylcarnitine the system should work as suggested. But the studies of Thomas and McNeil were done with organelles prepared in 0.4 M sucrose by differential centrifugations only; and from a tissue which is assumed to contain also glyoxysomes. If β-oxidation is closely geared to the glyoxylate cycle, as in glyoxysomes, there is no need for a short-chain acylcarnitine transferase, because butyryl-CoA is rapidly degraded to acetyl-CoA which is directly and in the same compartment used up in the glyoxylate cycle. If, however, only a peroxisome type of microbodies is present in a certain tissue, butyryl-CoA or hexanoyl-CoA may be the products of β-oxidation which cannot be further degraded in this organelle but are rather transferred to mitochondria via carnitine esters.

Several authors elaborated a theory [51] in which it was postulated that the peroxisomal membrane is impermeable to coenzyme A and acyl-CoA, but is permeable to carnitine and acyl-carnitines. Accordingly, shuttles of acetylcarnitine or acylcarnitines have to be assumed which allow the transfer of acyl groups from microbodies to mitochondria or plastids. Whether this sort of shuttle is also functioning in plant tissues lacking fully competent glyoxysomes but possessing peroxisomes of the liver type cooperating with mitochondria, is at present an unresolved question.

(iv) Degradation of unsaturated fatty acids

Unsaturated fatty acids seem to be oxidized by the same general pathway as saturated fatty acids, but several extra steps need to be included. If double bonds in the vicinity of the carboxyl group of unsaturated fatty acids are in *cis* configuration, isomerizations are obligate to lead to 2-*trans*-isomers which are required for the enoyl-CoA hydratase reaction.

Hence, during β-oxidation of oleic acid, linoleic acid, or 9-*cis*, 11-*trans*, 13-*trans*-octadecatrienoic acid (in cucurbitaceae), a *cis-trans* isomerase has to convert the 3-*cis*-acid into the 2-*trans*-isomer which only is further converted into the respective L-3-hydroxy acid.

$$cis\text{-}R\text{--}CH_2\text{--}CH{=}CH\text{--}CH_2\text{--}CO\text{--}SCoA$$

$$\rightarrow \quad trans\text{-}R\text{--}CH_2\text{--}CH_2\text{--}CH{=}CH\text{--}CO\text{--}SCoA$$

It is likely that glyoxysomes possess, like *E. coli* and rat liver, a 2,4-dienoyl-CoA reductase which is involved in degradation of unsaturated fatty acids [52,53].

$$2\text{-}trans,4\text{-}cis\text{-decadienoyl-CoA} \quad \rightarrow \quad 3\text{-decenoyl-CoA}$$

In this way, 4-*cis*-decanoyl-CoA, a metabolite of linoleic acid, would be converted by the acyl-CoA oxidase of peroxisomal oxidation into 2-*trans*,4-*cis*-decadienoyl-CoA. Via 3-decenoyl-CoA and 2-*trans*-decenoyl-CoA the main line of β-oxidation is reached.

Mobilization of ricinoleic acid, 12-hydroxy,9-*cis*-octadecenoic acid (main constituent in castor bean) requires isomerization of 3-*cis*-enoic acid into 2-*trans*-enoic acid at the level of C_{12}. At a later step, a 2-hydroxy acid (C_8) is formed which has to be further degraded by α-oxidation.

(c) α-Oxidation of fatty acids

α-Oxidation of fatty acids seems to play a central role in all the tissues that do not have a specialized β-oxidation system, tissues that lack glyoxysomes. In young leaf tissue, α-oxidation is more intensive than β-oxidation. Wounding, especially of rhizomes, tubers and other storage tissues, is usually followed by pronounced respiration which relies on fatty acid degradation via α-oxidation.

Furthermore, it is probable but not sufficiently established that α-oxidation supplements degradation of fatty acids if their chemical structure, substitution, kind of carbon chain etc., do not allow the machinery of β-oxidation to do the job alone.

(i) Mechanism of α-oxidation

α-Oxidation leads to α-hydroxycarboxylic acids and does not require coenzyme A for the activation of fatty acids. It is assumed that α-hydroperoxy acids are the primary products. They are then either reduced to the corresponding α-hydroxyacid or converted into the aldehyde with a carbon chain shortened by C_1. This step includes a decarboxylation and loss of the C_1 of the original fatty acids. The latter process, the CO_2 production, provides one of the means for assaying α-oxidation. Finally, an oxidoreductase and NAD^+ can oxidize the aldehyde to the acid which may be subjected to another α-oxidation [54].

Fig. 4 outlines the principal steps of α-oxidation, but leaves open the questions of

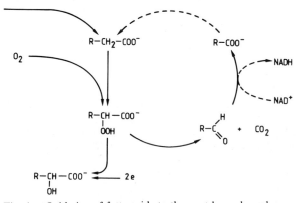

Fig. 4. α-Oxidation of fatty acids to the next lower homolog.

mechanism. Although there exists controversy as to whether O_2 or H_2O_2 is the substrate and which cofactors are involved, it is probable, at least for most α-oxidation systems, that O_2 is activated by a reduced flavoprotein, and a hydroperoxide intermediate at the enzyme is the active species which attacks the fatty acid.

Shine and Stumpf [54] demonstrated that only the D-isomer of α-hydroxyacid is formed. The formation of α-hydroxyacid outweighs the alternative step of decarboxylation (Fig. 4) when efficient reductants are present.

Two other processes with some similarities to respiratory processes sometimes are found to interfere with fatty acid α-oxidation: lipoxydation and CN^--resistant respiration. Lipoxygenase-mediated processes operate at a lower pH than the α-oxidation and are inactive toward saturated fatty acids. Fatty acid α-oxidation in combination with mitochondrial respiration also represent a fatty acid and O_2-dependent CO_2 production. Malonate inhibition of succinate respiration is coextensive with imidazole inhibition which is proposed to be typical of α-oxidation. As response to slicing, tubers not treated with ethylene exhibit α-oxidation which is inhibited by imidazole. At present, it is unclear whether induction of α-oxidation is related to the CN^--resistant alternative respiration [55].

The conversion of p-hydroxyphenylpropenoic acid to p-hydroxyphenylacetic acid and p-hydroxybenzoic acids takes place with the free fatty acid and is not dependent on coenzyme A [56,57]. It is clearly distinguishable from fatty acid β-oxidation.

In roots of cucumber seedlings, α-oxidation and β-oxidation take place in mitochondria. But while β-oxidation was dependent on CoA and localized in the mitochondrial matrix, the enzyme system forming p-hydroxybenzoate was clearly assigned to mitochondrial membranes [56]. Formation of p-hydroxybenzoic acid must be seen in relation to its further conversion into ubiquinones in the same organelle.

Another example demonstrating that a fatty acid not suitable for β-oxidation can be α-oxidized in mitochondria was studied by Tsai et al. [58]. 3,7,11,15-Tetramethyl-hexadecanoic acid was converted into the respective α-hydroxy acid and CO_2 by rat-liver mitochondria. Although this conversion has so far only been demonstrated in animals, the branched-chain compound mentioned should also be degraded by chlorophyll turnover in leaves. Tetramethyl hexadecanoic acid, also called phytanic acid, is a product of the phytol moiety of chlorophyll. α-Oxidation of phytanic acid yields 2,6,10,14-tetramethylpentadecanoic acid (pristanic acid), and this compound is subject to successive β-oxidation.

(ii) Intracellular location of α-oxidation

As most work on α-oxidation was performed using extracts from acetone powders (e.g. peanut seeds, pea leaf), reports on compartmentation of fatty acid α-oxidation are scarce [54]. In pea leaves, a high percentage of α-oxidation activity was found to be soluble. In peanut cotyledons, however, most activity was sedimentable at $100\,000 \times g$.

(d) ω-Oxidation of fatty acids

Free fatty acids were probably the substrates for ω-hydroxylation. Suggestive evidence was provided that this process takes place at the ER. The products should be further transported to the plasma membrane by membrane flow. ω-Hydroxylation, optimal at pH 8, requires NADPH and O_2 [59]. It is highly sensitive towards CO.

ω-Hydroxy acids, e.g. ω-hydroxypalmitic acid, the main products of ω-hydroxylation, can be subjected to further oxidation yielding dicarboxylic acids. Plants are unique in that they contain in their envelope polymers consisting of ω-hydroxy acids and corresponding dicarboxylic acids [60]. Cutin, as being present in the cuticular layers of seeds, fruits, or potato tubers primarily consists of C_{16} dihydroxy acids, whereas dicarboxylic acids dominate in suberins. ω-Hydroxypalmitic acid is a substrate for further hydroxylation, e.g. at C-10. Mid-chain hydroxylation requires O_2 and NADPH and is located at the endoplasmic reticulum [61]. The respective process in Pseudomonas species is catalyzed by a system consisting of iron-sulfur protein, NADH:iron-sulfur protein oxidoreductase and a Fe^{2+}-containing protein functioning as actual ω-hydroxylase [62,63].

(e) Lipoxidation

Lipoxidation of unsaturated fatty acids has to be seen in conjunction with the consecutive steps which lead to fragmentation of the carbon skeleton.

Lipoxygenases (linoleate:oxygen oxidoreductase, EC 1.13.11.12) catalyze the introduction of a hydroperoxy group into unsaturated fatty acids. Fig. 5 shows the principal scheme.

The reaction can be measured as linoleate-dependent O_2 uptake, or by estimating the peroxides produced, e.g. hydroperoxydienoic acid. Co-oxidation of cosubstrates,

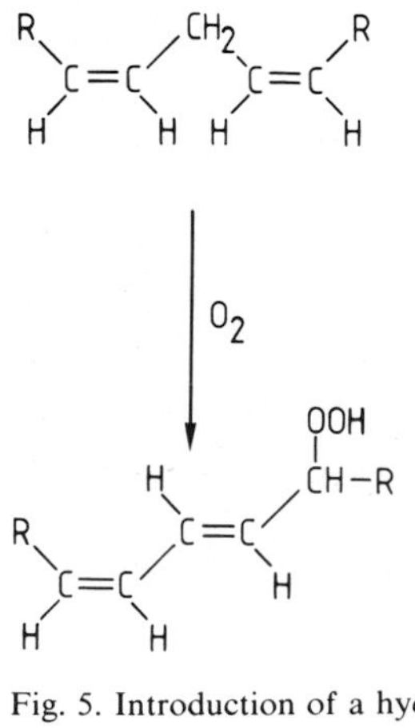

Fig. 5. Introduction of a hydroperoxy group by lipoxygenase.

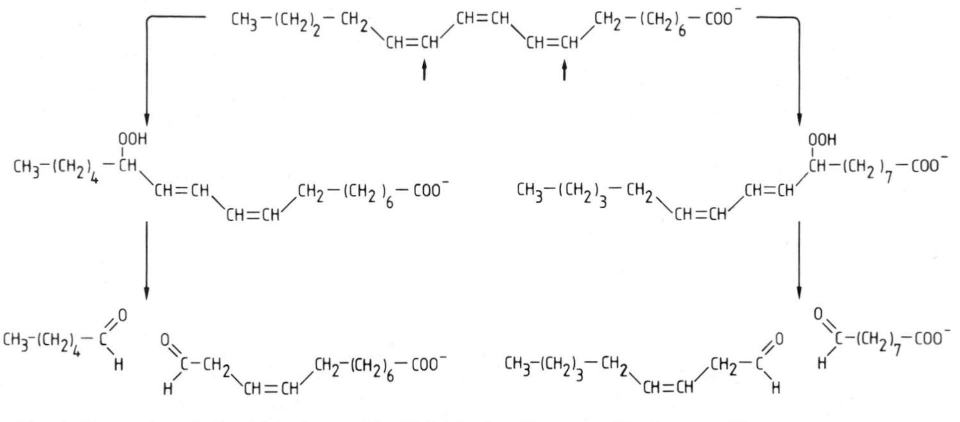

Fig. 6. Formation of C_6-aldehydes or C_9-aldehydes by cleavage of hydroperoxides.

another means of assaying lipoxygenase activity, is demonstrated by addition of carotenoids. Radical intermediates provided by the lipoxygenase reaction cause the oxidation of unsaturated compounds such as carotenoids.

Lipoxidation of linoleic acid can lead to 9-hydroperoxy- or to 12-hydroperoxy-dienoic acids as outlined in Fig. 6.

Products of lipoxygenase reaction can be further transformed into isomeric ketols. Hydroperoxide isomerases (EC 5.3.99.1) can convert hydroperoxydienes, e.g. 13-hydroperoxy-9-*cis*,11-*trans*-octa-decadienoic acid, into hydroxyoxoenes of the type R–CH$_2$–CO–CH=CH–CHOH–R without altering the carbon skeleton [64]. Mechanistic studies by Gardner and Jursinik [65] suggest radical intermediates and an additional attack by a radical oxygen species.

Cleavage of the carbon skeleton of linoleic acid can take place when a reactive oxygen species attack 9-hydroperoxides or the 13-hydroperoxide isomer. As outlined in Fig. 7, a radical derived from hydroperoxide is stabilized by breakage of a C–C bond, thus giving rise to an aldehyde and an alkene radical which can be further converted into the enol form of an aldehyde.

Unsaturated fatty acids can thus be the source of aldehyde with a C_6 or C_9 skeleton. They are the causing agents of characteristic odors and typical flavors. Leaf alcohol (*cis*-3-hexenol) and leaf aldehyde (*trans*-2-hexenol) are derived from C_{18}

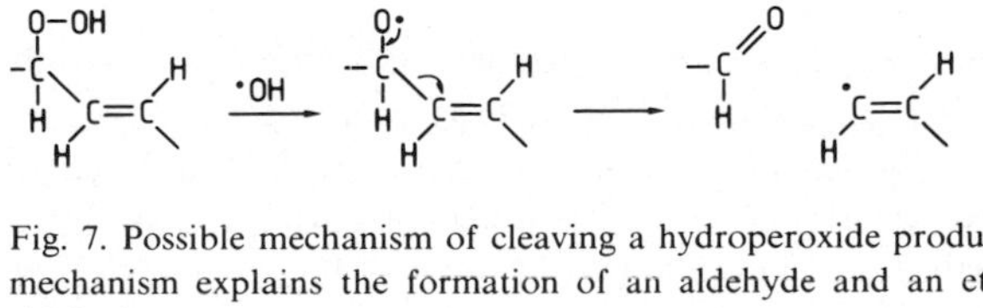

Fig. 7. Possible mechanism of cleaving a hydroperoxide produced by lipoxygenase reaction. The radical mechanism explains the formation of an aldehyde and an ethene radical which also gives rise to an aldehyde.

unsaturated fatty acids, with *cis*-3-hexenal being the product of oxidative split of linoleic acid (Fig. 6) and being the educt for isomerization or reduction steps. In tea leaves, Hatanaka et al. [66] found the enzyme responsible for the oxidative split of linoleic acid into *cis*-3-hexenal and 12-oxo-*cis*-9-dodecenoic acid, to be located at the thylakoid membrane.

A hydroperoxide-cleavage enzyme (or lyase) leading to C_6-aldehydes was also identified in etiolated seedlings and fruits. The 13-hydroperoxide of linoleic acid was converted into hexenals by a cleavage enzyme from apples or tomatoes. The membrane-bound enzyme could be solubilized [67] with 0.2% Triton X-100 and exhibited a rather high M_r of 200 000.

Galliard and coworkers [68,69] succeeded in characterizing a cleavage enzyme from cucumber fruits. It converts 9-hydroperoxyoctadecadienoic acid into *cis*-3-nonenal (Fig. 6) which can be further isomerized into the *trans*-2-enol. The subcellular location was studied with extracts which were prepared from flesh of cucumber fruits and subjected to isopycnic density gradient centrifugation. The activity of hydroperoxide cleavage was demonstrated to be attributable predominantly to plasma membrane and ER.

Lipoxygenases are widely distributed in higher plants. High activities are found in legume seeds, potato tubers and eggplant fruits. During development of *Phaseolus vulgaris* hypocotyls and young leaves were reported [70] to possess highest activities. Immature seeds were likewise distinguished by their high content of lipoxygenase and hydroperoxide lyase. As to the distribution of lipoxygenase among tissues, pronounced differences were also observed with many other systems. But we lack a more general concept as to why a certain distribution in plant parts occurs.

Equally undecided is the question where in the cell lipoxygenases are located. Plastids and lytic compartments may be candidates if we speculate about compartmentation of lipoxygenase.

Membrane lipids can also be attacked directly by $HO_2^{\cdot}$, the protonated form of $O_2^{\cdot-}$, which sufficiently occurs at pH lower than 5 and may, therefore, play a role in the lytic compartment. Lipoxygenases seem always to consist of a single polypeptide (M_r 100 000). The enzyme contains 1 non-heme iron and is characterized by a rather acidic isoelectric point, $pI = 5.5-6.0$. *Form 1* with an alkaline pH optimum (pH 9.0) and a selectivity in producing the 13-hydroperoxide is the classic soybean enzyme described by Theorell et al. [71]. In soybean, and in many other sources, *form 2* of lipoxygenase has been characterized by an acid pH optimum (pH 6.5) and by its lack of selectivity as far as 9- or 13-hydroperoxides as products are concerned. Both forms of lipoxygenase seem to occur in multiple forms distinguishable electrophoretically.

In crude mitochondrial pellets and in wounded tissues, lipoxygenase can be suspected to be responsible for the putative CN^--resistant respiration. Hydroxamates showing a relatively selective inhibition of CN^--resistant respiration have an exceedingly low K_i for lipoxygenase. Propyl gallate is another very effective inhibitor of CN^--insensitive respiration, and it is an excellent inhibitor of lipoxygenase [55]. Recent investigations [72] with mitochondria purified on a Percoll gradient seem to prove that CN^--insensitive O_2 consumption is indeed of mitochondrial origin while lipoxygenase activities found with crude mitochondrial preparations are contaminations.

We lack, at present, a unifying concept for the physiological role of lipoxygenase. Although the almost ubiquitous occurrence and the relation to membranes point to a general function of this enzyme in plants, we are left with suggestions. Most likely, lipoxygenases are involved in physiological response reactions to wounding of plants and microbial attack [73].

12-Oxo-*cis*-9-dodecenoic acid which is a product of hydroperoxide cleavage ($C_{18} \rightarrow C_6 + C_{12}$; Fig. 6) may be a precursor of 12-oxo-*trans*-10-dodecenoic acid, the precursor or active principle of traumatin. Traumatin [74] identified as C_{12}-dicarboxylic acid with a *trans*-2 double bond [75] and suggested to be a wound hormone, could thus be formed in parallel to the volatile leaf aldehyde. It is an attractive concept that wounding of plants by insects causes activation of the hydroperoxide cleavage process, and in this way not only provides a volatile repellent (C_6-aldehyde) but also a growth-inducing principle (C_{12}-carboxylic acid) which stimulates dividing and enlarging of cells.

4. Interrelationships to other pathways

Acetyl-CoA produced by fatty acid β-oxidation is fed into another pathway. This can be by transfer into other organelles, e.g. mitochondria running the citrate cycle, or without intraorganellar transfers, if acetyl-CoA produced in glyoxysomes is immediately used up in the glyoxylate cycle.

(a) Glyoxylate cycle

Two steps of the glyoxylate cycle take place in the matrix of glyoxysomes. Both, isocitrate lyase and aconitase are soluble enzymes and do not exhibit hydrophobic domains required to be attached to membranes nor do they have affinities towards membrane proteins such as malate synthase.

Malate synthase, malate dehydrogenase and citrate synthase are found, in most of the tissues investigated, to reside at the glyoxysomal membrane [78,79]. As they catalyze consecutive steps in the glyoxylate cycle and are located at the same intraorganellar site, it is conceivable to consider a close arrangement of the three enzymes. By this way, glyoxylate can be channeled into citrate, with malate and oxaloacetate being intermediates not fully equilibrating with the surrounding medium. For such an array, acetyl-CoA and NAD^+ have to be supplied while CoA and NADH leave the membrane-bound enzyme complex as products (Fig. 8).

Malate synthase converting glyoxylate, and acetyl-CoA furnished by fatty acid β-oxidation, occurs in the glyoxysomes as octamer [80] with M_r 540 000. The enzyme is distinguished by an alkaline isoelectric point pH = 9 and amphipathic properties. Under controlled conditions in vitro, monomeric, octameric and aggregated forms of

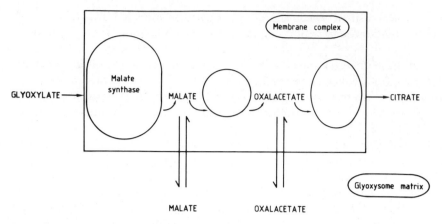

Fig. 8. Possible channeling by enzymes arranged as an array.

malate synthase exist all of which are enzymatically active [81,82]. As malate synthase does not shift from monomeric into octameric form or vice versa in the presence of Mg^{2+} and glyoxylate, the removal of malate synthase from the glyoxysomal membrane in the presence of Mg^{2+}/glyoxylate permits the examination of the enzyme's size without undertaking any risk to encounter artefacts. In the absence of cations, e.g. in a medium with the zwitter ion Tricine, malate synthase tends to aggregate. Under physiological conditions, spermidine or putrescine may assume the function of Mg^{2+} thus guaranteeing the occurrence of the octameric enzyme.

Malate dehydrogenase from glyoxysomes can be oligomerized to varying extent; dimers [82,83], tetramers and hexamers [80] being found. Malate dehydrogenase from leaf peroxisomes, and the other forms of malate dehydrogenase in plant cells, viz. in mitochondria and cytoplasm, occur exclusively as dimers. The glyoxysomal malate dehydrogenase [83] differs from the other malate dehydrogenase forms by its alkaline isoelectric point.

Malate dehydrogenase purified from glyoxysomes [85] exhibits affinities towards NAD^+ ($K_m = 0.46$ mM), NADH ($K_m = 0.13$ mM), malate ($K_m = 7$ mM), oxaloacetate ($K_m = 0.20$ mM), and various nucleotides. The enzyme can be bound e.g. to AMP-Sepharose. Unlike cytosolic forms of the enzyme, glyoxysomal malate dehydrogenase is more processed during biosynthesis and has a significantly lower subunit M_r, i.e. M_r 33 000 instead of 41 000 as found for the cytosolic forms or 38 000 for the mitochondrial form.

Citrate synthase resembles malate synthase in several respects. It can also be aggregated in the absence of Mg^{2+}. Dimeric and tetrameric forms co-occur in glyoxysomes [80]. With its high affinity towards oxaloacetate [86] ($K_m = 0.006$ mM), the enzyme can compete for the substrate with malate dehydrogenase. All three enzymes of the proposed channel (Fig. 8), malate synthase, malate dehydrogenase and citrate synthase, are distinguished by their relatively alkaline isoelectric point.

The resembling molecular properties, their common capability of binding to phospholipids or membranes, and the interaction between each other, predispose them to form complexes which may also be entities with respect to function.

Furthermore, it is remarkable that the various enzymes responsible for formation and channeling products of fatty acid β-oxidation (multifunctional protein, thiolase, malate synthase, and citrate synthase) are distinguished by their alkaline isoelectric point.

Aconitase is, as far as glyoxysomes are concerned, only poorly characterized [87]. In analogy to the mitochondrial counterpart, a highly oxygen-sensitive iron-sulfur protein is assumed to carry out the interconversion of citrate and isocitrate.

Isocitrate lyase as matrix enzyme [88] catalyzes the aldol reaction between isocitrate and succinate plus glyoxylate. The enzyme is a tetramer, and highly susceptible to proteolysis. This makes it rather difficult to decide whether or not more than one isoenzyme occurs in the seedling [89,90]. The in vitro equilibrium is in favor of isocitrate formation [91], and may also lead in vivo under steady-state conditions, together with the low velocity of the aconitase reaction, to tricarboxylic acids somewhat dammed up.

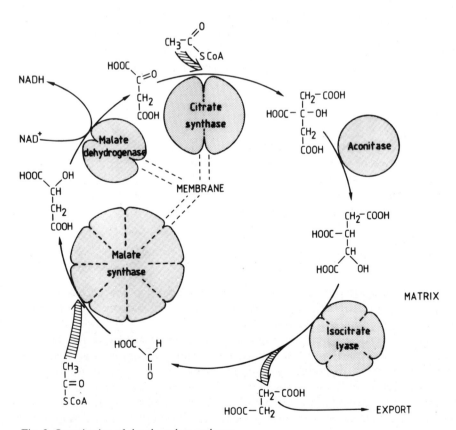

Fig. 9. Organization of the glyoxylate pathway.

Fig. 9 summarizes our present knowledge of how the glyoxylate pathway may be organized. It does not consider the comparative biochemistry when glyoxylate cycles are effective in different organisms and at different metabolic situations [92].

(b) Further conversions

If acetyl-CoA is not further metabolized by the glyoxylate cycle, e.g. because the microbodies producing acetyl-CoA are not competent anymore in the glyoxylate cycle or because acetyl-CoA is needed at another site in the cell, a few possible transfers can be envisaged.

An intensive production of membranes and lipids in the plastids during greening could be the reason that acetate units are transferred to chloroplasts. It is assumed that free acetic acid is generated and then moves to the chloroplast where acetyl-CoA synthetase converts it to acetyl-CoA [93]. Another example demonstrates the requirement for acetyl-CoA: when fungal attack elicits the biosynthesis of phytoalexins originating from acetyl-CoA. As exemplified by peanut cotyledons carrying out fatty acid β-oxidation and characterized by well developed glyoxysomes, acetyl-CoA is converted into phytoalexins derived from resveratrol [94].

Glyoxylate produced in glyoxysomes may be averted from malate synthase reaction and directed towards glycine and glycerate formation, when leaf peroxisomal activities emerge in the very same organelle [95]. A process like that undoubtedly drains the glyoxylate cycle of intermediates and should require, if effective, anaplerotic steps.

(c) Products of β-oxidation being used by citrate cycle

The transfer into mitochondria of succinate, and malate as vehicle of a shuttle for redox equivalents, seems to be indispensable. Only then the building blocks necessary for gluconeogenesis can be provided. This makes it highly likely that other biosynthetic routes starting from C_4 acids of the citrate cycle are supplied with carbon compounds furnished by fatty acid β-oxidation.

5. Control of fatty acid degradation and biosynthesis of glyoxysomes

The organelles that are primarily involved in plant lipid degradation are glyoxysomes [77]. The control of lipid oxidation is, therefore, first of all by regulating biosynthesis or degradation of glyoxysomes.

Glyoxysomes have rather similar morphological properties and specific activities of individual enzymes. When fat degradation is occurring most actively, glyoxysomes (0.2–1 μm in diameter, surrounded by a single unit membrane, equilibrium density $d = 1.25$ g/cm^3) are found closely associated with or even encircling lipid bodies. Some tissues housing the apparatus of degradation, e.g. castor bean endosperm, pine megagametophyte, maize scutellum, are existent only during lipid mobilization and are degraded as soon as the lipid storage compounds are depleted. Other tissues, e.g. cotyledons of cucurbitaceae, peanut, sunflower, persist after degradation of the main portion of lipid and take over biosynthetic functions as photoautotrophic tissues.

Rise of glyoxysomal activities is triggered by inhibition of fat-rich seeds and the fall of enzyme activities contributed by glyoxysomes parallels the depletion of fat. An enhanced decline in glyoxysome function is observed when tissues susceptible to light regulation are illuminated.

The molecular events which are necessary for assembly and turnover of organelles such as glyoxysomes are in many aspects only poorly understood. Following inhibition, transcription or post-transcriptional processes which are under the positive control of gibberellic acid and negative control of abscissic acid provide translatable mRNA. Martin and Northcote [96] observed an increase of poly A$^+$-mRNA coding for isocitrate lyase when they applied gibberellic acid to the storage tissue being active in fat mobilization. But there are proofs that, at least in a few cases, translatable mRNA and translation of glyoxysomal proteins can already take place at a late stage of seed maturation [97,98]. Hence, there is no principal but rather quantitative difference in biosynthesis of glyoxysomal components between seed maturation and seed germination. There is also no proof for a concerted and exactly balanced synthesis of the set of glyoxysomal proteins [99,100]. Several enzymes (catalase, β-oxidation enzymes) were found to be earlier synthesized than others (malate synthase).

Investigations both in vitro with cell-free translation systems [95,97,101–104] and in vivo by administration of radioactive precursors and analysis of the sequence of intracellular pools [105,106] provided strong evidence for a general statement: proteinaceous components of glyoxysomes are synthesized on free polysomes in the cytosol, a pool of precursors occurs in the cytosol determining the quality and quantity of precursor proteins to be imported into the organelles.

The means by which glyoxysomes selectively import the components destined to these organelles remain to be elucidated. It is not known whether specific receptors

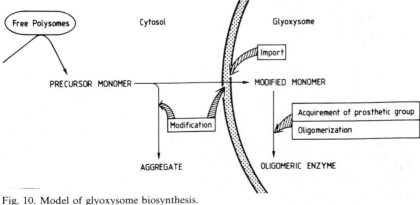

Fig. 10. Model of glyoxysome biosynthesis.

guarantee the uptake of the right precursors from the cytosol which contains also precursors for other organelles, e.g. mitochondria and plastids.

The model described for glyoxysome biosynthesis (Fig. 10) ought to be applicable to the biosynthesis of other microbodies [95], e.g. also for the transition state when glyoxysomes are replaced by leaf peroxisomes during greening of cotyledons (sunflower, cucumber). Qualitative changes in translatable mRNA may be the only process being switched. Uptake of precursors according to the quality and quantity of the cytosolic pools is assumed to proceed by the gradually changing microbodies without alterations of the principal mechanism [106a]. Several of the processes postulated for the biosynthesis of microbodies in higher plants will probably be identical or very similar to the one taking place in fungi [107,108].

Any model which allows for decline of glyoxysomal activities, either in castor bean endosperm after depletion of fat or in the cotyledons upon illumination, has to consider degradation of organelles or only of protein components housed in them. At present, we know that organelles can sometimes be degraded very rapidly, and the lytic compartment of plant cells is a likely candidate for this task, but we need considerably more investigations before a reliable description of the many processes and their regulation is possible.

References

1 Hitchcock, C. (1975) in: T. Galliard and E.I. Mercer (Eds.), Recent Advances in the Chemistry and Biochemistry of Plant Lipids, Academic Press, London, pp. 1–19.
2 Harwood, J.L. (1980) in: P.K. Stumpf and E.E. Conn (Eds.), Biochemistry of Plants, Academic Press, London, pp. 1–55.
3 Yatsu, L.Y., Jacks, T.J. and Hensarling, T.P. (1971) Plant Physiol. 48, 675–682.
4 Ory, R.L. (1969) Lipids 4, 177–185.
5 Yatsu, L.Y. and Jacks, T.J. (1972) Plant Physiol. 49, 937–943.
6 Slack, C.R. (1980) Biochem. J. 190, 551.
7 Kleinig, H., Steinki, E., Kopp, C. and Zaar, K. (1978) Planta 140, 233–237.
8 Bergfeld, R., Hong, Y.-N., Kuhne, T. and Schopfer, P. (1978) Planta 143, 297–307.
9 Wanner, G., Formanek, H. and Theimer, R.R. (1981) Planta 151, 109–123.
10 Wanner, G. and Theimer, R.R. (1978) Planta 140, 163–170.
11 Parker, M.L. and Murphy, G.J.P. (1981) Planta 152, 36–43.
12 Body, D.R. (1974) Phytochemistry 13, 1527–1530.
13 Lösel, D.M. (1978) New Phytol. 80, 167–174.
14 Burns, D.D., Galliard, T. and Harwood, J.L. (1977) Biochem. Soc. Trans. 5, 1302–1304.
15 Heinz, E., Bertrams, M., Joyard, J. and Douce, R. (1978) Z. Pflanzenphysiol. 87, 325–331.
16 Gerhardt, B. (1981) FEBS Lett. 126, 71–73.
17 Thomas, D.R. and McNeil, P.H. (1976) Planta 132, 61–63.
18 Laties, G.G. (1978) in: G. Kahl (Ed.), Biochemistry of Wounded Plant Tissues, de Gruyter, Berlin, pp. 421–466.
19 Moreau, R.A., Liu, K.D.F. and Huang, A.H.C. (1980) Plant Physiol. 65, 1176–1180.
20 Huang, A.H.C., Moreau, R.A. and Liu, K.D.F. (1978) Plant Physiol. 61, 339–341.
21 Sanders, T.H. and Pattee, H.E. (1975) Lipids 10, 50–54.
22 Huang, A.H.C. and Moreau, R.A. (1978) Planta 141, 111–116.
23 Muto, S. and Beevers, H. (1974) Plant Physiol. 54, 23–28.

24 Theimer, R.R. and Rosnitschek, I. (1978) Planta 139, 249–256.
25 Fujiki, Y., Aizono, Y. and Funatsu, M. (1978) Agric. Biol. Chem. 42, 599–606.
26 Hirayama, O., Matsuda, H., Takeda, H., Maenaka, K. and Takatsuka, H. (1975) Biochim. Biophys. Acta 384, 127–137.
27 Anderson, M.M., McCarty, R.E. and Zimmer, E.A. (1974) Plant Physiol. 53, 699–704.
28 Bligny, R. and Douce, R. (1978) Biochim. Biophys. Acta 529, 419–428.
29 Heller, M., Mozes, N. and Maes, E. (1975) Methods Enzymol. 35, 226–232.
30 Frevert, H. and Kindl, H. (1980) Eur. J. Biochem. 107, 79–86.
31 Osumi, T. and Hashimoto, T. (1979) Biochem. Biophys. Res. Commun. 89, 580–584.
32 Pawar, S. and Schulz, H. (1981) J. Biol. Chem. 256, 3894–3899.
33 Cooper, T.G. and Beevers, H. (1969) J. Biol. Chem. 244, 3514–3520.
34 Tolbert, N.E. (1982) Ann. N.Y. Acad. Sci. 386, 254–268.
35 Thomas, D.R., Jalil, M.N.H., Cooke, R.J., Yong, B.C.S., Ariffin, A., McNeil, P.H. and Wood, C. (1982) Planta 154, 60–65.
36 Cooper, T.G. (1971) J. Biol. Chem. 246, 3451–3455.
37 Mishina, M., Kamiryo, T., Tashiro, S., Hagihara, T., Tanaka, A., Fukui, S., Osumi, M. and Numa, S. (1978) Eur. J. Biochem. 89, 321–328.
38 Mishina, M., Kamiryo, T., Tashiro, S. and Numa, S. (1978) Eur. J. Biochem. 82, 347–354.
39 Kawamoto, S., Nozaki, C., Tanaka, A. and Fukui, S. (1978) Eur. J. Biochem. 83, 609–613.
40 Hashimoto, T. (1982) Ann. N.Y. Acad. Sci. 386, 5–12.
41 Gerdes, H.H., Behrends, W. and Kindl, H. (1982) Planta, 156, 571–578.
42 Furuta, S., Miyazawa, S., Osumi, T., Hashimoto, T. and Ui, N. (1980) J. Biochem. 88, 1059–1070.
43 Frevert, J. and Kindl, H. (1980) Hoppe Seyler's Z. Physiol. Chem. 361, 537–542.
44 Krahling, J.B. and Tolbert, N.E. (1981) Arch. Biochem. Biophys. 209, 100–110.
45 Miyazawa, S., Furuta, S., Osumi, T., Hashimoto, T. and Ui, N. (1981) J. Biochem. 90, 511–519.
46 Hicks, D.B. and Donaldson, R.P. (1982) Arch. Biochem. Biophys. 215, 280–288.
47 Mettler, I.J. and Beevers, H. (1980) Plant Physiol. 66, 555–560.
48 Beevers, H. (1982) Ann. N.Y. Acad. Sci. 386, 243–253.
49 Lord, J.M. and Beevers, H. (1972) Plant Physiol. 49, 249–251.
50 Blum, J.J. (1982) Ann. N.Y. Acad. Sci. 386, 217–227.
51 Leighton, F., Brandan, E., Lazo, O. and Bronfman, M. (1982) Ann. N.Y. Acad. Sci. 386, 62–80.
52 Dommes, V., Luster, W., Cvetanovic, M. and Kunau, W.-H. (1982) Eur. J. Biochem., in press.
53 Dommes, V., Baumgart, C. and Kunau, W.-H. (1981) J. Biol. Chem. 256, 8259–8262.
54 Shine, W.E. and Stumpf, P.K. (1974) Arch. Biochem. Biophys. 162, 147–157.
55 Laties, C.C. (1982) Annu. Rev. Plant Physiol. 33, 519–555.
56 Hagel, P. and Kindl, H. (1976) FEBS Lett. 59, 120–124.
57 French, C.J., Vance, C.P. and Towers, G.H.N. (1976) Phytochemistry 15, 564–566.
58 Tsai, S.-C., Stainberg, D., Avigan, J. and Fales, H.M. (1973) J. Biol. Chem. 248, 1091.
59 Soliday, C.L. and Kolattukudy, P.E. (1977) Plant Physiol. 59, 1116–1121.
60 Kolattukudy, P.E. (1977) in: M.E. Tevini and H.K. Lichtenthaler (Eds.), Lipids and Lipid Polymers in Higher PLants, Springer, Berlin, pp. 271–292.
61 Soliday, C.L. and Kolattukudy, P.E. (1978) Arch. Biochem. Biophys. 188, 338–347.
62 Gunsalus, I.C., Pederson, T.C. and Sligar, S.G. (1975) Annu. Rev. Biochem. 44, 377–407.
62 Peterson, J.A., Basu, D. and Coon, M.J. (1966) J. Biol. Chem. 241, 5162–5164.
64 Gerritsen, M., Veldink, G.A., Vliegenthart, J.F.G. and Boldingh, J. (1976) FEBS Lett. 67, 149–152.
65 Gardner, H.W. and Jursinik, P.A. (1981) Biochim. Biophys. Acta 665, 100–112.
66 Hatanaka, A., Sekiya, J., Kajiwara, T. and Miura, T. (1979) Agric. Biol. Chem. 43, 735–740.
67 Schreier, P. and Lorenz, G. (1982) Z. Naturforsch. 37c, 165–173.
68 Phillips, D.R. and Galliard, T. (1978) Phytochemistry 17, 355–358.
69 Wardale, D.A., Lambert, E.A. and Galliard, T. (1978) Phytochemistry 17, 205–212.
70 Sekiya, J., Kamiuchi, H. and Hatanaka, A. (1982) Plant Cell Physiol. 23, 631–638.
71 Theorell, H., Bergström, S. and Akeson, A. (1947) Acta Chem. Scand. 1, 571–576.

204

72   Shingles, R.M., Arron, G.P. and Hill, R.D. (1982) Plant Physiol. 69, 1435–1438.
73   Galliard, T. (1978) in: G. Kahl (Ed.), Biochemistry of Wounded Plant Storage Tissues, de Gruyter, Berlin, pp. 155–201.
74   Zimmerman, D.C. and Coudron, C.A. (1979) Plant Physiol. 63, 536–541.
75   English Jr., J., Bonner, J. and Haagen-Smit, A.J. (1939) Science 90, 329–331.
76   Tolbert, N.E. (1981) Annu. Rev. Biochem. 50, 133–157.
77   Beevers, H. (1979) Annu. Rev. Plant Physiol. 30, 159–193.
78   Huang, A.H.C. and Beevers, H. (1973) J. Cell Biol. 58, 379–389.
79   Bieglmayer, C., Graf, J. and Ruis, H. (1973) Eur. J. Biochem. 37, 553–562.
80   Köller, W. and Kindl, H. (1977) Arch. Biochem. Biophys. 181, 236–248.
81   Kindl, H. and Kruse, C. (1983) in: Methods in Enzymology, Vol. 3: Biogenesis of membranes, sorting and transport of membrane constituents, pp. 700–713.
82   Köller, W. and Kindl, H. (1978) FEBS Lett. 88, 83–86.
83   Hock, B. (1973) Planta 110, 329–344.
84   Walk, R.-A. and Hock, B. (1977) Planta 136, 211–220.
85   Hock, B. and Gietl, C. (1982) Ann. N.Y. Acad. Sci. 386, 350–361.
86   Schnarrenberger, C., Zehler, H. and Fitting, H.-H. (1980) Hoppe-Seyler's Z. Physiol. Chem. 361, 328–329.
87   Breidenbach, R.W. and Beevers, H. (1967) Biochem. Biophys. Res. Commun. 27, 462–469.
88   Frevert, J. and Kindl, H. (1978) Eur. J. Biochem. 92, 35–43.
89   Khan, F.R., Saleemuddin, M., Siddiqi, M. and McFadden, B.A. (1977) Arch. Biochem. Biophys. 183, 13–23.
90   Riezman, H., Weir, E.M., Leaver, C.J., Titus, D.E. and Becker, W.M. (1980) Plant Physiol. 65, 40–46.
91   McFadden, B.A. (1969) Methods Enzymol. 13, 163–170.
92   Cioni, M., Pinzauti, G. and Vanni, P. (1982) Comp. Biochem. Physiol. 70, 1–26.
93   Murphy, D.J. and Stumpf, P.K. (1981) Arch. Biochem. 212, 730–739.
94   Rolfs, C.H., Fritzemeier, K.H. and Kindl, H. (1981) Plant Cell Rep. 1, 83–85.
95   Kindl, H. (1982) Int. Rev. Cytol. 80, 193–229.
96   Martin, C. and Northcote, D.H. (1982) Planta 152, 174–183.
97   Kindl, H. (1982) Ann. N.Y. Acad. Sci. 386, 314–330.
98   Frevert, J., Köller, W. and Kindl, H. (1980) Hoppe-Seyler's Z. Physiol. Chem. 361, 1557–1565.
99   Choinski, J.S. and Trelease, R.N. (1978) Plant Physiol. 62, 141–145.
100 Miernyk, J.A. and Trelease, R.N. (1981) Plant Physiol. 67, 875–881.
101 Becker, W.M., Riezman, H., Weir, E.M., Titus, D.E. and Leaver, C.J. (1982) Ann. N.Y. Acad. Sci. 386, 329–349.
102 Riezman, H., Weir, E.M., Leaver, C.J., Titus, D.E. and Becker, W.M. (1980) Plant Physiol. 65, 40–46.
103 Kruse, C., Frevert, J. and Kindl, H. (1981) FEBS Lett. 129, 36–38.
104 Roberts, L.M. and Lord, J.M. (1982) Eur. J. Biochem. 119, 43–49.
105 Kindl, H., Köller, W. and Frevert, J. (1980) Hoppe-Seyler's Z. Physiol. Chem. 361, 465–467.
106 Köller, W. and Kindl, H. (1980) Hoppe-Seyler's Z. Physiol. Chem. 361, 1437–1444.
106a Kruse, C. and Kindl, H. (1983) Arch. Biochem. Biophys. 223, 629–638.
107 Zimmermann, R. and Neupert, W. (1980) Eur. J. Biochem. 112, 225–233.
108 Desel, H., Zimmermann, R., Jones, M., Miller, F. and Neupert, W. (1982) Ann. N.Y. Acad. Sci. 386, 377–389.

Subject Index